Guyton & Hall
Physiology Review

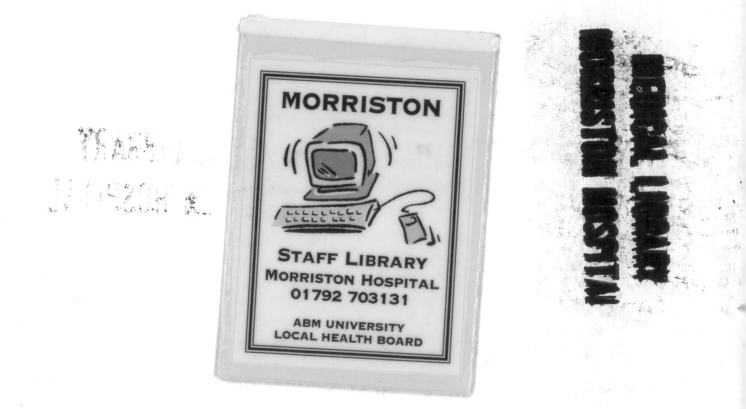

Guyton & Hall
Physiology Review

Second Edition

John E. Hall, PhD

Arthur C. Guyton Professor and Chair
Associate Vice Chancellor for Research
Department of Physiology and Biophysics
University of Mississippi Medical Center
Jackson, Mississippi

1600 John F. Kennedy Blvd., Ste. 1800
Philadelphia, PA 19103–2899

GUYTON & HALL PHYSIOLOGY REVIEW, SECOND EDITION   ISBN: 978-1-4160-5452-8

ISBN: 978-1-4160-5452-8

Acquisitions Editor: William R. Schmitt
Developmental Editors: Christine Abshire
Publishing Services Manager: Patricia Tannian
Senior Project Manager: Sarah Wunderly
Design Direction: Louis Forgione

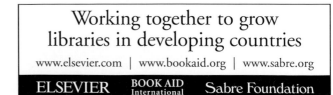

Printed in China

Last digit is the print number: 9   8   7   6   5   4   3   2   1

Contributors

Thomas H. Adair, PhD
Professor of Physiology and Biophysics
University of Mississippi Medical Center
Jackson, Mississippi
Unit II, Unit XII, and Unit XIII

David J. Dzielak, PhD
Professor of Surgery
Professor of Health Sciences
Associate Professor of Physiology and Biophysics
University of Mississippi Medical Center
Jackson, Mississippi
Unit IX, Unit X, and Unit XI

Joey P. Granger, PhD
Billy Guyton Professor of Physiology and Biophysics
    and Medicine
Dean of the School of Graduate Studies
University of Mississippi Medical Center
Jackson, Mississippi
Unit IV

John E. Hall, PhD
Arthur C. Guyton Professor and Chair
Associate Vice Chancellor for Research
Department of Physiology and Biophysics
University of Mississippi Medical Center
Jackson, Mississippi
Unit I, Unit V, and Unit XIII

Robert L. Hester, PhD
Professor of Physiology and Biophysics
University of Mississippi Medical Center
Jackson, Mississippi
Unit VI, Unit VII, and Unit VIII

Thomas E. Lohmeier, PhD
Professor of Physiology and Biophysics
University of Mississippi Medical Center
Jackson, Mississippi
Unit XIV

R. Davis Manning, PhD
Professor of Physiology and Biophysics
University of Mississippi Medical Center
Jackson, Mississippi
Unit III, Unit IV, and Unit XV

David B. Young, PhD
Professor Emeritus of Physiology and Biophysics
University of Mississippi Medical Center
Jackson, Mississippi
Unit XIV

Contributions

Preface

Self-assessment is an important component of effective learning, especially when studying a subject as complex as medical physiology. The *Guyton & Hall Physiology Review* is designed to provide a comprehensive review of medical physiology through multiple-choice questions and explanations of the answers. Medical students preparing for the United States Medical Licensure Examinations (USMLE) will also find this book useful, since test questions have been constructed according to the USMLE format.

The questions and answers in this review are based on *Guyton and Hall's Textbook of Medical Physiology*, twelfth edition (TMP 12). More than 1000 questions and answers are provided, and each answer is referenced to the *Textbook of Medical Physiology* to facilitate a more complete understanding of the topic and self-assessment of your knowledge. Illustrations are used to reinforce basic concepts. Some of the questions incorporate information from multiple chapters in the *Textbook of Medical Physiology* to test your ability to apply and integrate the principles necessary for the mastery of medical physiology.

An effective way to use the review is to allow an average of 1 minute for each question in a given unit, approximating the time limit for a question in the USMLE examination. As you proceed, indicate your answer next to each question. After finishing the questions and answers, spend as much time as necessary to verify your answers and to carefully read the explanations provided. Read the additional material referred to in the *Textbook of Medical* *Physiology*, especially for questions where incorrect answers were chosen.

Guyton & Hall Physiology Review should not be used as a substitute for the comprehensive information contained in the *Textbook of Medical Physiology*. It is intended mainly as a means of assessing your knowledge of physiology and of strengthening your ability to apply and integrate this knowledge.

We have attempted to make this review as accurate as possible, and we hope that it will be a valuable tool for your study of physiology. We invite you to send us your critiques, suggestions for improvement, and notifications of any errors.

I am grateful to each of the contributors for their careful work on this book. I also wish to express my thanks to William Schmitt, Rebecca Gruliow, Christine Abshire, and the rest of the Elsevier staff for their editorial and production excellence. I am especially indebted to the late Dr. Arthur C. Guyton, who wrote the first eight editions of the *Textbook of Medical Physiology*, beginning nearly 50 years ago. I had the privilege of working with him on the ninth and tenth editions and have attempted in the last two editions to continue his practice of accurately presenting the complex principles of physiology in language that is easy for students to read and understand.

John E. Hall, PhD
Jackson, Mississippi

Contents

Contents

The Cell and General Physiology

1. The term "glycocalyx" refers to

   A) the negatively charged carbohydrate chains that protrude into the cytosol from glycolipids and integral glycoproteins
   B) the negatively charged carbohydrate layer on the outer cell surface
   C) the layer of anions aligned on the cytosolic surface of the plasma membrane
   D) the large glycogen stores found in "fast" muscles
   E) a mechanism of cell–cell attachment

2. Messenger RNA (mRNA)

   A) carries the genetic code to the cytoplasm
   B) carries activated amino acids to the ribosomes
   C) is single-stranded RNA molecules of 21 to 23 nucleotides that can regulate gene transcription
   D) forms ribosomes

3. Which of the following statements is true for **both** pinocytosis and phagocytosis?

   A) Involves the recruitment of actin filaments
   B) Occurs spontaneously and non-selectively
   C) Endocytotic vesicles fuse with ribosomes that release hydrolases into the vesicles
   D) Is only observed in macrophages and neutrophils
   E) Does not require ATP

4. In comparing two types of cells from the same person, the variation in the proteins expressed by each cell type reflects

   A) differences in the DNA contained in the nucleus of each cell
   B) differences in the numbers of specific genes in their genomes
   C) cell-specific expression and repression of specific genes
   D) differences in the number of chromosomes in each cell
   E) the age of the cells

5. Micro RNAs (miRNAs)

   A) are formed in the cytoplasm and repress translation or promote degradation of mRNA before it can be translated
   B) are formed in the nucleus and then processed in the cytoplasma by the dicer enzyme
   C) are short (21 to 23 nucleotides) double-stranded RNA fragments that regulate gene expression
   D) repress gene transcription

Questions 6–8

A) Nucleolus
B) Nucleus
C) Agranular endoplasmic reticulum
D) Granular endoplasmic reticulum
E) Golgi apparatus
F) Endosomes
G) Peroxisomes
H) Lysosomes
I) Cytosol
J) Cytoskeleton
K) Glycocalyx
L) Microtubules

For each of the scenarios described below, identify the most likely subcellular site listed above for the deficient or mutant protein.

6. Studies completed on a 5-year-old boy show an accumulation of cholesteryl esters and triglycerides in his liver, spleen, and intestines and calcification of both adrenal glands. Additional studies indicate the cause to be a deficiency in acid lipase A activity.

7. The abnormal cleavage of mannose residues during the post-translational processing of glycoproteins results in the development of a lupus-like autoimmune disease in mice. The abnormal cleavage is due to a mutation of the enzyme α-mannosidase II.

8. The observation that abnormal cleavage of mannose residues from glycoproteins causes an autoimmune disease in mice supports the role of this structure in the normal immune response.

Questions 9–11

A) Nucleolus
B) Nucleus
C) Agranular endoplasmic reticulum
D) Granular endoplasmic reticulum
E) Golgi apparatus
F) Endosomes
G) Peroxisomes
H) Lysosomes
I) Cytosol
J) Cytoskeleton
K) Glycocalyx
L) Microtubules

Match the cellular location for each of the steps involved in the synthesis and packaging of a secreted protein listed below with a term listed above.

9. Initiation of translation

10. Protein condensation and packaging

11. Gene transcription

12. "Redundancy" or "degeneration" of the genetic code occurs during which of the following steps of protein synthesis?

A) DNA replication
B) Transcription
C) Post-transcriptional modification
D) Translation
E) Protein glycosylation

13. Which of the following does not play a direct role in the process of transcription?

A) Helicase
B) RNA polymerase
C) Chain-terminating sequence
D) "Activated" RNA molecules
E) Promoter sequence

14. Which of the following proteins is most likely to be the product of a proto-oncogene?

A) Growth factor receptor
B) Cytoskeletal protein
C) Na^+ channel
D) Ca^{++}-ATPase
E) Myosin light chain

15. Which of the following events does not occur during the process of mitosis?

A) Condensation of the chromosomes
B) Replication of the genome
C) Fragmentation of the nuclear envelope
D) Alignment of the chromatids along the equatorial plate
E) Separation of the chromatids into two sets of 46 "daughter" chromosomes

16. Which of the following characteristics of a biological membrane is most influenced by its cholesterol content?

A) Thickness
B) Ion permeability
C) Fluidity
D) Glycosylation
E) Hydrophobicity

17. The appearance of which of the following distinguishes eukaryotic cells from lower units of life?

A) DNA
B) RNA
C) Membranes
D) Protein
E) Nucleus

18. Assume that excess blood is transfused into a patient whose arterial baroreceptors are nonfunctional and blood pressure increases from 100 to 150 mm Hg. Then, assume that the same volume is blood is infused into the same patient under conditions where his arterial baroreceptors are functioning normally and blood pressure increases from 100 to 125 mm Hg. What is the approximate feedback "gain" of the arterial baroreceptors in this patient when they are functioning normally?

A) −1.0
B) −2.0
C) 0.0
D) +1.0
E) +2.0

1. **B)** The cell "glycocalyx" is the loose negatively charged carbohydrate coat on the outside of the surface of the cell membrane. The membrane carbohydrates usually occur in combination with proteins or lipids in the form of glycoproteins or glycolipids, and the "glyco" portion of these molecules almost invariably protrudes to the outside of the cell.
   TMP12 14

2. **A)** mRNA molecules are long, single RNA strands that are suspended in the cytoplasm, and are composed of several hundred to several thousand RNA nucleotides in unpaired strands. The mRNA carries the genetic code to the cytoplasm for controlling the type of protein formed. The *transfer RNA* (tRNA) transports activated amino acids to the ribosomes. *Ribosomal RNA*, along with about 75 different proteins, forms ribosomes. MicroRNAs are single-stranded RNA molecules of 21 to 23 nucleotides that regulate gene transcription and translation.
   TMP12 31

3. **A)** Both pinocytosis and phagocytosis involve movement of the plasma membrane. Pinocytosis involves invagination of the cell membrane whereas phagocytosis involves evagination. Both events require the recruitment of actin and other cytoskeleton elements. Phagocytosis is not spontaneous and is selective, being triggered by specific receptor-ligand interactions.
   TMP12 19

4. **C)** The variation in proteins expressed by each cell reflects cell-specific expression and repression of specific genes. Each cell contains the same DNA in the nucleus and the same number of genes. So differentiation results not from differences in the genes but from selective repression and /or activation of different gene promoters.
   TMP12 39–40

5. **A)** MicroRNAs (miRNA) are formed in the cytoplasm from pre-miRNAs and processed by the enzyme dicer that ultimately assembles RNA-induced silencing complex (RISC), which then generates miRNAs. The miRNAs regulate gene expression by binding to the complementary region of the RNA and repressing translation or promoting degradation of mRNA before it can be translated by the ribosome.
   TMP 12 32–33

6. **H)** Acid lipases, along with other acid hydrolases, are localized to lysosomes. Fusion of endocytotic and autolytic vesicles with lysosomes initiates the intracellular process that allows cells to digest cellular debris and particles ingested from the extracellular milieu, including bacteria. In the normal acidic environment of the lysosome, acid lipases use hydrogen to convert lipids into fatty acids and glycerol. Other acid lipases include a variety of nucleases, proteases, and polysaccharide-hydrolyzing enzymes.
   TMP12 15

7. **E)** Membrane proteins are glycosylated during their synthesis in the lumen of the rough endoplasmic reticulum. Most post-translational modification of the oligosaccharide chains, however, occurs during the transport of the protein through the layers of the Golgi apparatus matrix, where enzymes such as α-mannosidase II are localized.
   TMP12 15

8. **K)** The oligosaccharide chains that are added to glycoproteins on the luminal side of the rough endoplasmic reticulum, and subsequently modified during their transport through the Golgi apparatus, are attached to the extracellular surface of the cell. This negatively charged layer of carbohydrate moieties is collectively called the glycocalyx. It participates in cell–cell interactions, cell–ligand interactions, and the immune response.
   TMP12 14; see also Chapter 34

9. **I)** Initiation of translation, whether of a cytosolic protein, a membrane-bound protein, or a secreted protein, occurs in the cytosol and involves a common pool of ribosomes. Only after the appearance of the N-terminus of the polypeptide is it identified as a protein destined for secretion. At this point, the ribosome attaches to the cytosolic surface of the rough endoplasmic reticulum. Translation continues, and the new polypeptide is extruded into the matrix of the endoplasmic reticulum.
   TMP12 32–33

10. **E)** Secreted proteins are condensed, sorted, and packaged into secretory vesicles in the terminal portions of the Golgi apparatus, also known as the trans-Golgi network. It is here that proteins destined for secretion are separated from those destined for intracellular compartments or cellular membranes.
    TMP12 15

11. **B)** All transcription events occur in the nucleus, regardless of the final destination of the protein product. The resulting messenger RNA molecule is transported through the nuclear pores in the nuclear membrane and translated into either the cytosol or the lumen of the rough endoplasmic reticulum.

    TMP12 31

12. **D)** During both replication and transcription, the new nucleic acid molecule is an exact complement of the parent DNA molecule. This is a result of predictable, specific, one-to-one base pairing. During the process of translation, however, each amino acid in the new polypeptide is encoded by a codon, a series of three consecutive nucleotides. Whereas each codon encodes a specific amino acid, most amino acids can be encoded for by multiple codons. Redundancy results because 60 codons encode a mere 20 amino acids.

    TMP12 31

13. **A)** Helicase is one of the many proteins involved in the process of DNA replication. It does not play a role in transcription. RNA polymerase binds to the promoter sequence and facilitates the addition of "activated" RNA molecules to the growing RNA molecule until the polymerase reaches the chain-terminating sequence on the template DNA molecule.

    TMP12 30–31

14. **A)** An oncogene is a gene that is either abnormally activated or mutated in such a way that its product causes uncontrolled cell growth. A proto-oncogene is simply the "normal" version of an oncogene. By definition, proto-oncogenes are divided into several families of proteins, all of which participate in the control of cell growth. These families include, but are not limited to, growth factors and their receptors, protein kinases, transcription factors, and proteins that regulate cell proliferation.

    TMP12 40–41

15. **B)** DNA replication occurs during the S phase of the cell cycle and precedes mitosis. Condensation of the chromosomes occurs during the prophase of mitosis. Fragmentation of the nuclear envelope occurs during the prometaphase of mitosis. The chromatids align at the equatorial plate during metaphase and separate into two complete sets of daughter chromosomes during anaphase.

    TMP12 37

16. **C)** The cholesterol content of a membrane determines the packing density of phospholipids. The higher the cholesterol content, the more fluid the membrane and the greater the lateral mobility of membrane components, including proteins and phospholipid molecules themselves. To a lesser extent, cholesterol content also affects the "leakiness" of a membrane to water-soluble molecules.

    TMP12 13

17. **E)** Nucleic acids and proteins, together, constitute the fundamental replicable unit of life, exemplified by viruses. Membranes and even organelles appear in prokaryotic cells, but only eukaryotic cells possess a nucleus.

    TMP12 17–18

18. **A)** The feedback gain of the control system is calculated as the amount of correction divided by the remaining error of the system. In this example, blood pressure increased from 100 to 150 mm Hg when the baroreceptors were not functioning. When the baroreceptors were functioning, the pressure increased only 25 mm Hg. Therefore, the feedback system caused a "correction" of −25 mm Hg, from 150 to 125 mm Hg. The remaining increase in pressure of +25 mm is called the "error." In this example the correction is therefore −25 mm Hg and the remaining error is +25 mm Hg. Thus, the feedback gain of the baroreceptors in this person is −1, indicating a negative feedback control system.

    TMP 12 7–8

Membrane Physiology, Nerve, and Muscle

1. Which of the following best describes the changes in cell volume that will occur when red blood cells (previously equilibrated in a 280-milliosmolar solution of NaCl) are placed in a solution of 140 millimolar NaCl containing 20 millimolar urea, a relatively large but permeant molecule?

    A) Cells shrink initially, then swell over time and lyse
    B) Cells shrink transiently and return to their original volume over time
    C) Cells swell and lyse
    D) Cells swell transiently and return to their original volume over time
    E) No change in cell volume will occur

2. What is the calculated osmolarity of a solution containing 12 millimolar NaCl, 4 millimolar KCl, and 2 millimolar $CaCl_2$ (in mOsm/L)?

    A) 16
    B) 26
    C) 29
    D) 32
    E) 38
    F) 42

Questions 3–6

Intracellular (mM)	Extracellular (mM)
140 K^+	14 K^+
10 Na^+	100 Na^+
11 Cl^-	110 Cl^-
$10-4$ Ca^{++}	2 Ca^{++}

The table shows the concentrations of four ions across the plasma membrane of a model cell. Refer to this table when answering the following four questions.

3. What is the equilibrium potential for Cl^- across the plasma membrane of this cell?

    A) 0 millivolts
    B) 122 millivolts
    C) -122 millivolts
    D) 61 millivolts
    E) -61 millivolts

4. What is the equilibrium potential for K^+ across the plasma membrane of this cell?

    A) 0 millivolts
    B) 122 millivolts
    C) -122 millivolts
    D) 61 millivolts
    E) -61 millivolts

5. If the membrane potential of this cell is -80 millivolts, the driving force is greatest for which ion?

    A) Ca^{++}
    B) Cl^-
    C) K^+
    D) Na^+

6. If this cell were permeable only to K^+, what would be the effect of reducing the extracellular K^+ concentration from 14 to 1.4 millimolar?

    A) 10 millivolts depolarization
    B) 10 millivolts hyperpolarization
    C) 122 millivolts depolarization
    D) 122 millivolts hyperpolarization
    E) 61 millivolts depolarization
    F) 61 millivolts hyperpolarization

7. The diagram shows the length–tension relationship for a single sarcomere. (Data from Gordon AM, Huxley AF, Julian FJ: The length–tension diagram of single vertebrate striated muscle fibers. *J Physiol* 171:28P, 1964.) Why is the tension development maximal between points B and C?

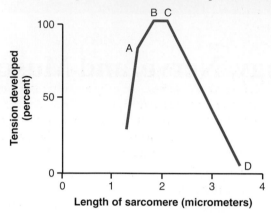

Length of sarcomere (micrometers)

A) Actin filaments are overlapping each other
B) Myosin filaments are overlapping each other
C) The myosin filament is at its minimal length
D) The Z discs of the sarcomere abut the ends of the myosin filament
E) There is optimal overlap between the actin and myosin filaments
F) There is minimal overlap between the actin and myosin filaments

8. Simple diffusion and facilitated diffusion share which of the following characteristics?

A) Can be blocked by specific inhibitors
B) Do not require adenosine triphosphate (ATP)
C) Require transport protein
D) Saturation kinetics
E) Transport solute against concentration gradient

9. Excitation–contraction coupling in skeletal muscle involves all of the following events EXCEPT one. Which one is this EXCEPTION?

A) ATP hydrolysis
B) Binding of Ca^{++} to calmodulin
C) Conformational change in dihydropyridine receptor
D) Depolarization of the transverse tubule (T tubule) membrane
E) Increased Na^+ conductance of sarcolemma

10. A single contraction of skeletal muscle is most likely to be terminated by which of the following actions?

A) Closure of the postsynaptic nicotinic acetylcholine receptor
B) Removal of acetylcholine from the neuromuscular junction
C) Removal of Ca^{++} from the terminal of the motor neuron
D) Removal of sarcoplasmic Ca^{++}
E) Return of the dihydropyridine receptor to its resting conformation

11. Which of the following statements about smooth muscle contraction is most accurate?

A) Ca^{++} independent
B) Does not require an action potential
C) Requires more energy compared to skeletal muscle
D) Shorter in duration compared to skeletal muscle

12. Which of the following best describes an attribute of visceral smooth muscle not shared by skeletal muscle?

A) Contraction is ATP dependent
B) Contracts in response to stretch
C) Does not contain actin filaments
D) High rate of cross-bridge cycling
E) Low maximal force of contraction

13. The resting potential of a myelinated nerve fiber is primarily dependent on the concentration gradient of which of the following ions?

A) Ca^{++}
B) Cl^-
C) HCO_3^-
D) K^+
E) Na^+

14. Calmodulin is most closely related, both structurally and functionally, to which of the following proteins?

A) G-actin
B) Myosin light chain
C) Tropomyosin
D) Troponin C

15. Which of the following is a consequence of myelination in large nerve fibers?

A) Decreased velocity of nerve impulses
B) Generation of action potentials only at the nodes of Ranvier
C) Increased energy requirement to maintain ion gradients
D) Increased membrane capacitance
E) Increased nonselective diffusion of ions across the axon membrane

16. During a demonstration for medical students, a neurologist uses magnetic cortical stimulation to trigger firing of the ulnar nerve in a volunteer. At relatively low-amplitude stimulation, action potentials are recorded only from muscle fibers in the index finger. As the amplitude of the stimulation is increased, action potentials are recorded from muscle fibers in both the index finger and the biceps muscle. What is the fundamental principle underlying this amplitude-dependent response?

A) Large motor neurons that innervate large motor units require a larger depolarizing stimulus
B) Recruitment of multiple motor units requires a larger depolarizing stimulus
C) The biceps muscle is innervated by more motor neurons
D) The motor units in the biceps are smaller than those in the muscles of the fingers
E) The muscles in the fingers are innervated only by the ulnar nerve

17. Similarities between smooth and cardiac muscle include which of the following?

A) Ability to contract in the absence of an action potential
B) Dependence of contraction on Ca^{++} ions
C) Presence of a T tubule network
D) Role of myosin kinase in muscle contraction
E) Striated arrangement of the actin and myosin filaments

18. In a normal, healthy muscle, what occurs as a result of propagation of an action potential to the terminal membrane of a motor neuron?

A) Opening of voltage-gated Ca^{++} channels in the presynaptic membrane
B) Depolarization of the T tubule membrane follows
C) Always results in muscle contraction
D) Increase in intracellular Ca^{++} concentration in the motor neuron terminal
E) All of the above are correct

19. Which of the following decreases in length during the contraction of a skeletal muscle fiber?

A) A band of the sarcomere
B) I band of the sarcomere
C) Thick filaments
D) Thin filaments
E) Z discs of the sarcomere

20. A cross-sectional view of a skeletal muscle fiber through the H zone would reveal the presence of what?

A) Actin and titin
B) Actin, but no myosin
C) Actin, myosin, and titin
D) Myosin and actin
E) Myosin, but no actin

21. Tetanic contraction of a skeletal muscle fiber results from a cumulative increase in the intracellular concentration of which of the following?

A) ATP
B) Ca^{++}
C) K^+
D) Na^+
E) Troponin

22. Malignant hyperthermia is a potentially fatal genetic disorder characterized by a hyper-responsiveness to inhaled anesthetics and results in elevated body temperature, skeletal muscle rigidity, and lactic acidosis. Which of the following molecular changes could account for these clinical manifestations?

A) Decreased voltage sensitivity of the dihydropyridine receptor
B) Enhanced activity of the sarcoplasmic reticulum Ca^{++}-ATPase
C) Prolonged opening of the ryanodine receptor channel
D) Reduction in the density of voltage-sensitive Na^+ channels in the T tubule membrane

23. Weightlifting can result in a dramatic increase in skeletal muscle mass. This increase in muscle mass is primarily attributable to which of the following?

A) Fusion of sarcomeres between adjacent myofibrils
B) Hypertrophy of individual muscle fibers
C) Increase in skeletal muscle blood supply
D) Increase in the number of motor neurons
E) Increase in the number of neuromuscular junctions

24. Which of the following transport mechanisms is not rate limited by an intrinsic V_{max}?

A) Facilitated diffusion via carrier proteins
B) Primary active transport via carrier proteins
C) Secondary co-transport
D) Secondary counter-transport
E) Simple diffusion through protein channels

25. Assuming complete dissociation of all solutes, which of the following solutions would be hyperosmotic relative to 1 millimolar NaCl?

A) 1 millimolar $CaCl_2$
B) 1 millimolar glucose
C) 1 millimolar KCl
D) 1 millimolar sucrose
E) 1.5 millimolar glucose

Questions 26 and 27

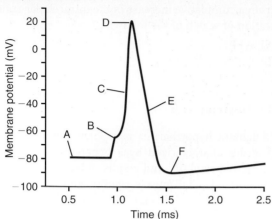

The diagram shows the change in membrane potential during an action potential in a giant squid axon. Refer to it when answering the next two questions.

26. Which of the following is primarily responsible for the change in membrane potential between points B and D?

    A) Inhibition of the Na^+, K^+-ATPase
    B) Movement of K^+ into the cell
    C) Movement of K^+ out of the cell
    D) Movement of Na^+ into the cell
    E) Movement of Na^+ out of the cell

27. Which of the following is primarily responsible for the change in membrane potential between points D and E?

    A) Inhibition of the Na^+, K^+-ATPase
    B) Movement of K^+ into the cell
    C) Movement of K^+ out of the cell
    D) Movement of Na^+ into the cell
    E) Movement of Na^+ out of the cell

28. The delayed onset and prolonged duration of smooth muscle contraction, as well as the greater force generated by smooth muscle compared with skeletal muscle, are all consequences of which of the following?

    A) Greater amount of myosin filaments present in smooth muscle
    B) Higher energy requirement of smooth muscle
    C) Physical arrangement of actin and myosin filaments
    D) Slower cycling rate of the smooth muscle myosin cross-bridges
    E) Slower uptake of Ca^{++} ions following contraction

29. An experimental drug is being tested as a potential therapeutic treatment for asthma. Preclinical studies have shown that this drug induces the relaxation of cultured porcine tracheal smooth muscle cells pre-contracted with acetylcholine. Which of the following mechanisms of action is most likely to induce this effect?

    A) Decreased affinity of troponin C for Ca^{++}
    B) Decreased plasma membrane K^+ permeability
    C) Increased plasma membrane Na^+ permeability
    D) Inhibition of the sarcoplasmic reticulum Ca^{++}-ATPase
    E) Stimulation of adenylate cyclase

Questions 30 and 31

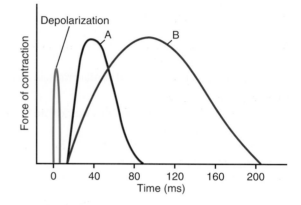

The diagram illustrates the single isometric twitch characteristics of two skeletal muscles, A and B, in response to a depolarizing stimulus. Refer to it when answering the next two questions.

30. Which of the following best describes muscle B, when compared to muscle A?

    A) Adapted for rapid contraction
    B) Composed of larger muscle fibers
    C) Fewer mitochondria
    D) Innervated by smaller nerve fibers
    E) Less extensive blood supply

31. The delay between the termination of the transient depolarization of the muscle membrane and the onset of muscle contraction observed in both muscles A and B reflects the time necessary for which of the following events to occur?

    A) ADP to be released from the myosin head
    B) ATP to be synthesized
    C) Ca^{++} to accumulate in the sarcoplasm
    D) G-actin to polymerize into F-actin
    E) Myosin head to complete one cross-bridge cycle

Questions 32–34

A 55-year-old woman visits her physician because of double vision, eyelid droop, difficulty chewing and swallowing, and general weakness in her limbs. All these symptoms are made worse with exercise and occur more frequently late in the day. The physician suspects myasthenia gravis and orders a Tensilon test. The test is positive.

32. The increased muscle strength observed during the Tensilon test is due to an increase in which of the following?

   A) Amount of acetylcholine (ACh) released from the motor nerves
   B) Levels of ACh at the muscle end-plates
   C) Number of ACh receptors on the muscle end-plates
   D) Synthesis of norepinephrine

33. What is the most likely basis for the symptoms described in this patient?

   A) Autoimmune response
   B) Botulinum toxicity
   C) Depletion of voltage-gated Ca^{++} channels in certain motor neurons
   D) Development of macro motor units following recovery from poliomyelitis
   E) Overexertion

34. Which of the following drugs would likely alleviate this patient's symptoms?

   A) Atropine
   B) Botulinum toxin antiserum
   C) Curare
   D) Halothane
   E) Neostigmine

35. The diagrams depict rigid containers composed of two aqueous chambers, A and B, each containing a Na^+ solution and separated by a Na^+-permeable membrane. The panel on the left represents the distribution of Na^+ ions at rest in the absence of any electrical potential. In this scenario, the concentration of Na^+ ions in chamber A equals the concentration of Na^+ ions in chamber B ($[Na]_A = [Na]_B$). The panel on the right illustrates the effect of a +60-millivolt potential applied across the membrane (chamber B relative to chamber A). Assuming a temperature of 37°C, which of the following expressions best describes the resulting distribution of Na^+ ions between the two chambers?

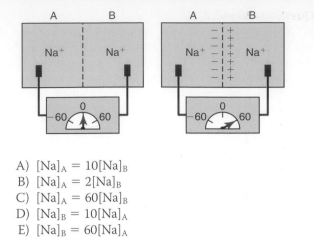

   A) $[Na]_A = 10[Na]_B$
   B) $[Na]_A = 2[Na]_B$
   C) $[Na]_A = 60[Na]_B$
   D) $[Na]_B = 10[Na]_A$
   E) $[Na]_B = 60[Na]_A$

Questions 36–38

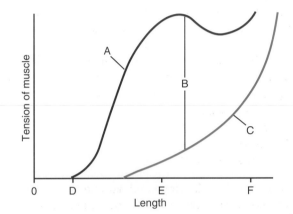

The diagram illustrates the isometric length-tension relationship in a representative intact skeletal muscle. When answering the following three questions, use the letters in the diagram to identify each of the following.

36. So-called "active" or contraction-dependent tension.

37. The muscle length at which active tension is maximal.

38. The contribution of non-contractile muscle elements to total tension.

39. Smooth muscle contraction is terminated by which of the following?

   A) Dephosphorylation of myosin kinase
   B) Dephosphorylation of myosin light chain
   C) Efflux of Ca^{++} ions across the plasma membrane
   D) Inhibition of myosin phosphatase
   E) Uptake of Ca^{++} ions into the sarcoplasmic reticulum

Questions 40–42

A 56-year-old man sees a neurologist because of weakness in his legs that improves over the course of the day or with exercise. Extracellular electrical recordings from a single skeletal muscle fiber reveal normal minia-ture end-plate potentials. Low-frequency electrical stimulation of the motor neuron, however, elicits an abnormally small depolarization of the muscle fibers. The amplitude of the depolarization is increased after exercise.

40. Based on these findings, which of the following is the most likely cause of this patient's leg weakness?

 A) Acetylcholinesterase deficiency
 B) Blockade of postsynaptic acetylcholine receptors
 C) Impaired presynaptic voltage-sensitive Ca^{++} influx
 D) Inhibition of Ca^{++} re-uptake into the sarcoplasmic reticulum
 E) Reduced acetylcholine synthesis

41. A preliminary diagnosis is confirmed by the presence of which of the following?

 A) Antibodies against the acetylcholine receptor
 B) Antibodies against the voltage-sensitive Ca^{++} channel
 C) Mutation in the gene that codes for the ryanodine receptor
 D) Relatively few vesicles in the presynaptic terminal
 E) Residual acetylcholine in the neuromuscular junction

42. The molecular mechanism underlying these symptoms is most similar to which of the following?

 A) Acetylcholine
 B) Botulinum toxin
 C) Curare
 D) Neostigmine
 E) Tetrodotoxin

Questions 43–45

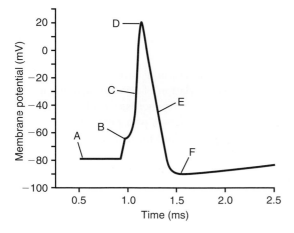

Match each of the descriptions to one of the points of the nerve action potential shown in the diagram.

43. Point at which the membrane potential (V_m) is closest to the Na^+ equilibrium potential.

44. Point at which the driving force for Na^+ is the greatest.

45. Point at which the ratio of K^+ permeability to Na^+ permeability (P_K/P_{Na}) is the greatest.

46. ATP is used directly for each of the following processes EXCEPT one. Which one is this EXCEPTION?

 A) Accumulation of Ca^{++} by the sarcoplasmic reticulum
 B) Transport of glucose into muscle cells
 C) Transport of H^+ from the parietal cells into the lumen of the stomach
 D) Transport of K^+ from the extracellular to intracel-lular fluid
 E) Transport of Na^+ from the intracellular to extracel-lular fluid

47. In the experiment illustrated in diagram A, equal vol-umes of solutions X, Y, and Z are placed into the com-partments of the two U-shaped vessels shown. The two compartments of each vessel are separated by semiper-meable membranes (i.e., impermeable to ions and large polar molecules). Diagram B illustrates the fluid distribu-tion across the membranes at equilibration. Assuming complete dissociation, identify each of the solutions shown.

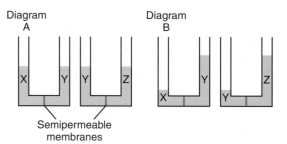

	Solution X	Solution Y	Solution Z
A)	1 M CaCl$_2$	1 M NaCl	1 M glucose
B)	1 M glucose	1 M NaCl	1 M CaCl$_2$
C)	1 M NaCl	2 M glucose	3 M CaCl$_2$
D)	2 M NaCl	1 M NaCl	Pure water
E)	Pure water	1 M CaCl$_2$	2 M glucose

48. The force produced by a single skeletal muscle fiber can be increased by which of the following?

 A) Decreasing extracellular K^+ concentration
 B) Increasing the amplitude of the depolarizing stimulus
 C) Increasing the frequency of stimulation of the fiber
 D) Increasing the number of voltage-gated Na^+ chan-nels in the sarcolemma
 E) Increasing the permeability of the sarcolemma to K^+

Questions 49 and 50

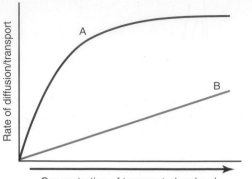

49. Trace A best describes the kinetics of which of the following events?

   A) Movement of CO_2 across the plasma membrane
   B) Movement of O_2 across a lipid bilayer
   C) Na^+ flux through an open nicotinic acetylcholine receptor channel
   D) Transport of K^+ into a muscle cell
   E) Voltage-dependent movement of Ca^{++} into the terminal of a motor neuron

50. Trace B best describes the kinetics which of the following events?

   A) Na^+-dependent transport of glucose into an epithelial cell
   B) Transport of Ca^{++} into the sarcoplasmic reticulum of a smooth muscle cell
   C) Transport of K^+ into a muscle cell
   D) Transport of Na^+ out of a nerve cell
   E) Transport of O_2 across an artificial lipid bilayer

51. Trace A represents a typical action potential recorded under control conditions from a normal nerve cell in response to a depolarizing stimulus. Which of the following perturbations would explain the conversion of the response shown in trace A to the action potential shown in trace B?

   A) Blockade of voltage-sensitive Na^+ channels
   B) Blockade of voltage-sensitive K^+ channels
   C) Blockade of Na-K "leak" channels
   D) Replacement of the voltage-sensitive K^+ channels with "slow" Ca^{++} channels
   E) Replacement of the voltage-sensitive Na^+ channels with "slow" Ca^{++} channels

52. Which of the following perturbations would account for the failure of the same stimulus to elicit an action potential in trace C?

   A) Blockade of voltage-sensitive Na^+ channels
   B) Blockade of voltage-sensitive K^+ channels
   C) Blockade of Na-K "leak" channels
   D) Replacement of the voltage-sensitive K^+ channels with "slow" Ca^{++} channels
   E) Replacement of the voltage-sensitive Na^+ channels with "slow" Ca^{++} channels

Questions 51 and 52

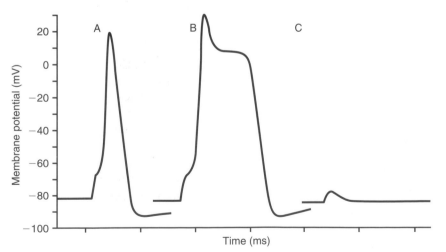

53. A 17-year-old soccer player suffered a fracture to the left tibia. After her lower leg has been in a cast for 8 weeks, she is surprised to find that the left gastrocnemius muscle is significantly smaller in circumference than it was before the fracture. What is the most likely explanation?

   A) Decrease in the number of individual muscle fibers in the left gastrocnemius
   B) Decrease in blood flow to the muscle caused by constriction from the cast
   C) Temporary reduction in actin and myosin protein synthesis
   D) Increase in glycolytic activity in the affected muscle
   E) Progressive denervation

54. Smooth muscle that exhibits rhythmical contraction in the absence of external stimuli also necessarily exhibits which of the following?

   A) "Slow" voltage-sensitive Ca^{++} channels
   B) Intrinsic pacemaker wave activity
   C) Higher resting cytosolic Ca^{++} concentration
   D) Hyperpolarized membrane potential
   E) Action potentials with "plateaus"

Questions 55–59

   A) Simple diffusion
   B) Facilitated diffusion
   C) Primary active transport
   D) Co-transport
   E) Counter-transport

Match each of the processes described below with the correct type of transport listed above (each answer may be used more than once).

55. Ouabain-sensitive transport of Na^+ ions from the cytosol to the extracellular fluid

56. Glucose uptake into skeletal muscle

57. Na^+-dependent transport of Ca^{++} from the cytosol to the extracellular fluid

58. Transport of glucose from the intestinal lumen into an intestinal epithelial cell

59. Movement of Na^+ ions into a nerve cell during the upstroke of an action potential

60. Traces A, B, and C in the diagram summarize the changes in membrane potential (V_m) and the underlying membrane permeabilities (P) that occur in a nerve cell over the course of an action potential. Choose the combination of labels below that accurately identifies each of the traces.

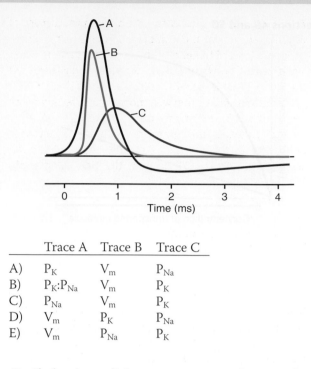

	Trace A	Trace B	Trace C
A)	P_K	V_m	P_{Na}
B)	P_K:P_{Na}	V_m	P_K
C)	P_{Na}	V_m	P_K
D)	V_m	P_K	P_{Na}
E)	V_m	P_{Na}	P_K

61. If the intracellular concentration of a membrane-permeant substance doubles from 10 to 20 millimolar and the extracellular concentration remains at 5 millimolar, the rate of diffusion of that substance across the plasma membrane will increase by a factor of how much?

   A) 2
   B) 3
   C) 4
   D) 5
   E) 6

62. Which of the following pairs of aqueous solutions will exert equal osmotic pressures across a normal cell membrane once steady-state conditions have been established?

	Solution A	Solution B
A)	10% albumin	10% IgG
B)	100 mmol/L NaCl	100 mOsm/L $CaCl_2$
C)	300 mOsm/L glucose	300 mOsm/L urea
D)	300 mOsm/L glycerol	300 mOsm/L NaCl
E)	300 mOsm/L glycerol	300 mOsm/L urea

63. A 12-year-old boy presents with a 4-month history of diminished vision and diplopia. He also experiences tiredness toward the end of the day. There are no other symptoms. On examination, the patient has ptosis of the left eye that improves after a period of sleep. Clinical examination is otherwise normal. There is no evidence of weakness of any other muscles. Additional testing indicates the presence of anti-acetylcholine antibodies in the plasma, a normal thyroid function test, and a normal CT scan of the brain and orbit. What is the initial diagnosis?

A) Astrocytoma
B) Graves disease
C) Hashimoto thyroiditis
D) Juvenile myasthenia gravis
E) Multiple sclerosis

64. The length–tension diagram shown here was obtained from a skeletal muscle with equal numbers of red and white fibers. Supramaximal tetanic stimuli were used to initiate an isometric contraction at each muscle length studied. The resting length was 20 cm. What is the maximum amount of active tension that the muscle is capable of generating at a preload of 100 grams?

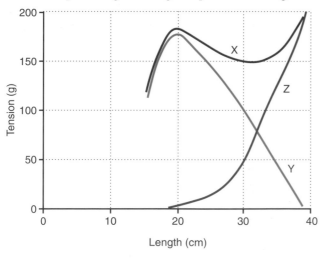

A) 145–155 grams
B) 25–35 grams
C) 55–65 grams
D) 95–105 grams
E) Cannot be determined

65. The sensitivity of the smooth muscle contractile apparatus to calcium is known to increase in the steady-state under normal conditions. This increase in calcium sensitivity can be attributed to a decrease in the levels of which of the following substances?

A) Actin
B) Adenosine Triphosphate (ATP)
C) Calcium-calmodulin complex
D) Calmodulin
E) Myosin light chain phosphatase (MLCP)

66. The diagram shows the force–velocity relationship for isotonic contractions of skeletal muscle. The differences in the three curves result from differences in which of the following?

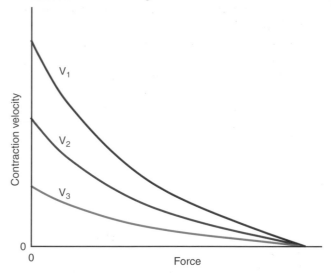

A) Frequency of muscle contraction
B) Hypertrophy
C) Muscle mass
D) Myosin ATPase activity
E) Recruitment of motor units

67. A 24-year-old woman is admitted as an emergency to University Hospital following an automobile accident in which severe lacerations to the left wrist severed a major muscle tendon. The severed ends of the tendon were overlapped by 6 cm to facilitate suturing and reattachment. Which of the following would be expected after 6 weeks compared to the preinjured muscle? Assume that series growth of sarcomeres cannot be completed within 6 weeks.

	Passive tension	Maximal active tension
A)	decrease	decrease
B)	decrease	increase
C)	increase	increase
D)	increase	decrease
E)	no change	no change

ANSWERS

1. B) A solution of 140 millimolar NaCl has an osmolarity of 280 milliosmoles, which is iso-osmotic relative to "normal" intracellular osmolarity. If red blood cells were placed in 140 millimolar NaCl alone, there would be no change in cell volume because intracellular and extracellular osmolarities are equal. The presence of 20 millimolar urea, however, increases the solution's osmolarity and makes it hypertonic relative to the intracellular solution. Water will initially move out of the cell, but because the plasma membrane is permeable to urea, urea will diffuse into the cell and equilibrate across the plasma membrane. As a result, water will re-enter the cell, and the cell will return to its original volume.
TMP12 52

2. E) A 1 millimolar solution has an osmolarity of 1 milliosmole when the solute molecule does not dissociate. However, NaCl and KCl both dissociate into two molecules, and $CaCl_2$ dissociates into three molecules. Therefore, 12 millimolar NaCl has an osmolarity of 24 milliosmoles, 4 millimolar KCl has an osmolarity of 8 milliosmoles, and 2 millimolar $CaCl_2$ has an osmolarity of 6 milliosmoles. These add up to 38 milliosmoles.
TMP12 52

3. E) The equilibrium potential for chloride (E_{Cl}^-), a monovalent anion, can be calculated using the Nernst equation: E_{Cl}^- (in millivolts) $= 61 \times \log (C_i/C_o)$, where C_i is the intracellular concentration and C_o is the extracellular concentration. In this case, $E_{Cl}^- = 61 \times \log (11/110) = -61$ millivolts.
TMP12 58

4. E) The equilibrium potential for potassium (E_K^+), a monovalent cation, can be calculated using the Nernst equation: E_K^+ (in millivolts) $= -61 \times \log (C_i/C_o)$. Here, $E_K^+ = -61 \times \log (140/14) = -61$ millivolts.
TMP12 58

5. A) Quantitatively, the driving force on any given ion is the difference in millivolts between the membrane potential (V_m) and the equilibrium potential for that ion (E_{ion}). In this cell, $E_K = -61$ millivolts, $E_{Cl} = -61$ millivolts, $E_{Na} = +61$ millivolts, and $E_{Ca} = 525$ millivolts. Therefore, Ca^{++} is the ion with the equilibrium potential farthest from V_m. This means that Ca^{++} would have the greatest tendency to cross the membrane through an open channel (in this particular example).
TMP12 58

6. F) If a membrane is permeable to only a single ion, V_m is equal to the equilibrium potential for that ion. In this cell, $E_K = -61$ millivolts. If the extracellular K^+ concentration is reduced 10-fold, $E_K = 61 \times \log (1.4/140) = -122$ millivolts, which is a hyperpolarization of 61 millivolts.
TMP12 58

7. E) Tension development in a single sarcomere is directly proportional to the number of active myosin cross-bridges attached to actin filaments. Overlap between the myosin and actin filaments is optimal at sarcomere lengths of about 2.0 to 2.5 micrometers, which allows maximal contact between myosin heads and actin filaments. At lengths less than 2.0 micrometers, the actin filaments protrude into the H band, where no myosin heads exist. At lengths greater than 2.5 micrometers, the actin filaments are pulled toward the ends of the myosin filaments, again reducing the number of possible cross-bridges.
TMP12 77

8. B) In contrast to primary and secondary active transport, neither facilitated diffusion nor simple diffusion requires additional energy and, therefore, can work in the absence of ATP. Only facilitated diffusion displays saturation kinetics and involves a carrier protein. By definition, neither simple nor facilitated diffusion can move molecules from low to high concentration. The concept of specific inhibitors is not applicable to simple diffusion that occurs through a lipid bilayer without the aid of protein.
TMP12 46

9. B) Excitation–contraction coupling in skeletal muscle begins with an excitatory depolarization of the muscle fiber membrane (sarcolemma). This depolarization triggers the all-or-none opening of voltage-sensitive Na^+ channels and an action potential that travels deep into the muscle fiber via the T tubule network. At the T tubule–sarcoplasmic reticulum "triad," the depolarization of the T tubule causes a conformational change in the dihydropyridine receptor and subsequently in the ryanodine receptor on the sarcoplasmic reticulum. The latter causes the release of Ca^{++} into the sarcoplasm and the binding of Ca^{++} to troponin C (not to calmodulin) on the actin filament.
TMP12 88

10. **D)** Skeletal muscle contraction is tightly regulated by the concentration of Ca^{++} in the sarcoplasm. As long as sarcoplasmic Ca^{++} is sufficiently high, none of the remaining events—removal of acetylcholine from the neuromuscular junction, removal of Ca^{++} from the presynaptic terminal, closure of the acetylcholine receptor channel, and return of the dihydropyridine receptor to its resting conformation—would have any effect on the contractile state of the muscle.
    TMP12 88

11. **B)** In contrast to skeletal muscle, smooth muscle can be stimulated to contract without the generation of an action potential. For example, smooth muscle contracts in response to any stimulus that increases the cytosolic Ca^{++} concentration. This includes Ca^{++} channel openers, subthreshold depolarization, and a variety of tissue factors and circulating hormones that stimulate the release of intracellular Ca^{++} stores. Smooth muscle contraction uses less energy and lasts longer compared to that of skeletal muscle. Smooth muscle contraction is heavily Ca^{++} dependent.
    TMP12 96

12. **B)** An important characteristic of visceral smooth muscle is its ability to contract in response to stretch. Stretch results in depolarization and potentially the generation of action potentials. These action potentials, coupled with normal slow-wave potentials, stimulate rhythmical contractions. Like skeletal muscle, smooth muscle contraction is both actin and ATP dependent. However, the cross-bridge cycle in smooth muscle is considerably slower than in skeletal muscle, which allows for a higher maximal force of contraction.
    TMP12 93

13. **D)** The resting potential of any cell is dependent on the concentration gradients of the permeant ions and their relative permeabilities (Goldman equation). In the myelinated nerve fiber, as in most cells, the resting membrane is predominantly permeable to K^+. The negative membrane potential observed in most cells (including nerve cells) is due primarily to the relatively high intracellular concentration and high permeability of K^+.
    TMP12 58

14. **D)** In smooth muscle, the binding of four Ca^{++} ions to the protein calmodulin permits the interaction of the Ca^{++}-calmodulin complex with myosin light chain kinase. This interaction activates myosin light chain kinase, resulting in the phosphorylation of the myosin light chains and, ultimately, muscle contraction. In skeletal muscle, the activating Ca^{++} signal is received by the protein troponin C. Like calmodulin, each molecule of troponin C can bind with up to four Ca^{++} ions. Binding results in a conformational change in the troponin C protein that dislodges the tropomyosin molecule and exposes the active sites on the actin filament.
    TMP12 93

15. **B)** Myelination of the axons of large nerve fibers has several consequences. It provides insulation to the axon membrane, decreasing membrane capacitance and thereby decreasing the "leakage" of ions across the cell membrane. Action potentials in myelinated axons occur only at the periodic breaks in the myelin sheath, called *nodes of Ranvier*. Voltage-gated Na^+ channels are concentrated at these nodes. This arrangement both increases the velocity of the nerve impulses along the axon and minimizes the number of charges that cross the membrane during an impulse, thereby minimizing the energy required by Na^+, K^+-ATPase to re-establish the relative concentration gradients for Na^+ and K^+.
    TMP12 67

16. **A)** Muscle fibers involved in fine motor control are generally innervated by small motor neurons with relatively small motor units, including those that innervate single fibers. These neurons fire in response to a smaller depolarizing stimulus compared with motor neurons with larger motor units. As a result, during weak contractions, increases in muscle contraction can occur in small steps, allowing for fine motor control. This concept is called the *size principle*.
    TMP12 80

17. **B)** The strongest common denominator among smooth, skeletal, and cardiac muscle contraction is their shared dependence on Ca^{++} for the initiation of contraction. Cardiac and skeletal muscles exhibit several characteristics not shared by smooth muscle. For example, the contractile proteins in both cardiac and skeletal muscles are organized into discrete sarcomeres. Both muscle types also possess some semblance of a T tubule system and are dependent on the generation of action potentials for their contraction. Smooth muscle, in contrast, is relatively less organized, is uniquely regulated by myosin light chain phosphorylation, and can contract in vivo in the absence of action potentials.
    TMP12 93

18. **E)** The neuromuscular junction is equipped with a so-called safety factor that ensures that every nerve impulse that travels to the terminal of a motor neuron results in an action potential in the sarcolemma. Given a normal, healthy muscle, contraction is also ensured. The voltage sensitivity of the Ca^{++} channels in the presynaptic membrane and the high concentration of extracellular Ca^{++} ensure an influx of Ca^{++} sufficient to stimulate the fusion of synaptic vesicles to the presynaptic membrane and the release of acetylcholine. The overabundance of acetylcholine released guarantees a depolarization of the postsynaptic membrane and the firing of an action potential.
    TMP12 85

19. **B)** The physical lengths of the actin and myosin filaments do not change during contraction. Therefore,

the A band, which is composed of myosin filaments, does not change either. The distance between Z discs decreases, but the Z discs themselves do not change. Only the I band decreases in length as the muscle contracts.

TMP12 74

20. **E)** The H zone is the region in the center of the sarcomere composed of the lighter bands on either side of and including the M line. In this region, the myosin filaments are centered on the M line, and there are no overlapping actin filaments. Therefore, a cross-section through this region would reveal only myosin.

TMP12 72

21. **B)** Muscle contraction is dependent on an elevation of intracellular Ca^{++} concentration. As the twitch frequency increases, the initiation of a subsequent twitch can occur before the previous twitch has subsided. As a result, the amplitude of the individual twitches is summed. At very high twitch frequencies, the muscle exhibits tetanic contraction. Under these conditions, intracellular Ca^{++} accumulates and supports sustained maximal contraction.

TMP12 80

22. **C)** As long as the ryanodine receptor channel on the sarcoplasmic reticulum remains open, Ca^{++} will continue to flood the sarcoplasm and stimulate contraction. This prolonged contraction results in heat production, muscle rigidity, and lactic acidosis. In contrast, factors that either inhibit Ca^{++} release or stimulate Ca^{++} uptake into the sarcoplasmic reticulum, or that prevent either the depolarization of the T tubule membrane or the transduction of the depolarization into Ca^{++} release, would favor muscle relaxation.

TMP12 88

23. **B)** Prolonged or repeated maximal contraction results in a concomitant increase in the synthesis of contractile proteins and an increase in muscle mass. This increase in mass, or hypertrophy, is observed at the level of individual muscle fibers.

TMP12 81

24. **E)** Facilitated diffusion and both primary and secondary active transport all involve protein transporters or carriers that must undergo some rate-limited conformational change. The rate of simple diffusion is linear with solute concentration.

TMP12 46

25. **A)** The term "hyperosmotic" refers to a solution that has a higher osmolarity relative to another solution. The osmolarity of a 1-millimolar NaCl solution is 2 mOsm/L. The osmolarity of a 1-millimolar solution of either glucose or sucrose is only 1 mOsm/L. The osmolarity of a 1.5-millimolar glucose solution is 1.5 mOsm/L. These solutions are all "hypo-osmotic" relative to 1 millimolar

NaCl. The osmolarity of a 1-millimolar KCl solution is 2 mOsm/L. It is "iso-osmotic" relative to 1 millimolar NaCl. Only 1 millimolar $CaCl_2$, with an osmolarity of 3 mOsm/L is hyperosmotic relative to 1 millimolar NaCl.

TMP12 52

26. **D)** At point B in this action potential, V_m has reached threshold potential and has triggered the opening of voltage-gated Na^+ channels. The resulting Na^+ influx is responsible for the rapid, self-perpetuating depolarization phase of the action potential.

TMP12 63

27. **C)** The rapid depolarization phase is terminated at point D by the inactivation of the voltage-gated Na^+ channels and the opening of the voltage-gated K^+ channels. The latter results in the efflux of K^+ from the cytosol into the extracellular fluid and repolarization of the cell membrane.

TMP12 63

28. **D)** The slower cycling rate of the cross-bridges in smooth muscle means that a higher percentage of possible cross-bridges is active at any point in time. The more active cross-bridges there are, the greater the force that is generated. Although the relatively slow cycling rate means that it takes longer for the myosin head to attach to the actin filament, it also means that the myosin head remains attached longer, prolonging muscle contraction. Because of the slow cross-bridge cycling rate, smooth muscle actually requires less energy to maintain a contraction compared with skeletal muscle.

TMP12 92

29. **E)** The stimulation of either adenylate or guanylate cyclase induces smooth muscle relaxation. The cyclic nucleotides produced by these enzymes stimulate cAMP- and cGMP-dependent kinases, respectively. These kinases phosphorylate, among other things, enzymes that remove Ca^{++} from the cytosol, and in doing so they inhibit contraction. In contrast, either a decrease in K^+ permeability or an increase in Na^+ permeability results in membrane depolarization and contraction. Likewise, inhibition of the sarcoplasmic reticulum Ca^{++}-ATPase, one of the enzymes activated by cyclic nucleotide-dependent kinases, would also favor muscle contraction. Smooth muscle does not express troponin.

TMP12 97

30. **D)** Muscle B is characteristic of a slow twitch muscle (Type 1) composed of predominantly slow twitch muscle fibers. These fibers are smaller in size and are innervated by smaller nerve fibers. They typically have a more extensive blood supply, a greater number of mitochondria, and large amounts of myoglobin, all of which support high levels of oxidative phosphorylation.

TMP12 79

31. C) Muscle contraction is triggered by an increase in sarcoplasmic Ca^{++} concentration. The delay between the termination of the depolarizing pulse and the onset of muscle contraction, also called the "lag," reflects the time necessary for the depolarizing pulse to be translated into an increase in sarcoplasmic Ca^{++} concentration. This process involves a conformational change in the voltage-sensing, or dihydropyridine receptor, located on the T tubule membrane; the subsequent conformational change in the ryanodine receptor on the sarcoplasmic reticulum; and the release of Ca^{++} from the sarcoplasmic reticulum.

TMP12 88

32. B) Myasthenia gravis is an autoimmune disease in which antibodies damage postsynaptic nicotinic acetylcholine receptors. This damage prevents the firing of an action potential in the postsynaptic membrane. Tensilon is a readily reversible acetylcholinesterase inhibitor that increases acetylcholine levels in the neuromuscular junction, thereby increasing the strength of muscle contraction.

TMP12 86

33. A) Myasthenia gravis is an autoimmune disease characterized by the presence of anti–acetylcholine receptor antibodies in the plasma. Overexertion can cause junction fatigue, and both a decrease in the density of voltage-sensitive Ca^{++} channels in the presynaptic membrane and botulinum toxicity can cause muscle weakness. However, these effects are presynaptic and therefore would not be reversed by acetylcholinesterase inhibition. Although the macro-motor units formed during reinnervation following poliomyelitis compromise the patient's fine motor control, they do not affect muscle strength.

TMP12 86

34. E) Neostigmine is an acetylcholinesterase inhibitor. Administration of this drug would increase the amount of acetylcholine (ACh) present in the synapse and its ability to sufficiently depolarize the postsynaptic membrane and trigger an action potential. Botulinum toxin antiserum is effective only against botulinum toxicity. Curare blocks the nicotinic ACh receptor and causes muscle weakness. Atropine is a muscarinic ACh receptor antagonist, and halothane is an anesthetic gas. Neither atropine nor halothane has any effect on the neuromuscular junction.

TMP12 86

35. D) When a positive electrical charge of 60 millivolts is applied to chamber B, the positively charged Na^+ ions are repelled from chamber B into chamber A until the diffusional force from the concentration gradient is sufficient to counter the electromotive force. Using the Nernst equation, a 60-millivolt electromotive force would be offset by a 10-fold Na^+ concentration gradient.

Therefore, at the new steady state, the $[Na]_A$ would be 10 times the $[Na]_B$.

TMP12 58

36. B) In this diagram, "active" or contraction-dependent tension is the difference between total tension (trace A) and the passive tension contributed by noncontractile elements (trace C). The length-tension relationship in intact muscle resembles the biphasic relationship observed in individual sarcomeres and reflects the same physical interactions between actin and myosin filaments.

TMP12 77

37. E) "Active" tension is maximal at normal physiological muscle lengths. At this point, there is optimal overlap between actin and myosin filaments to support maximal cross-bridge formation and tension development.

TMP12 77

38. C) Trace C represents the passive tension contributed by noncontractile elements, including fascia, tendons, and ligaments. This passive tension accounts for an increasingly large portion of the total tension recorded in intact muscle as it is stretched beyond its normal length.

TMP12 77

39. B) Smooth muscle contraction is regulated by both Ca^{++} and myosin light chain phosphorylation. When the cytosolic Ca^{++} concentration decreases following the initiation of contraction, myosin kinase becomes inactivated. However, cross-bridge formation continues, even in the absence of Ca^{++}, until the myosin light chains are dephosphorylated through the action of myosin light chain phosphatase.

TMP12 94

40. C) The normal miniature end-plate potentials indicate sufficient synthesis and packaging of ACh and the presence and normal function of ACh receptor channels. The most likely explanation for this patient's symptoms is a presynaptic deficiency—in this case, an impairment of the voltage-sensitive Ca^{++} channels responsible for the increase in cytosolic Ca^{++} that triggers the release of ACh into the synapse. The increase in postsynaptic depolarization observed after exercise is indicative of an accumulation of Ca^{++} in the presynaptic terminal after multiple action potentials have reached the nerve terminal.

TMP12 85

41. B) Inhibition of the presynaptic voltage-sensitive Ca^{++} channels is most consistent with the presence of antibodies against this channel. Antibodies against the ACh receptor, a mutation in the ryanodine receptor, and residual ACh in the junction are all indicative of postsynaptic defects. Although it is a presynaptic defect, a deficit of ACh vesicles is unlikely in this scenario, given the normal miniature end-plate potentials recorded in the postsynaptic membrane.

TMP12 83

42. **B)** Botulinum toxin inhibits muscle contraction presynaptically by decreasing the amount of ACh released into the neuromuscular junction. In contrast, curare acts post-synaptically, blocking the nicotinic ACh receptors and preventing the excitation of the muscle cell membrane. Tetrodotoxin blocks voltage-sensitive Na^+ channels, impacting both the initiation and the propagation of action potentials in the motor neuron. Both ACh and neostigmine stimulate muscle contraction.

TMP12 85

43. **D)** During an action potential in a nerve cell, V_m approaches E_{Na} during the rapid depolarization phase when the permeability of the membrane to Na^+ (P_{Na}) increases relative to its permeability to K^+ (P_K). In a "typical" cell, E_{Na} is close to 60 millivolts. V_m is closest to E_{Na} at point D in this diagram. At this point, the ratio of P_{Na} to P_K is the greatest.

TMP12 63

44. **F)** The driving force for Na^+ is greatest at the point at which V_m is the farthest from E_{Na}. If E_{Na} is very positive (approximately 60 millivolts), V_m is farthest from E_{Na} at point F, or when the cell is the most hyperpolarized.

TMP12 63

45. **F)** Generally, V_m is closest to the equilibrium potential of the most permeant ion. In nerve cells, $P_K >> P_{Na}$ at rest. As a result, V_m is relatively close to E_K. During the after-potential or the hyperpolarization phase of the action potential, the ratio of P_K to P_{Na} is even greater than it is at rest. This is due to the residual opening of voltage-gated K^+ channels and the inactivation of the voltage-gated Na^+ channels. P_K:P_{Na} is greatest at point F, at which point V_m comes closest to E_K.

TMP12 63

46. **B)** The accumulation of Ca^{++} by the sarcoplasmic reticulum, the transport of Na^+ into and K^+ out of a cell, and the transport of H^+ from parietal cells all occur through primary active transport mechanisms involving ATPase enzymes. In this case, only glucose transport, which occurs via facilitated diffusion in muscle, does not directly utilize ATP.

TMP12 50

47. **B)** The redistribution of fluid volume shown in diagram B reflects the net diffusion of water, or osmosis, due to differences in the osmolarity of the solutions on either side of the semipermeable membrane. Osmosis occurs from solutions of high water concentration to low water concentration or from low osmolarity to high osmolarity. In diagram B, osmosis has occurred from X to Y and from Y to Z. Therefore, the osmolarity of solution Z is

higher than that of solution Y, and the osmolarity of solution Y is higher than that of solution X.

TMP12 51

48. **C)** Increasing the sarcoplasmic Ca^{++} concentration can increase force generation in a single muscle fiber. This can be accomplished by increasing the frequency of stimulation of the fiber. Neither increasing the amplitude of the depolarization at the postsynaptic membrane of the neuromuscular junction nor increasing the number of voltage-gated Na^+ channels is likely to affect the release of Ca^{++} from the sarcoplasmic reticulum. In contrast, both a decrease in the extracellular K^+ concentration and an increase in the permeability of the muscle membrane to K^+ would decrease excitability of the muscle cell.

TMP12 80

49. **D)** Trace A reflects the kinetics of a process that is limited by an intrinsic V_{max}. Of the choices provided, only the transport of K^+, which occurs through the activity of the Na^+, K^+-ATPase, is the result of an active transport event. The movement of CO_2 and O_2 through a biological membrane and the movement of Ca^{++} and Na^+ through ion channels are all examples of simple diffusion.

TMP12 49

50. **E)** Trace B is indicative of a process not limited by an intrinsic V_{max}. This excludes active transport and facilitated diffusion. Therefore, of the choices provided, only the rate of transport of O_2 across an artificial lipid bilayer via simple diffusion would be accurately reflected by trace B.

TMP12 49

51. **E)** These so-called slow Ca^{++} channels have a slower inactivation rate, thereby lengthening the time during which they are open. This, in turn, delays the repolarization phase of the action potential, creating a "plateau" before the channels inactivate.

TMP12 63; see also Chapter 9

52. **A)** In the absence of hyperpolarization, the inability of an otherwise excitatory stimulus to initiate an action potential is most likely the result of the blockade of the voltage-gated channels responsible for the generation of the all-or-none depolarization. In nerve cells, these are the voltage-gated Na^+ channels.

TMP12 62

53. **C)** Skeletal muscle continuously remodels in response to its level of use. When a muscle is inactive for an extended period, the rate of synthesis of the contractile proteins in individual muscle fibers decreases, resulting in an overall reduction in muscle mass. This reversible reduction in muscle mass is called *atrophy*.

TMP12 81

54. B) For a muscle to contract spontaneously and rhythmically, there must be an intrinsic rhythmical "pacemaker." Intestinal smooth muscle, for example, exhibits a rhythmical slow-wave potential that transiently depolarizes and repolarizes the muscle membrane. This slow wave does not stimulate contraction itself, but if the amplitude is sufficient, it can trigger one or more action potentials that result in Ca^{++} influx and contraction. Although they are typical of smooth muscle, neither "slow" voltage-sensitive Ca^{++} channels nor action potentials with "plateaus" play a necessary role in rhythmical contraction. A high resting cytosolic Ca^{++} concentration would support a sustained contraction, and hyperpolarization would favor relaxation.

TMP12 96

55. C) Ouabain inhibits Na^+, K^+-ATPase. This ATP-dependent enzyme transports three Na^+ ions out of the cell for every two K^+ ions it transports into the cell. It is a classic example of primary active transport.

TMP12 53

56. B) Glucose is transported into skeletal muscle cells via insulin-dependent facilitated diffusion.

TMP12 50; see also Chapter 78

57. E) The activity of Na^+, K^+-ATPase maintains the relatively high K^+ concentration inside the cell and the relatively high Na^+ concentration in the extracellular fluid. This large concentration gradient for Na^+ across the plasma membrane, together with the net negative charge on the inside of the cell, continuously drives Na^+ ions from the extracellular fluid into the cytosol. This energy is used to transport other molecules, such as Ca^{++}, against their concentration gradients. Because ATP is required to maintain the Na^+ gradient that drives this counter-transport, this type of transport is called *secondary active transport.*

TMP12 52

58. D) Much like Na^+-Ca^{++} counter-transport, the strong tendency for Na^+ to move across the plasma membrane into the cytosol can be harnessed by transport proteins and used to co-transport molecules against their concentration gradients into the cytosol. An example of this type of secondary co-transport is the transport of glucose into intestinal epithelial cells.

TMP12 52

59. A) During the rapid depolarization phase of a nerve action potential, voltage-sensitive $Na+$ channels open and allow the influx of Na^+ ions into the cytosol. Transport through membrane channels is an example of simple diffusion.

TMP12 46; see also Chapter 5

60. E) Trace A exhibits the characteristic shape of an action potential, including the rapid depolarization followed by a rapid repolarization that temporarily overshoots the resting potential. Trace B best illustrates the change in P_{Na} that occurs during an action potential. The rapid increase in P_{Na} closely parallels the rapid depolarization phase of the action potential. Trace C best illustrates the slow onset of the increase in P_K that reflects the opening of the voltage-gated K^+ channels.

TMP12 63

61. B) Net diffusion of a substance across a permeable membrane is proportional to the concentration difference of the substance on either side of the membrane. Initially, the concentration difference is 5 millimolar (10 millimolar − 5 millimolar). When the intracellular concentration doubles to 20 millimolar, the concentration difference becomes 15 millimolar (20 millimolar − 5 millimolar). The concentration difference has tripled; therefore, the rate of diffusion would also increase by a factor of 3.

TMP12 50

62. E) Glycerol and urea are both permeant molecules, which means that both will diffuse through the cell membrane until the intracellular and extracellular concentrations are identical. Thus, during steady-state conditions the intracellular and extracellular osmolarity is 600 mOsm/L (300 mOsm/L from urea and 300 mOsm/L from glycerol). Choice A is not correct because albumin is a smaller molecule compared to IgG. This difference in molecular weight means that a 10% solution of albumin will contain more molecules per unit volume compared to a 10% solution of IgG and thus exert a greater osmotic effect. Choice B: A solution of 100 mmol/L NaCl has an osmolarity of 200 mOsm/L because Na and Cl dissociate. Thus, the osmolarity of solution A will be two times greater than solution B. Choices C and D: Both solutions have equal osmolarities; however, both urea and glycerol are permeant molecules (whereas glucose and NaCl are not), which means that urea and glycerol will diffuse into the cell and effectively cancel their osmotic effects across the cell membrane.

TMP12 52

63. D) Myasthenia gravis is an acquired autoimmune disease causing skeletal muscle fatigue and weakness. The disease is associated with (caused by) IgG antibodies to acetylcholine receptors at post-synaptic membranes of neuromuscular junctions. The major symptom is muscle weakness, which gets worse with activity. Patients often feel well in the morning, but become weaker as the day goes on. The muscle weakness usually causes symptoms of double vision (diplopia) and drooping eyelids (ptosis). The presence of anti-acetylcholine antibodies in the plasma is specific for myasthenia gravis and thus rules out the other answer choices. In addition, the normal CT scan of the brain and orbit specifically rules out the possibility of an astrocytoma (choice A), that is, brain tumor, that could compress cranial nerves. Double vision commonly occurs in Graves disease (choice B); however, the thyroid test was normal (which also rules out Hashimoto thyroiditis, choice C). Multiple sclerosis (choice E) is commonly associated with a spastic weakness of the legs, but, again, the presence of anti-acetylcholine antibodies is specific for myasthenia gravis.

   TMP12 86

64. **C)** The diagram shows the relationship between preload or passive tension (curve Z), total tension (curve X), and active tension (curve Y). Active tension cannot be measured directly: it is the difference between total tension and passive tension. To answer this question, the student must first find where 100 grams intersects the preload curve (passive tension curve) and then move down to the active tension curve. One can see that a preload of 100 grams is associated with a total tension of a little more than 150 grams, and an active tension of a little more than 50 grams. Note that active tension equals total tension minus passive tension, as discussed above. Drawing these three curves in a manner that is mathematically correct is not an easy task. The student should thus recognize that active tension may not equal total tension minus passive tension at all points on the diagram shown here as well as on USMLE diagrams.

   TMP12 77

65. **E)** Smooth muscle is unique in its ability to generate various degrees of tension at a constant concentration of intracellular calcium. This change in calcium sensitivity of smooth muscle can be attributed to differences in the activity of MLCP. Smooth muscle contracts when the myosin light chain is phosphorylated by the actions of myosin light chain kinase (MLCK). MLCP is a phosphatase that can dephosphorylate the myosin light chain, rendering it inactive and therefore attenuating the muscle contraction. Choice A: Both actin and myosin are important components of the smooth muscle contractile apparatus much like that of skeletal muscle and cardiac muscle, but these do not play a role in calcium sensitivity. Choice B: ATP is required for smooth muscle contraction. Decreased ATP levels would be expected to decrease the ability of smooth muscle to contract even in the face of high calcium levels. Choice C: The calcium–calmodulin complex binds with MLCK, which leads to phosphorylation of the myosin light chain. A decrease in the calcium–calmodulin complex should attenuate the contraction of smooth muscle. Choice D: Again, the binding of calcium ions to calmodulin is an initial step in the activation of the smooth muscle contractile apparatus.

   TMP12 93-94

66. **D)** The diagram shows that the maximum velocity of shortening (V_{max}) occurs when there is no afterload on the muscle (force = 0). Increasing afterload decreases the velocity of shortening until a point is reached where shortening does not occur (isometric contraction) and contraction velocity is thus 0 (where curves intersect X-axis). The maximum velocity of shortening is dictated by the ATPase activity of the muscle, increasing to high levels when the ATPase activity is elevated. Choice A: Increasing the frequency of muscle contraction will increase the load that a muscle can lift within the limits of the muscle, but will not affect the velocity of contraction. Choices B, C, and E: Muscle hypertrophy, increasing muscle mass, and recruiting additional motor units will increase the maximum load that a muscle can lift, but these will not affect the maximum velocity of contraction.

   TMP12 77

67. **D)** Stretching the muscle to facilitate reattachment of the tendons leads to an increase in passive tension or preload. This increase in passive tension increases the muscle length beyond its ideal length, which in turn leads to a decrease in the maximal active tension that can be generated by the muscle. The reason that maximal active tension decreases is that interdigitation of actin and myosin filaments decreases when the muscle is stretched; the interdigitation of a muscle is normally optimal at its resting length.

   TMP12 77

Questions 1–4

A 60-year-old woman has a resting heart rate of 70 beats/min, arterial pressure is 130/85 mm Hg, and body temperature is normal. Her pressure-volume diagram of the left ventricle is shown above.

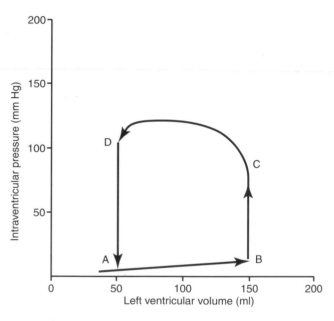

1. What is her cardiac output in milliliters per minute?

   A) 2000
   B) 3000
   C) 4000
   D) 6000
   E) 7000

2. When does the second heart sound occur in the ventricular pressure–volume relationship?

   A) At point D
   B) Between point A and point B
   C) Between point B and point C
   D) Between point C and point D
   E) Between point D and point A

3. When does the third heart sound occur in the ventricular pressure–volume relationship?

   A) At point D
   B) Between point A and point B
   C) Between point B and point C
   D) Between point C and point D
   E) Between point D and point A

4. What is her ventricular ejection fraction?

   A) 33%
   B) 50%
   C) 60%
   D) 67%
   E) 80%

5. In which phase of the ventricular muscle action potential is the potassium permeability the highest?

   A) 0
   B) 1
   C) 2
   D) 3
   E) 4

6. In a resting adult, the typical ventricular ejection fraction has what value?

   A) 20%
   B) 30%
   C) 40%
   D) 60%
   E) 80%

7. A 30-year-old man has an ejection fraction of 0.25 and an end systolic volume of 150 ml. What is his end diastolic volume?

   A) 50 ml
   B) 100 ml
   C) 125 ml
   D) 200 ml
   E) 250 ml

8. Which of the following statements about cardiac muscle is most accurate?

   A) The T-tubules of cardiac muscle can store much less calcium than T-tubules in skeletal muscle
   B) The strength and contraction of cardiac muscle depends on the amount of calcium surrounding cardiac myocytes
   C) In cardiac muscle the initiation of the action potential causes an immediate opening of slow calcium channels
   D) Cardiac muscle repolarization is caused by opening of sodium channels
   E) Mucopolysaccharides inside the T-tubules bind chloride ions

9. A 60-year-old man's EKG shows that he has an R-R interval of 0.55 sec. Which of the following best explains his condition?

   A) He has fever
   B) He has a normal heart rate
   C) He has excess parasympathetic stimulation of the S-A node
   D) He is a trained athlete at rest
   E) He has hyperpolarization of the S-A node

10. Which of the following is most likely to cause the heart to go into spastic contraction?

    A) Increased body temperature
    B) Increased sympathetic activity
    C) Decreased extracellular fluid potassium ions
    D) Excess extracellular fluid potassium ions
    E) Excess extracellular fluid calcium ions

11. Which of the following events occurs at the end of the period of ventricular ejection?

    A) A-V valves close
    B) Aortic valve opens
    C) Aortic valve remains open
    D) A-V valves open
    E) Pulmonary valve closes

12. Which of the following phases of the cardiac cycle follows immediately after the beginning of the QRS wave?

    A) Isovolumic relaxation
    B) Ventricular ejection
    C) Atrial systole
    D) Diastasis
    E) Isovolumic contraction

13. Which of the following conditions will result in a dilated, flaccid heart?

    A) Excess calcium ions in the blood
    B) Excess potassium ions in the blood
    C) Excess sodium ions in the blood
    D) Increased sympathetic stimulation
    E) Increased norepinephrine concentration in the blood

14. A 25-year-old, well-conditioned athlete weighs 80 kg (176 lb). During maximal sympathetic stimulation, what is the plateau level of his cardiac output function curve?

    A) 3 L/min
    B) 5 L/min
    C) 10 L/min
    D) 13 L/min
    E) 25 L/min

15. Which of the following events is associated with the first heart sound?

    A) Closing of the aortic valve
    B) Inrushing of blood into the ventricles during diastole
    C) Beginning of diastole
    D) Opening of the A-V valves
    E) Closing of the A-V valves

16. Which of the following conditions at the A-V node will cause a decrease in heart rate?

    A) Increased sodium permeability
    B) Decreased acetylcholine levels
    C) Increased norepinephrine levels
    D) Increased potassium permeability
    E) Increased calcium permeability

17. Sympathetic stimulation of the heart

    A) Releases acetylcholine at the sympathetic endings
    B) Decreases sinus nodal discharge rate
    C) Decreases excitability of the heart
    D) Releases norepinephrine at the sympathetic endings
    E) Decreases cardiac contractility

18. What is the normal total delay of the cardiac impulse in the A-V node plus bundle?

    A) 0.22 sec
    B) 0.18 sec
    C) 0.16 sec
    D) 0.13 sec
    E) 0.09 sec

19. Which of the following best explains how sympathetic stimulation affects the heart?

    A) Permeability of the S-A node to sodium decreases
    B) Permeability of the A-V node to sodium decreases
    C) Permeability of the S-A node to potassium increases
    D) There is an increased rate of upward drift of the resting membrane potential of the S-A node
    E) Permeability of the cardiac muscle to calcium decreases

20. Which of the following structures will have the slowest rate of conduction of the cardiac action potential?

    A) Atrial muscle
    B) Anterior internodal pathway
    C) A-V bundle fibers
    D) Purkinje fibers
    E) Ventricular muscle

21. If the S-A node discharges at 0.00 seconds, when will the action potential normally arrive at the epicardial surface at the base of the left ventricle?

    A) 0.22 sec
    B) 0.18 sec
    C) 0.16 sec
    D) 0.12 sec
    E) 0.09 sec

22. If the S-A node discharges at 0.00 seconds, when will the action potential normally arrive at the A-V bundle (bundle of His)?

    A) 0.22 sec
    B) 0.18 sec
    C) 0.16 sec
    D) 0.12 sec
    E) 0.09 sec

23. Which of the following conditions at the S-A node will cause heart rate to decrease?

    A) Increased norepinephrine levels
    B) Increased sodium permeability
    C) Increased calcium permeability
    D) Increased potassium permeability
    E) Decreased acetylcholine levels

24. Which of the following are caused by acetylcholine?

    A) Hyperpolarization of the S-A node
    B) Depolarization of the A-V node
    C) Decreased permeability of the S-A node to potassium ions
    D) Increased heart rate
    E) Increased permeability of the cardiac muscle to calcium ions

25. What is the membrane potential (threshold level) at which the S-A node discharges?

    A) −40 mV
    B) −55 mV
    C) −65 mV
    D) −85 mV
    E) −105 mV

26. Which of the following conditions at the A-V node will cause a decrease in heart rate?

    A) Increased sodium permeability
    B) Decreased acetylcholine levels
    C) Increased norepinephrine levels
    D) Increased potassium permeability
    E) Increased calcium permeability

27. If the ventricular Purkinje fibers become the pacemaker of the heart, what is the expected heart rate?

    A) 30/min
    B) 50/min
    C) 65/min
    D) 75/min
    E) 85/min

28. What is the normal total delay of the cardiac impulse in the A-V node and the A-V bundle system?

    A) 0.03 sec
    B) 0.06 sec
    C) 0.09 sec
    D) 0.13 sec
    E) 0.17 sec

29. What is the resting membrane potential of the sinus nodal fibers?

    A) −100 mV
    B) −90 mV
    C) −80 mV
    D) −55 mV
    E) −20 mV

30. If the Purkinje fibers, situated distal to the A-V junction, become the pacemaker of the heart, what is the expected heart rate?

    A) 30/min
    B) 50/min
    C) 60/min
    D) 70/min
    E) 80/min

31. Sympathetic stimulation of the heart normally causes which of the following conditions?

    A) Acetylcholine release at the sympathetic endings
    B) Decreased heart rate
    C) Decreased rate of conduction of the cardiac impulse
    D) Decreased force of contraction of the atria
    E) Increased force of contraction of the ventricles

32. When recording lead I on an EKG, the right arm is the negative electrode, and the positive electrode is the

    A) left arm
    B) left leg
    C) right leg
    D) left arm + left leg
    E) right arm + left leg

33. When recording lead aVL on an EKG, the positive electrode is the

    A) left arm
    B) left leg
    C) right leg
    D) left arm + left leg
    E) right arm + left leg

34. A 70-year-old man was had the following EKG during his annual physical exam. What is his Q-T interval?

    A) 0.12 sec
    B) 0.16 sec
    C) 0.22 sec
    D) 0.30 sec
    E) 0.40 sec

35. What is the heart rate in the following EKG?

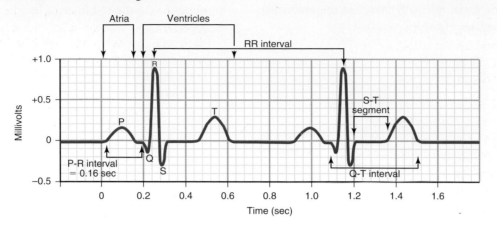

A) 64
B) 70
C) 88
D) 94
E) 104

36. What is the normal QT interval?

A) 0.03 seconds
B) 0.13 seconds
C) 0.16 seconds
D) 0.20 seconds
E) 0.35 seconds

37. When recording lead II on an EKG, the positive electrode is the

A) left arm
B) left leg
C) right leg
D) left arm + left leg
E) right arm + left leg

38. When recording lead III on an EKG, the negative electrode is the

A) left arm
B) left leg
C) right leg
D) left arm + left leg
E) right arm + left leg

39. A 65-year-old man had an EKG recorded at a local emergency room following a biking accident. His weight was 80 kg and his aortic blood pressure was 160/90 mm Hg. The QRS voltage was 0.5 mV in lead I and 1.5 mV in lead III. What is the QRS voltage in lead II?

A) 0.5 mV
B) 1.0 mV
C) 1.5 mV
D) 2.0 mV
E) 2.5 mV

40. A ventricular depolarization wave when traveling −90° in the frontal plane will cause a large negative deflection in which lead?

A) aVR
B) aVL
C) Lead II
D) Lead III
E) aVF

Questions 41-43
A 60-year-old woman had the following EKG recorded at a local emergency room following an automobile accident. Her weight was 70 kg and her aortic blood pressure was 140/80 mm Hg.

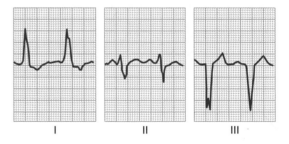

41. What is the mean electrical axis calculated from standard leads I, II, and III shown in her EKG?

A) −90°
B) −50°
C) −12°
D) +100°
E) +170°

42. What is the heart rate using lead I for the calculation?

A) 70
B) 88
C) 100
D) 112
E) 148

43. What is her likely diagnosis?

   A) Mitral valve stenosis
   B) Left bundle branch block
   C) Pulmonary valve stenosis
   D) Right bundle branch block
   E) Left ventricular hypertrophy

44. Which of the following conditions will usually result in right axis deviation in an EKG?

   A) Systemic hypertension
   B) Aortic valve stenosis
   C) Aortic valve regurgitation
   D) Excess abdominal fat
   E) Pulmonary hypertension

45. A ventricular depolarization wave when traveling 60° in the frontal plane will cause a large positive deflection in which of the following leads?

   A) aVR
   B) aVL
   C) Lead I
   D) Lead II
   E) aVF

Questions 46 and 47

A male long-term smoker who is 62 years old weighs 250 lb. He had the following EKG recorded at his local hospital.

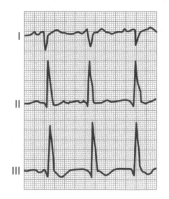

46. Which of the following is the mean electrical axis calculated from standard leads I, II, and III shown in his EKG?

   A) −110°
   B) −20°
   C) +90°
   D) +105°
   E) +180°

47. Which of the following is the likely diagnosis?

   A) Left ventricular hypertrophy
   B) Left bundle branch block
   C) Tricuspid stenosis
   D) Right bundle branch block
   E) Right ventricular hypertrophy

48. A 60-year-old woman has lost some ability to perform normal household tasks and is not feeling well. An EKG shows a QRS complex with a width of 0.20 sec, the T wave is inverted in lead I, and the R wave has a large negative deflection in lead III. Which of the following is the likely diagnosis?

   A) Right ventricular hypertrophy
   B) Left bundle branch block
   C) Pulmonary valve stenosis
   D) Right bundle branch block
   E) Left ventricular hypertrophy

49. A 70-year-old woman sought assistance at a hospital emergency department because she is experiencing chest pain. Based on the following EKG tracing, which of the following is the likely diagnosis?

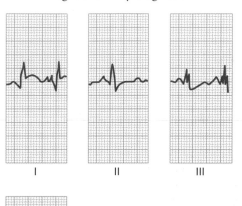

I   II   III

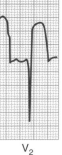

V₂

   A) Acute anterior infarction in the left ventricle of the heart
   B) Acute anterior infarction in the right ventricle of the heart
   C) Acute posterior infarction in the left ventricle of the heart
   D) Acute posterior infarction in the right ventricle of the heart
   E) Right ventricular hypertrophy

50. A 30-year-old man had his EKG measured at his physician's office, but his records were lost. The EKG technician remembered that the QRS deflection was large and positive in lead aVF and 0 in lead I. What is the mean electrical axis in the frontal plane?

    A) 90°
    B) 60°
    C) 0°
    D) −60°
    E) −90°

51. Which of the following is most likely at the "J point" in an EKG of a patient with a damaged cardiac muscle?

    A) Entire heart is depolarized
    B) All the heart is depolarized except for the damaged cardiac muscle
    C) About half the heart is depolarized
    D) All of the heart is repolarized
    E) All of the heart is repolarized except for the damaged cardiac muscle

52. A 50-year-old man is a new employee at ABC Software. The EKG shown here was recorded during a routine physical examination. His likely diagnosis is which of the following?

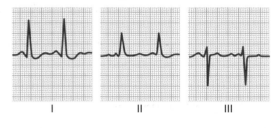

    A) Chronic systemic hypertension
    B) Chronic pulmonary hypertension
    C) Second-degree heart block
    D) Paroxysmal tachycardia
    E) Tricuspid valve stenosis

53. A 55-year-old man had his EKG measured at an annual physical, and his net deflection (R wave minus Q or S wave) in standard limb lead I is −1.2 mV. Standard limb lead II has a net deflection of +1.2 mV. What is the mean electrical axis of his QRS?

    A) −30°
    B) +30°
    C) +60°
    D) +120°
    E) −120°

54. A 65-year-old patient with a heart murmur has a mean QRS axis of 120°, and the QRS complex lasts 0.18 sec. Which of the following is the likely diagnosis?

    A) Aortic valve stenosis
    B) Aortic valve regurgitation
    C) Pulmonary valve stenosis
    D) Right bundle branch block
    E) Left bundle branch block

55. A 60-year-old woman tires easily. Her EKG shows a QRS complex that is positive in the aVF lead and negative in standard limb lead I. A likely cause of this condition is which of the following?

    A) Chronic systemic hypertension
    B) Pulmonary hypertension
    C) Aortic valve stenosis
    D) Aortic valve regurgitation

56. A 60-year-old woman came to the hospital emergency department and complained of chest pain. Based on the EKG tracing shown here, which of the following is the most likely diagnosis?

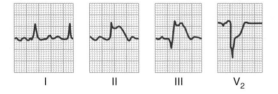

    A) Acute anterior infarction in the base of the heart
    B) Acute anterior infarction in the apex of the heart
    C) Acute posterior infarction in the base of the heart
    D) Acute posterior infarction in the apex of the heart
    E) Right ventricular hypertrophy

57. A 50-year-old man has a blood pressure of 140/85 and weighs 200 lb. He reports that he is not feeling well, his EKG has no P-waves, he has a heart rate of 46, and the QRS complexes occur regularly. What is his likely condition?

    A) First-degree heart block
    B) Second-degree heart block
    C) Third-degree heart block
    D) Sinoatrial heart block
    E) Sinus bradycardia

58. An 80-year-old man had an EKG taken at his local doctor's office, and the diagnosis was atrial fibrillation. Which of the following statements are likely conditions in someone with atrial fibrillation?

    A) Ventricular fibrillation normally accompanies atrial fibrillation
    B) P waves of the EKG are strong
    C) Rate of ventricular contraction is irregular and fast
    D) Atrial "a" wave is normal
    E) Atria have a smaller volume than normal

59. Circus movements in the ventricle can lead to ventricular fibrillation. Which of the following conditions in the ventricular muscle will increase the tendency for circus movements?

    A) Decreased refractory period
    B) Low extracellular potassium concentration
    C) Increased refractory period
    D) Shorter conduction pathway (decreased ventricular volume)
    E) Increase in parasympathetic impulses to the heart

60. A 75-year-old man goes to the hospital emergency department and faints. Five minutes later he is alert. An EKG shows 75 P waves per minute and 35 QRS waves per minute with a normal QRS width. Which of the following is the likely diagnosis?

   A) First-degree A-V block
   B) Stokes-Adams syndrome
   C) Atrial paroxysmal tachycardia
   D) Electrical alternans
   E) Atrial premature contractions

61. A 60-year-old man weighing 220 lb had the following EKG, which shows the standard lead II. What is his diagnosis?

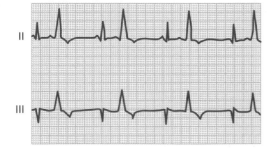

   A) A-V nodal rhythm
   B) First-degree A-V heart block
   C) Second-degree A-V heart block
   D) Third-degree A-V heart block
   E) Atrial flutter

62. A 35-year-old woman had unusual sensations in her chest after she smoked a cigarette. Her EKG is shown here. Which of the following is the likely diagnosis?

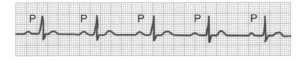

   A) Premature contraction originating in the atrium
   B) Premature contraction originating high in the A-V node
   C) Premature contraction originating low in the A-V node
   D) Premature contraction originating in the apex of the ventricle
   E) Premature contraction originating in the base of the ventricle

Questions 63 and 64

A 55-year-old man had the following EKG recorded at his doctor's office during a routine physical examination.

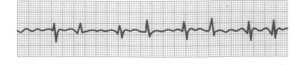

63. What is his diagnosis?

   A) Normal EKG
   B) Atrial flutter
   C) High A-V junctional pacemaker
   D) Middle A-V junctional pacemaker
   E) Low A-V junctional pacemaker

64. What is his ventricular heart rate in beats per minute?

   A) 37.5
   B) 60
   C) 75
   D) 100
   E) 120

65. A 60-year-old woman has been diagnosed with atrial fibrillation. Which of the following statements best describe this condition?

   A) Ventricular rate of contraction is 140 beats/min
   B) P waves of the EKG are pronounced
   C) Ventricular contractions occur at regular intervals
   D) QRS waves are more pronounced than normal
   E) Atria are smaller than normal

66. Which of the following is most characteristic of atrial fibrillation?

   A) Occurs less frequently in patients with atrial enlargement
   B) Ventricular heart rate is about 40 beats per min
   C) Efficiency of ventricular pumping is decreased 20 to 30 percent
   D) Ventricular beat is regular
   E) Atrial P wave is easily seen

67. A 65-year-old woman who had a myocardial infarction 10 days ago returns to her family physician's office and reports that her pulse rate may be rapid. Based on the above EKG, which of the following is the likely diagnosis?

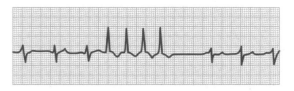

   A) Stokes-Adams syndrome
   B) Atrial fibrillation
   C) A-V nodal tachycardia
   D) Atrial paroxysmal tachycardia
   E) Ventricular paroxysmal tachycardia

68. A 65-year-old man had the EKG shown here recorded at his annual physical examination. Which of the following is the likely diagnosis?

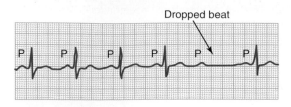

Dropped beat

A) Atrial paroxysmal tachycardia
B) First-degree A-V block
C) Second-degree A-V block
D) Third-degree A-V block
E) Atrial flutter

69. Which of the following decreases the risk of ventricular fibrillation?

A) Dilated heart
B) Increased ventricular refractory period
C) Decreased electrical conduction velocity
D) Exposure of the heart to 60-cycle alternating current
E) Epinephrine administration

70. Which of the following occurs after the heart is stimulated with a 60-cycle alternating current?

A) Velocity of conduction through the heart muscle decreases
B) Longer ventricular refractory period
C) Decreased tendency for circus movements
D) Decreased tendency for ventricular fibrillation

71. Which of the following statements best describes a patient with premature atrial contraction?

A) Pulse taken from the radial artery immediately following the premature contraction will be weak
B) Stroke volume immediately following the premature contraction will be increased
C) P wave is never seen
D) Probability of these premature contractions occurring is decreased in people with a large caffeine intake
E) Causes the QRS interval to be lengthened

Questions 72 and 73
A male patient had a myocardial infarction at age 55. He is now 63 years old. Standard limb lead I is shown here.

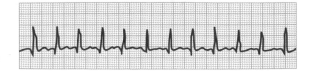

72. What is his heart rate?

A) 40 beats/min
B) 50 beats/min
C) 75 beats/min
D) 100 beats/min
E) 150 beats/min

73. What is his current diagnosis?

A) Sinus tachycardia
B) First-degree heart block
C) Second-degree heart block
D) ST segment depression
E) Third-degree heart block

74. A 55-year-old man has been diagnosed with Stokes-Adams syndrome. Two minutes after the syndrome starts to cause active blockade of the cardiac impulse, which of the following is the pacemaker of the heart?

A) Sinus node
B) A-V node
C) Purkinje fibers
D) Cardiac septum
E) Left atrium

75. If the origin of the stimulus that causes atrial paroxysmal tachycardia is near the A-V node, which of the following statements about the P-wave in standard limb lead I is most accurate?

A) P wave will originate in the sinus node
B) It will be upright
C) It will be inverted
D) P wave will be missing

76. A 45-year-old man had the EKG below recorded at his annual physical. Which of the following is the likely diagnosis?

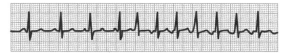

A) Atrial paroxysmal tachycardia
B) First-degree A-V block
C) Second-degree A-V block
D) Ventricular paroxysmal tachycardia
E) Atrial flutter

77. A 60-year-old woman sees her physician for her annual physical examination. The physician orders an EKG, which is shown below. Which of the following is the likely diagnosis?

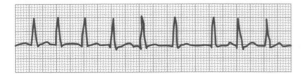

A) First-degree A-V block
B) Second-degree A-V block
C) Third-degree A-V block
D) Atrial paroxysmal tachycardia
E) Atrial fibrillation

Questions 78 and 79
An 80-year-old man went to his family physician for his annual checkup, and his EKG tracing is shown here.

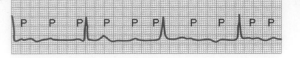

78. What is his heart rate?
A) 105
B) 95
C) 85
D) 75
E) 40

79. Which of the following is the likely diagnosis?
A) Left bundle branch block
B) First-degree A-V block
C) Second-degree A-V block
D) Electrical alternans
E) Complete A-V block

1. **E)** This patient has a heart rate of 70 beats/, and you can determine the cardiac output by using the following formula: cardiac output = heart rate × stroke volume. The stroke volume can be determined from the figure, which is 100 ml, the volume change during the C-D segment. Using this you can determine that the cardiac output is 7000 ml/min.
   TMP12 109

2. **A)** During the ejection phase, the aortic and pulmonary valves open and blood flows into the aorta and pulmonary artery. The ejection phase is between C and D, so the aortic and pulmonary valves open at C and then close at D. The closing of these valves causes the second heart sound.
   TMP12 105

3. **B)** Between points A and B is the period of ventricular filling. The vibration of the ventricular walls makes this sound after sufficient blood has entered the ventricular chambers.
   TMP12 105

4. **D)** The ejection fraction is the stroke volume/end diastolic volume. Stroke volume is 100 ml, and the end systolic volume at point D is 150 ml. This gives you an ejection fraction of 0.667 or in terms of percentage 66.7%.
   TMP12 109

5. **D)** During phase 3 of the ventricular muscle action potential, the potassium permeability of ventricular muscle greatly increases, which causes a more negative membrane potential.
   TMP12 102

6. **D)** The typical ejection fraction is 60%, and lower values are indicative of a weakened heart.
   TMP12 109

7. **D)** The end diastolic volume is always greater than the end systolic volume. Multiplication of the ejection fraction by the end diastolic volume gives you the stroke volume, which is 50 ml in this problem. Therefore, the end diastolic volume is 50 ml greater than the end systolic volume and has a value of 200 ml.
   TMP12 109

8. **B)** The cardiac muscle stores much more calcium in its tubular system than skeletal muscle and is much more dependent on extracellular calcium than the skeletal muscle. An abundance of calcium is bound by the mucopolysaccharides inside the T-tubule. This calcium is necessary for contraction of cardiac muscle, and its strength of contraction depends on the calcium concentration surrounding the cardiac myocytes. At the initiation of the action potential, the fast sodium channels open first, followed later by the opening of the slow calcium channels.
   TMP12 102–103

9. **A)** Heart rate is determined by the formula 60/R-R interval, and the heart rate for this patient is 109 beats/min. This is a fast heart rate, which would occur during fever. A trained athlete has a low heart rate. Excess parasympathetic stimulation and hyperpolarization of the S-A node both decrease heart rate.
   TMP12 112

10. **E)** The heart goes into spastic contraction following a large increase in the calcium ion concentration surrounding the cardiac myofibrils, and this occurs if extracellular fluid calcium ion concentration increases too much. An excess potassium concentration in the extracellular fluids causes the heart to become dilated because of the more positive resting membrane potential of the cardiac muscle fibers.
    TMP12 112

11. **E)** At the end of ventricular ejection, both the aortic valves and the pulmonary valves close. This is followed by the period of isovolumic relaxation.
    TMP12 108

12. **E)** Immediately after the QRS wave, the ventricles begin to contract and the first phase that occurs is isovolumic contraction. This occurs before the ejection phase and increases the ventricular pressure enough to mechanically open the aortic and pulmonary valves.
    TMP12 108

13. **B)** Excess potassium ions in the blood and extracellular fluid cause the heart to become dilated and flaccid as well as slowing the heart. This effect is important due to a more positive resting membrane potential in the cardiac muscle fibers. As the membrane potential becomes more positive, the intensity of the action potential decreases, which makes the contraction of the heart progressively weaker. Excess calcium ions in the blood and sympathetic stimulation and increased norepinephrine concentration of the blood all cause the heart to contract vigorously.
    TMP12 112

14. **E)** The normal plateau level of the cardiac output function curve is 13 L/min. This level decreases in any kind of cardiac failure and increases markedly during sympathetic stimulation.
    TMP12 111

15. **E)** As seen in Chapter 9, the first heart sound by definition occurs just after the ventricular pressure exceeds the atrial pressure. This causes the A-V valves to mechanically close. The second heart sound occurs when the aortic and pulmonary valves close.
    TMP12 105

16. **D)** The increase in potassium permeability causes a hyperpolarization of the A-V node, and this will decrease the heart rate. Increases in sodium permeability will actually partially depolarize the A-V node, and an increase in norepinephrine levels increases the heart rate.
    TMP12 102

17. **D)** Increased sympathetic stimulation of the heart increases heart rate, atrial contractility, and ventricular contractility and also increases norepinephrine release at the ventricular sympathetic nerve endings. It does not release acetylcholine. It does cause an increased sodium permeability of the A-V node, which increases the rate of upward drift of the membrane potential to the threshold level for self-excitation, thus increasing heart rate.
    TMP12 111 and 120

18. **D)** The impulse from the S-A node travels rapidly through the internodal pathways and arrives at the A-V node at 0.03 sec, at the A-V bundle at 0.12 sec and at the ventricular septum at 0.16 sec. The total delay is thus 0.13 sec.
    TMP12 118

19. **D)** During sympathetic stimulation, the permeabilities of the S-A node and the A-V node increase. Also, the permeability of cardiac muscle to calcium increases resulting in an increased contractile strength. In addition, there is an upward drift of the resting membrane potential of the S-A node. Increased permeability of the S-A node to potassium does not occur during sympathetic stimulation.
    TMP12 120

20. **C)** The atrial and ventricular muscles have a relatively rapid rate of conduction of the cardiac action potential, and the anterior internodal pathway also has fairly rapid conduction of the impulse. However, the A-V bundle myofibrils have a slow rate of conduction because their sizes are considerably smaller than the sizes of the normal atrial and ventricular muscle. Also, their slow conduction is partly caused by diminished numbers of gap junctions between successive muscle cells in the conducting pathway, causing a great resistance to conduction of the excitatory ions from one cell to the next.
    TMP12 117

21. **A)** After the S-A node discharges, the action potential travels through the atria, through the A-V bundle system and finally to the ventricular septum and throughout the ventricle. The last place that the impulse arrives is at the epicardial surface at the base of the left ventricle, which requires a transit time of 0.22 sec.
    TMP12 118

22. **D)** The action potential arrives at the A-V bundle at 0.12 sec. It arrives at the A-V node at 0.03 sec and is delayed 0.09 sec in the A-V node, which results in an arrival time at the bundle of His of 0.12 sec.
    TMP12 118

23. **D)** Increases in sodium and calcium permeability at the S-A node result in an increased heart rate. An increased potassium permeability causes a hyperpolarization of the S-A node, which causes the heart rate to decrease.
    TMP12 120

24. **A)** Acetylcholine does not depolarize the A-V node or increase permeability of the cardiac muscle to calcium ions but causes hyperpolarization of the S-A node and the A-V node by increasing permeability to potassium ions. This results in a decreased heart rate.
    TMP12 120

25. **A)** The normal resting membrane potential of the S-A node is -55 mV. As the sodium leaks into the membrane an upward drift of the membrane potential occurs until it reaches -40 mV. This is the threshold level that initiates the action potential at the S-A node.
    TMP12 116

26. **D)** An increase in potassium permeability causes a decrease in the membrane potential of the A-V node. Thus, it will be extremely hyperpolarized, making it much more difficult for the membrane potential to reach its threshold level for conduction. This results in a decrease in heart rate. Increases in sodium and calcium permeability and norepinephrine levels increase the membrane potential, causing a tendency to increase the heart rate.
    TMP12 120

27. **A)** If there is a failure in conduction of the S-A nodal impulse to the A-V node or if the S-A node stops firing, the A-V node will take over as the pacemaker of the heart. The intrinsic rhythmical rate of the A-V node is 40 to 60 times per minute. If the Purkinje fibers take over as pacemakers, the heart rate will be between 15 and 40 beats/min.
    TMP12 119

28. **D)** The impulse coming from the S-A node to the A-V node arrives at 0.03 sec. Then there is a total delay of 0.13

sec in the A-V node and bundle system allowing the impulse to arrive at the ventricular septum at 0.16 sec.
TMP12 118

29. **D)** The resting membrane potential of the sinus nodal fibers is −55 mV, and this is in contrast with the −85 to −90 mV membrane potential of cardiac muscle. Other major differences between the sinus nodal fibers and ventricular muscle fibers are that the sinus fibers exhibit self-excitation from inward leaking of sodium ions.
TMP12 116

30. **A)** If the Purkinje fibers are the pacemaker of the heart, the heart rate ranges between 15 and 40 beats/min. In contrast, the rate of firing of the A-V nodal fibers are 40 to 60 times a minute, and the sinus node fires at 70 to 80 times per minute. If the sinus node is blocked for some reason, the A-V node will take over as the pacemaker; and if the A-V node is blocked, the Purkinje fibers will take over as the pacemaker of the heart.
TMP12 119

31. **E)** Sympathetic stimulation of the heart normally causes an increased heart rate, increased rate of conduction of the cardiac impulse and increased force of contraction in the atria and ventricles. However, it does not cause acetylcholine release at the sympathetic endings because they contain norepinephrine. Parasympathetic stimulation causes acetylcholine release. The sympathetic nervous system firing increases the permeability of the cardiac muscle fibers, the S-A node, and the A-V node to sodium and calcium.
TMP12 120

32. **A)** By convention, the left arm is the positive electrode for lead I of an EKG.
TMP12 125

33. **A)** By convention, the left arm is the positive electrode for lead aVL of an EKG.
TMP12 126

34. **E)** The contraction of the ventricles lasts almost from the beginning of the Q wave and continues to the end of the T wave. This interval is called the Q-T interval and ordinarily lasts about 0.35 sec. In this particular example the Q-T interval is a little bit longer than average and equals 0.40 sec.
TMP12 123

35. **B)** The heart rate can be calculated by 60 divided by the R-R interval, which is 0.86 sec. This results in a heart rate of 70 beats/min.
TMP12 121, 123

36. **E)** The contraction of the ventricles lasts almost from the beginning of the Q wave and continues to the end of the T wave. This interval is called the Q-T interval and ordinarily lasts about 0.35 sec.
TMP12 123

37. **B)** By convention, the left leg is the positive electrode for lead II of an EKG.
TMP12 125

38. **A)** By convention, the left arm is the negative electrode for lead III of an EKG.
TMP12 125

39. **D)** Einthoven's law states that the voltage in lead I plus the voltage in lead III is equal to the voltage in lead II, which in this case is 2.0 mV.
TMP12 125

40. **E)** As can be seen in Figure 12-3 (TMP12), the positive portion of lead aVF has an axis of 90° and the negative part of this lead has an axis of −90°. Note the difference between the positive and the negative ends of this vector is 180°.
TMP12 130

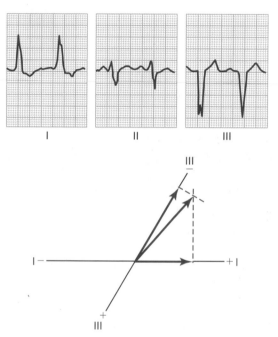

41. **B)** The mean electrical axis can be determined plotting the resultant voltage of the QRS for leads I, II, and III. The result is as is shown above and has a value of −50°.
TMP12 134

42. **A)** The heart rate can be calculated by 60 divided by the R-R interval, which is 0.68 sec. This results in a heart rate of 88 beats/min.
TMP12 123

43. **B)** Note in Figure 12-14 (TMP12), which is shown above, that there is a QRS width greater than 0.12 sec. This indicates a bundle branch block. There is also a left axis deviation, which is consistent with a left bundle branch block.
TMP12 136

44. **E)** Systemic hypertension results in a left axis deviation because of the enlargement of the left ventricle. Aortic valve stenosis and aortic valve regurgitation also result in a large left ventricle and left axis deviation. Excessive abdominal fat, because of the mechanical pressure of the fat, causes a rotation of the heart to the left resulting in a leftward shift of the mean electrical axis. Pulmonary hypertension causes enlargement of the right heart and thus causes right axis deviation.
    TMP12 136

45. **D)** Lead II has a positive vector at the 60° angle. The positive end of lead II is at −120°.
    TMP12 130

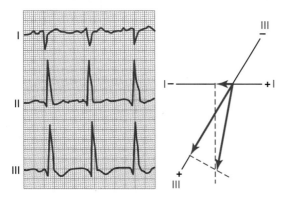

46. **D)** Note that lead III has the strongest vector, therefore the mean electrical axis will be closer to this lead than to leads I or II. The angle of lead III is 120°, and the resultant vector (mean electrical axis) is close to that lead and has a value of +105°.
    TMP12 134

47. **D)** The diagnosis is right bundle branch block. This can be determined by a rightward shift in mean electrical axis as well as the greatly prolonged QRS complex. In right ventricular hypertrophy, the QRS complex is only moderately prolonged.
    TMP12 137

48. **D)** The patient has a left axis deviation because of the large negative deflection of the R wave in lead III. Also, her T wave was inverted in lead I, which means that it is in the opposite direction of the QRS complex. This is characteristic of bundle branch block. Also, the QRS complex had a width of 0.20 sec, a very prolonged QRS complex. A QRS complex that has a width greater than 0.12 sec is normally caused by a conduction block. All these factors indicate that this patient has a left bundle branch block.
    TMP12 136

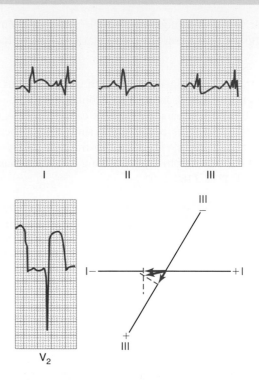

49. **A)** This patient has an acute anterior infarction in the left ventricle of the heart. This can be determined by plotting the currents of injury from the different leads. The limb leads are used to determine whether the infarction is coming from the left or right side of the heart and from the base or apex of the heart. The chest leads are used to determine whether it is an anterior or posterior infarct. When we analyze the currents of injury, a negative potential, caused by the current of injury, occurs in lead I and a positive potential, caused by the current of injury, occurs in lead III. This is determined by subtracting the J point from the TP segment. The negative end of the resultant vector originates in the ischemic area, which is therefore the left side of the heart. In lead V_2, the chest lead, the electrode is in a field of very negative potential, which occurs in patients with an anterior lesion.
    TMP12 140

50. **A)** Since the deflection in this EKG is 0 in lead I, the axis has to be 90° away from this lead. Therefore, the mean electrical axis has to be +90° or −90°. Since the aVF lead has a positive deflection, the mean electrical axis must be at +90°.
    TMP12 134

51. **A)** At the J point the entire heart is depolarized in a patient with a damaged cardiac muscle or a patient with a normal cardiac muscle. The area of the heart that is damaged will not repolarize, but remains depolarized at all times.
    TMP12 139

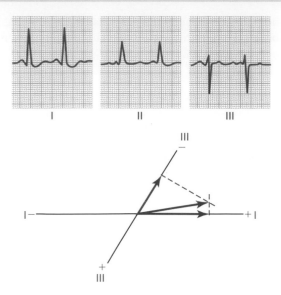

vertical. The negative end of the vector points to where the current of injury originated, which is in the apex of the heart. The elevation of the TP segment above the J point indicates a posterior lesion. Therefore, the EKG is consistent with acute posterior infarction in the apex of the heart.

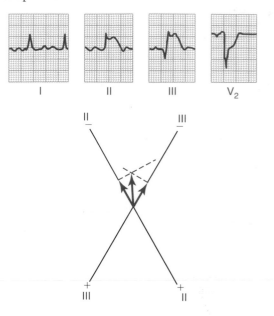

TMP12 140

52. A) Note that the QRS complex has a positive deflection in lead I and a negative in lead III, which indicates that there is a leftward axis deviation. This occurs during chronic systemic hypertension. Pulmonary hypertension increases the ventricular mass on the right side of the heart, which gives a right axis deviation.

   TMP12 135

53. D) The QRS wave plotted on lead I was −1.2 mV and lead II was +1.2 mV so the absolute value of the deflections were the same. Therefore, the mean electrical axis has to be exactly halfway in between these two leads, which is halfway between the lead II axis of 60° and the lead I negative axis of 180°, resulting in a value of 120°.

   TMP12 134

54. D) A QRS axis of 120° indicates a rightward shift. Since the QRS complex is 0.18 sec, this indicates a conduction block. Therefore, this EKG, which fits with these characteristics, is a right bundle branch block.

   TMP12 137

55. B) The EKG from this patient has a positive deflection in aVF and a negative deflection in standard limb lead I. Therefore, the mean electrical axis is between 90° and 180°, which is a rightward shift in the EKG mean electrical axis. Systemic hypertension, aortic valve stenosis, and aortic valve regurgitation cause hypertrophy of the left ventricle and thus a leftward shift in the mean electrical axis. Pulmonary hypertension causes a rightward shift in the axis, and is therefore characterized by this EKG.

   TMP12 136

56. D) Note in the following figure that the current of injury is plotted on the graph at the bottom. This is not a plot of the QRS voltages but the current of injury voltages. They are plotted for leads II and III, which are both negative, and the resultant vector is nearly

57. D) When a patient has no P waves and a low heart rate, it is likely that the impulse leaving the sinus node is totally blocked before entering the atrial muscle. This is called sinoatrial block. The ventricles pick up the new rhythm usually initiated in the A-V node at this point, which results in a heart rate of 40 to 60 beats/min. In contrast, during sinus bradycardia you still have P waves associated with each QRS complex. In first-, second-, and third-degree heart block, you have P waves in each of these instances, although some are not associated with QRS complex.

   TMP12 144

58. C) Atrial fibrillation has a rapid irregular heart rate. The P waves are missing or are very weak. The atria exhibit circus movements, and atrial volume is often increased, causing the atrial fibrillation.

   TMP12 151–152

59. A) Circus movements occur in ventricular muscle particularly if you have a dilated heart or decreases in conduction velocity. High extracellular potassium and sympathetic stimulation, not parasympathetic stimulation, increase the tendency for circus movements. A longer refractory period tends to prevent circus movements of the heart, because when the impulses travel around the heart and contact the area of ventricular muscle that has a longer refractory period, the action potential stops at this point.

   TMP12 150

60. B) A sudden onset of A-V block that comes and goes is called the Stokes-Adams syndrome. The patient depicted here has about 75 P-waves/min, which means that the atria are contracting normally. But the A-V block that occurs allows only 35 QRS waves to occur each minute.

   TMP12 145

61. D) By definition, first-degree A-V heart block occurs when the P-R interval exceeds a value of 0.20 sec, but without any dropped QRS waves. In the following figure, the P-R interval is about 0.30 sec, which is considerably prolonged. However, there are no dropped QRS waves. During second-degree A-V block or third-degree A-V block, QRS waves are dropped.

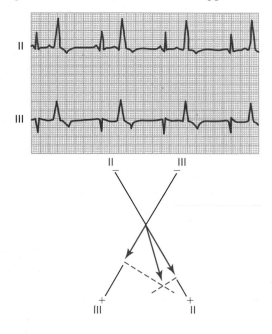

   TMP12 144

62. E) Note that the premature ventricular contractions (PVCs) have wide and tall QRS waves in the EKG. The mean electrical axis of the premature contraction can be determined by plotting these large QRS complexes on the standard limb leads. The PVC originates at the negative end of the resultant mean electrical axis, which is at the base of the ventricle. Note that the QRS of the PVC is wider and much taller than the normal QRS waves in this EKG.

   TMP12 147

63. B) This patient has atrial flutter characterized by several P waves for each QRS complex. In this EKG, you see some areas that have two P waves for every QRS and other areas that have three P waves for each QRS. Note the rapid heart rate, which is characteristic of atrial flutter, and the irregular R-R intervals.

   TMP12 152

64. E) The average ventricular rate is 120 beats/min in this EKG, which is typical of atrial flutter. Once again,

note that the heart rate is irregular due to the inability of the impulses to quickly pass through the A-V node because of its refractory period.

   TMP12 123

65. A) Atrial fibrillation has a rapid irregular heart rate. The P waves are missing or are very weak. The atria exhibit circus movements, and often are very enlarged, causing the atrial fibrillation.

   TMP12 151–152

66. C) Atrial fibrillation occurs often with patients with an atrial enlargement. This causes an increased tendency for circus movements to occur. The ventricular beat is irregular because impulses are rapidly arriving at the A-V node; however, many times the A-V node is in a refractory period. Therefore the A-V node will not pass a second impulse until about 0.35 sec elapses after the previous one. There is also a variable interval between when the atrial impulses reach the A-V node. This results in a very irregular heartbeat but one that is very rapid with a rate of 125 to 150 beats/min.

   TMP12 151–152

67. E) The term paroxysmal means that the heart rate becomes rapid in paroxysms, with the paroxysm beginning suddenly and lasting for a few seconds, a few minutes, a few hours, or much longer. Then the paroxysm usually ends as suddenly as it began and the pacemaker shifts back to the S-A node. The mechanism by which this is believed to occur is by a re-entrant circus movement feedback pathway that sets up an area of local repeated self-re-excitation. The EKG shown is ventricular paroxysmal tachycardia. That the origin is in the ventricles can be determined because of the changes in the QRS complex that have high voltages and look much different than the preceding normal QRS complexes. This is very characteristic of a ventricular irritable locus.

   TMP12 149

68. C) Note in this EKG that a P wave precedes each of the first four QRS complexes. After that we see a P wave but a dropped QRS wave. This is characteristic of second-degree A-V block.

   TMP12 145

69. B) A dilated heart increases the risk of occurrence of ventricular fibrillation because of an increase in likelihood of circus movements. Also, if the conduction velocity decreases, it will take longer for the impulse to travel around the heart, which decreases the risk of ventricular fibrillation. Exposure of the heart to 60-cycle alternating current or epinephrine administration increases the irritability of the heart. If the refractory period is long, the likelihood of the re-entrant type of pathways decreases, because when the impulse travels around the heart, the ventricles remain in a refractory period.

   TMP12 149

70. A) The risk of occurrence of ventricular fibrillation increases in a heart exposed to a 60-cycle alternating current. A shortened ventricular refractory period and a decreased conduction through the heart muscle occur, which increases the probability of re-entrant pathways. Therefore, when the electrical stimulus travels around the heart and reaches the ventricular muscle that was again initially stimulated, the risk of ventricular fibrillation increases if this muscle has a short refractory period.
TMP12 150

71. A) The heartbeat immediately following a premature atrial contraction weakens because the diastolic period is very short in this condition. Therefore, the ventricular filling time is very short, and thus the stroke volume decreases. The P wave is usually visible in this arrhythmia unless it coincides with the QRS complex. The probability of these premature contractions increases in people with toxic irritation of the heart and local ischemic areas.
TMP12 146

72. E) The heart rate can be determined by 60 divided by the R-R interval, which gives you a value of 150 beats/min. This is tachycardia, defined as a heart rate greater than 100 beats/min.
TMP12 123

73. A) The relationship between the P waves and the QRS complexes appears to be normal and there are no missing beats. Therefore, this patient has a sinus rhythm, and there is no heart block. There is also no ST segment depression in this patient. Since we have normal P and QRS and T waves, this condition is sinus tachycardia.
TMP12 143

74. B) During a Stokes-Adams syndrome attack total A-V block suddenly begins, and the duration of the block may be a few seconds or even several weeks. The new pacemaker of the heart is distal to the point of blockade but is usually the A-V node or the A-V bundle.
TMP12 143

75. C) During atrial paroxysmal tachycardia the impulse is initiated by an ectopic focus somewhere in the atria. If the point of initiation is near the A-V node the P wave travels backward toward the S-A node and then forward into the ventricles at the same time. Therefore, the P wave will be inverted.
TMP12 146

76. A) This EKG has characteristics of atrial paroxysmal tachycardia. This means the tachycardia may come and go at random times. The basic shape of the QRS complex and its magnitude are virtually unchanged from the normal QRS complexes, which eliminates the possibility of ventricular paroxysmal tachycardia. This EKG is not characteristic of atrial flutter since there is only one P wave for each QRS complex.
TMP12 148

77. E) First-, second-, and third-degree heart blocks as well as atrial paroxysmal tachycardia all have P waves in the EKG. However, there are usually no evident P waves during atrial fibrillation, and the heart rate is irregular. Therefore, this EKG is characteristic of atrial fibrillation.
TMP12 151-152

78. E) This patient's heart rate is 40 beats/min, which can be determined by dividing 60 by the R-R interval. This is characteristic of some type of A-V block.
TMP12 123

79. E) This EKG is characteristic of complete A-V block, which is also called third-degree A-V block. The P waves seem to be totally dissociated from the QRS complexes, since sometimes there are three P waves and sometimes two P waves between QRS complexes. First-degree A-V block causes a lengthened P-R interval, and second-degree A-V block has long P-R intervals with dropped beats. However, this does not seem to be occurring in this EKG, since there is no relationship between the ORS waves and the P waves.
TMP12 145

The Circulation

1. A healthy 28-year-old woman stands up from a supine position. Which of the following sets of cardiovascular changes is most likely to occur?

	Heart rate	Renal blood flow	Total peripheral resistance
A)	↑	↑	↑
B)	↑	↓	↑
C)	↑	↓	↓
D)	↑	↑	↓
E)	↓	↓	↓
F)	↓	↑	↓
G)	↓	↑	↑
H)	↓	↓	↑

2. A healthy 25-year-old male medical student has an exercise stress test at a local health club. Which of the following sets of physiological changes is most likely to occur in this man's skeletal muscles during exercise?

	Arteriolar resistance	Adenosine concentration	Vascular conductance
A)	↑	↑	↑
B)	↑	↓	↑
C)	↑	↓	↓
D)	↑	↑	↓
E)	↓	↓	↓
F)	↓	↑	↓
G)	↓	↑	↑
H)	↓	↓	↑

3. A 60-year-old woman has experienced dizziness for the past 6 months when getting out of bed in the morning and when standing up. Her mean arterial pressure is 130/90 mm Hg lying down and 95/60 sitting. Which of the following sets of physiological changes would be expected in response to moving from a supine to an upright position?

	Parasympathetic nerve activity	Plasma renin activity	Sympathetic activity
A)	↑	↑	↑
B)	↑	↓	↑
C)	↑	↓	↓
D)	↑	↑	↓
E)	↓	↓	↓
F)	↓	↑	↓
G)	↓	↑	↑
H)	↓	↓	↑

4. Which of the following sets of physiological changes would be expected to occur in response to an increase in atrial natriuretic peptide?

	Angiotensin II	Aldosterone	Sodium excretion
A)	↑	↑	↑
B)	↑	↓	↑
C)	↑	↓	↓
D)	↑	↑	↓
E)	↓	↓	↓
F)	↓	↑	↓
G)	↓	↑	↑
H)	↓	↓	↑

5. Listed below are the hydrostatic and oncotic pressures within a microcirculatory bed:

Plasma colloid osmotic pressure = 25 mm Hg
Capillary hydrostatic pressure = 25 mm Hg
Venous hydrostatic pressure = 5 mm Hg
Arterial pressure = 80 mm Hg
Interstitial fluid hydrostatic pressure = −5 mm Hg
Interstitial colloid osmotic pressure = 10 mm Hg
Capillary filtration coefficient = 10 ml/min/mm Hg
What is the rate of net fluid movement across the capillary wall?

A) 25 ml/min
B) 50 ml/min
C) 100 ml/min
D) 150 ml/min
E) 200 ml/min

6. Listed below are the hydrostatic and oncotic pressures and filtration rate across a muscle capillary wall:

Capillary hydrostatic pressure (P_c) = 25 mm Hg
Plasma colloid osmotic pressure (Π_p) = 25 mm Hg
Interstitial colloid osmotic pressure (Π_I) = 10 mm Hg
Interstitial hydrostatic pressure (P_I) = −5 mm Hg
Capillary filtration rate = 150 ml/min
What is the capillary filtration coefficient?

A) 0
B) 5
C) 10
D) 15
E) 20

7. Administration of a drug decreases the diameter of arterioles in the muscle bed of an experimental animal. Which of the following sets of physiological changes would be expected to occur in response to the decrease in diameter?

	Vascular conductance	Capillary filtration	Blood flow
A)	↑	↑	↑
B)	↑	↓	↑
C)	↑	↓	↓
D)	↑	↑	↓
E)	↓	↓	↓
F)	↓	↑	↓
G)	↓	↑	↑
H)	↓	↓	↑

8. A 35-year-old woman visits her family practitioner for an examination. She has a blood pressure of 160/75 mm Hg and a heart rate of 74 beats/min. Further tests by a cardiologist reveal that the patient has moderate aortic regurgitation. Which of the following sets of changes would be expected in this patient?

	Pulse pressure	Systolic pressure	Stroke volume
A)	↑	↑	↑
B)	↑	↓	↑
C)	↑	↓	↓
D)	↑	↑	↓
E)	↓	↓	↓
F)	↓	↑	↓
G)	↓	↑	↑
H)	↓	↓	↑

9. A 65-year-old man with a 5-year history of congestive heart failure is being treated with an angiotensin-converting enzyme (ACE) inhibitor. Which of the following sets of changes would be expected to occur in response to the ACE inhibitor drug therapy?

vasoconstrictor

	Arterial pressure	Angiotensin II	Total peripheral resistance
A)	↑	↑	↑
B)	↑	↓	↑
C)	↑	↓	↓
D)	↑	↑	↓
E)	↓	↓	↓
F)	↓	↑	↓
G)	↓	↑	↑
H)	↓	↓	↑

10. Cognitive stimuli such as reading, problem solving, and talking all result in significant increases in cerebral blood flow. Which of the following changes in cerebral tissue concentrations is the most likely explanation for the increase in cerebral blood flow?

	Carbon dioxide	pH	Adenosine
A)	↑	↑	↑
B)	↑	↓	↑
C)	↑	↓	↓
D)	↑	↑	↓
E)	↓	↓	↓
F)	↓	↑	↓
G)	↓	↑	↑
H)	↓	↓	↑

11. A 55-year-old man with a history of normal health visits his physician for a checkup. The physical examination reveals that his blood pressure is 170/98 mm Hg. Further tests indicate that he has renovascular hypertension as a result of stenosis in the left kidney. Which of the following sets of findings would be expected in this man with renovascular hypertension?

	Total peripheral resistance	Plasma renin activity	Plasma aldosterone concentration
A)	↑	↑	↑
B)	↑	↓	↑
C)	↑	↓	↓
D)	↑	↑	↓
E)	↓	↓	↓
F)	↓	↑	↓
G)	↓	↑	↑
H)	↓	↓	↑

12. Histamine is infused into the brachial artery. Which of the following sets of microcirculatory changes would be expected in the infused arm?

	Capillary water permeability	Capillary hydrostatic pressure	Capillary filtration rate
A)	↑	↑	↑
B)	↑	↑	↓
C)	↑	↓	↓
D)	↑	↓	↑
E)	↓	↓	↓
F)	↓	↓	↑
G)	↓	↑	↑
H)	↓	↑	↓

13. Bradykinin is infused into the brachial artery of a 22-year-old man. Which of the following sets of microcirculatory changes would be expected in the infused arm?

	Capillary hydrostatic pressure	Interstitial hydrostatic pressure	Lymph flow
A)	↑	↑	↑
B)	↑	↑	↓
C)	↑	↓	↓
D)	↑	↓	↑
E)	↓	↓	↓
F)	↓	↓	↑
G)	↓	↑	↑
H)	↓	↑	↓

14. An increase in shear stress in a blood vessel results in which of the following changes?
   A) Decreased endothelin production
   B) Decreased cyclic guanosine monophosphate production
   C) Increased nitric oxide release
   D) Increased renin production
   E) Decreased prostacyclin production

15. A 72-year-old man had surgery to remove an abdominal tumor. Pathohistologic studies reveal that the tumor mass contains a large number of blood vessels. An increase in which of the following is the most likely stimulus for the growth of vessels in a solid tumor?
   A) Growth hormone
   B) Plasma glucose concentration
   C) Angiostatin growth factor
   D) Tissue oxygen concentration
   E) Vascular endothelial growth factor

16. The diameter of a precapillary arteriole is increased in a muscle vascular bed. A decrease in which of the following would be expected?
   A) Capillary filtration rate
   B) Vascular conductance
   C) Capillary blood flow
   D) Capillary hydrostatic pressure
   E) Arteriolar resistance

17. Under control conditions, flow through a blood vessel is 100 ml/min with a pressure gradient of 50 mm Hg. What would be the approximate flow through the vessel after increasing the vessel diameter by 50%, assuming the pressure gradient is maintained at 100 mm Hg?
   A) 100 ml/min
   B) 150 ml/min
   C) 300 ml/min
   D) 500 ml/min
   E) 700 ml/min

18. A 24-year-old woman delivers a 6-lb, 8-oz female baby. The newborn is diagnosed as having patent ductus arteriosus. Which of the following sets of changes would be expected in this baby?

	Pulse pressure	Stroke volume	Systolic pressure
A)	↑	↑	↑
B)	↑	↓	↑
C)	↑	↓	↓
D)	↑	↑	↓
E)	↓	↓	↓
F)	↓	↑	↓
G)	↓	↑	↑
H)	↓	↓	↑

19. Which of the following sets of changes would be expected to cause the greatest increase in the net movement of sodium across a muscle capillary wall?

	Wall permeability to sodium	Wall surface area	Concentration difference across wall
A)	↑	↑	↑
B)	↑	↑	↓
C)	↑	↓	↓
D)	↑	↓	↑
E)	↓	↓	↓
F)	↓	↓	↑
G)	↓	↑	↑
H)	↓	↑	↓

20. A 60-year-old man visits his family practitioner for an annual examination. He has a mean blood pressure of 130 mm Hg and a heart rate of 78 beats/min. His plasma cholesterol level is in the upper 25th percentile, and he is diagnosed as having atherosclerosis. Which of the following sets of changes would be expected in this patient?

	Pulse pressure	Arterial compliance	Systolic pressure
A)	↑	↑	↑
B)	↑	↓	↑
C)	↑	↓	↓
D)	↑	↑	↓
E)	↓	↓	↓
F)	↓	↑	↓
G)	↓	↑	↑
H)	↓	↓	↑

21. While participating in a cardiovascular physiology laboratory, a medical student isolates the carotid artery of an animal and partially constricts the artery with a tie around the vessel. Which of the following sets of changes would be expected to occur in response to constriction of the carotid artery?

	Sympathetic nerve activity	Renal blood flow	Total peripheral resistance
A)	↑	↑	↑
B)	↑	↓	↑
C)	↑	↓	↓
D)	↑	↑	↓
E)	↓	↓	↓
F)	↓	↑	↓
G)	↓	↑	↑
H)	↓	↓	↑

22. A balloon catheter is advanced from the superior vena cava into the heart and inflated to increase atrial pressure by 5 mm Hg. An increase in which of the following would be expected to occur in response to the elevated atrial pressure?

A) Atrial natriuretic peptide
B) Angiotensin II
C) Aldosterone
D) Renal sympathetic nerve activity

23. The diameter of a precapillary arteriole is decreased in a muscle vascular bed. Which of the following changes in the microcirculation would be expected?

A) Decreased capillary filtration rate
B) Increased interstitial volume
C) Increased lymph flow
D) Increased capillary hydrostatic pressure
E) Decreased arteriolar resistance

24. A 50-year-old man has a 3-year history of hypertension. He complains of fatigue and occasional muscle cramps. There is no family history of hypertension. The patient has not had any other significant medical problems in the past. Examination reveals a blood pressure of 168/104 mm Hg. Additional laboratory tests indicate that the patient has primary hyperaldosteronism. Which of the following sets of findings would be expected in this man with primary hyperaldosteronism hypertension?

	Extracellular fluid volume	Plasma renin activity	Plasma potassium concentration
A)	↑	↑	↑
B)	↑	↓	↑
C)	↑	↓	↓
D)	↑	↑	↓
E)	↓	↓	↓
F)	↓	↑	↓
G)	↓	↑	↑
H)	↓	↓	↑

25. A 72-year-old man had surgery to remove an abdominal tumor. Pathohistologic studies revealed that the tumor mass contained a large number of vessels. A decrease in which of the following is the most likely stimulus for the growth of vessels in a solid tumor?

A) Growth hormone
B) Plasma glucose concentration
C) Angiostatin growth factor
D) Vascular endothelial growth factor
E) Tissue oxygen concentration

26. Under control conditions, flow through a blood vessel is 100 ml/min under a pressure gradient of 50 mm Hg. What would be the approximate flow through the vessel after increasing the vessel diameter to four times normal, assuming that the pressure gradient was maintained at 50 mm Hg?

A) 300 ml/min
B) 1600 ml/min
C) 1000 ml/min
D) 16,000 ml/min
E) 25,600 ml/min

27. While participating in a cardiovascular physiology laboratory, a medical student isolates an animal's carotid artery proximal to the carotid bifurcation and partially constricts the artery with a tie around the vessel. Which of the following sets of changes would be expected to occur in response to constriction of the carotid artery?

	Mean carotid sinus nerve impulses	Parasympathetic nerve activity	Total peripheral resistance
A)	↑	↑	↑
B)	↑	↓	↑
C)	↑	↓	↓
D)	↑	↑	↓
E)	↓	↓	↓
F)	↓	↑	↓
G)	↓	↑	↑
(H)	↓	↓	↑

28. A 22-year-old man enters the hospital emergency room after severing a major artery in a motorcycle accident. It is estimated that he has lost approximately 700 ml of blood. His blood pressure is 90/55 mm Hg. Which of the following sets of changes would be expected in response to hemorrhage in this man?

	Heart rate flow	Sympathetic nerve activity	Total peripheral resistance
(A)	↑	↑	↑
B)	↑	↓	↑
C)	↑	↓	↓
D)	↑	↑	↓
E)	↓	↓	↓
F)	↓	↑	↓
G)	↓	↑	↑
H)	↓	↓	↑

29. A 22-year-old man has a muscle blood flow of 250 ml/min and a hematocrit of 50. He has a mean arterial pressure of 130 mm Hg, a muscle venous pressure of 5 mm Hg, and a heart rate of 80 beats/min. Which of the following is the approximate vascular resistance in the muscle of this man?

A) 0.10 mm Hg/ml/min
B) 0.20 mm Hg/ml/min
C) 0.50 mm Hg/ml/min
D) 1.00 mm Hg/ml/min
E) 2.50 mm Hg/ml/min

30. A healthy 28-year-old woman stands up from a supine position. Moving from a supine to a standing position results in a transient decrease in arterial pressure that is detected by arterial baroreceptors located in the aortic arch and carotid sinuses. Which of the following sets of cardiovascular changes is most likely to occur in response to activation of the baroreceptors?

	Mean circulatory filling pressure	Strength of cardiac contraction	Sympathetic nerve activity
A)	↑	↑	↑
B)	↑	↓	↑
C)	↑	↓	↓
D)	↑	↑	↓
E)	↓	↓	↓
F)	↓	↑	↑
G)	↓	↑	↑
H)	↓	↓	↑

31. A 35-year-old woman visits her family practice physician for an examination. She has a mean arterial blood pressure of 105 mm Hg and a heart rate of 74 beats/min. Further tests by a cardiologist reveal that the patient has moderate aortic valve stenosis. Which of the following sets of changes would be expected in this patient?

	Pulse pressure	Stroke volume	Systolic pressure
A)	↑	↑	↑
B)	↑	↓	↑
C)	↑	↓	↓
D)	↑	↑	↓
(E)	↓	↓	↓
F)	↓	↑	↓
G)	↓	↑	↑
H)	↓	↓	↑

32. A 25-year-old man enters the hospital emergency room after severing a major artery during a farm accident. It is estimated that the patient has lost approximately 800 ml of blood. His mean blood pressure is 65 mm Hg, and his heart rate is elevated as a result of activation of the chemoreceptor reflex. Which of the following sets of changes in plasma concentration would be expected to cause the greatest activation of the chemoreceptor reflex?

	Oxygen	Carbon dioxide	Hydrogen
A)	↑	↑	↑
B)	↑	↓	↑
C)	↑	↓	↓
D)	↑	↑	↓
E)	↓	↓	↓
F)	↓	↑	↓
(G)	↓	↑	↑
H)	↓	↓	↑

33. An increase in which of the following would tend to increase lymph flow?

    A) Hydraulic conductivity of the capillary wall
    B) Plasma colloid osmotic pressure
    C) Capillary hydrostatic pressure
    D) Arteriolar resistance
    E) A and C

34. Under normal physiological conditions, blood flow to the skeletal muscles is determined mainly by which of the following?

    A) Sympathetic nerves
    B) Angiotensin II
    C) Vasopressin
    D) Metabolic needs
    E) Capillary osmotic pressure

35. Which of the following substances in plasma is the major factor that contributes to plasma colloid osmotic pressure?

    A) Sodium chloride
    B) Glucose
    C) Albumin
    D) Cholesterol
    E) Potassium

36. A healthy 22-year-old female medical student has an exercise stress test at a local health club. An increase in which of the following is most likely to occur in this woman's skeletal muscles during exercise?

    A) Vascular conductance
    B) Blood flow
    C) Carbon dioxide concentration
    D) Arteriolar diameter
    E) All of the above

37. Assuming that vessels A to D are the same length, which one has the greatest flow?

Blood vessel	Pressure gradient	Radius	Viscosity
A)	100	1	10
B)	50	2	5
C)	25	4	2
D)	10	6	1

38. Which blood vessel has the highest vascular resistance?

Blood vessel	Blood flow (ml/min)	Pressure gradient (mm Hg)
A)	1000	100
B)	1200	60
C)	1400	20
D)	1600	80
E)	1800	40

39. A twofold increase in which of the following would result in the greatest increase in the transport of oxygen across the capillary wall?

    A) Capillary hydrostatic pressure
    B) Intercellular clefts in the capillary wall
    C) Oxygen concentration gradient
    D) Plasma colloid osmotic pressure
    E) Capillary wall hydraulic permeability

40. Which of the following vessels has the greatest total cross-sectional area in the circulatory system?

    A) Aorta
    B) Small arteries
    C) Capillaries
    D) Venules
    E) Vena cava

41. Which of the following components of the circulatory system contains the largest percentage of the total blood volume?

    A) Arteries
    B) Capillaries
    C) Veins
    D) Pulmonary circulation
    E) Heart

42. An increase in which of the following would be expected to decrease blood flow in a vessel?

    A) Pressure gradient across the vessel
    B) Radius of the vessel
    C) Plasma colloid osmotic pressure
    D) Viscosity of the blood
    E) Plasma sodium concentration

43. Which of the following segments of the circulatory system has the highest velocity of blood flow?

    A) Aorta
    B) Arteries
    C) Capillaries
    D) Venules
    E) Veins

44. A decrease in which of the following tends to increase pulse pressure?

    A) Systolic pressure
    B) Stroke volume
    C) Arterial compliance
    D) Venous return
    E) Plasma volume

45. An increase in which of the following tends to decrease capillary filtration rate?

    A) Capillary hydrostatic pressure
    B) Plasma colloid osmotic pressure
    C) Interstitial colloid osmotic pressure
    D) Venous hydrostatic pressure
    E) Arteriolar diameter

46. An increase in which of the following tends to increase capillary filtration rate?

    A) Capillary wall hydraulic conductivity
    B) Arteriolar resistance
    C) Plasma colloid osmotic pressure
    D) Interstitial hydrostatic pressure
    E) Plasma sodium concentration

47. A decrease in which of the following tends to increase lymph flow?

    A) Capillary hydrostatic pressure
    B) Interstitial hydrostatic pressure
    C) Plasma colloid osmotic pressure
    D) Lymphatic pump activity
    E) Arteriolar diameter

48. Which of the following capillaries has the lowest capillary permeability to plasma molecules?

    A) Glomerular
    B) Liver
    C) Muscle
    D) Intestinal
    E) Brain

49. Which of the following tends to increase the net movement of glucose across a capillary wall?

    A) Increase in plasma sodium concentration
    B) Increase in the concentration difference of glucose across the wall
    C) Decrease in wall permeability to glucose
    D) Decrease in wall surface area without an increase in the number of pores
    E) Decrease in plasma potassium concentration

50. A 65-year-old man is suffering from congestive heart failure. He has a cardiac output of 4 L/min, arterial pressure of 115/85 mm Hg, and a heart rate of 90 beats/min. Further tests by a cardiologist reveal that the patient has a right atrial pressure of 10 mm Hg. An increase in which of the following would be expected in this patient?

    A) Plasma colloid osmotic pressure
    B) Interstitial colloid osmotic pressure
    C) Arterial pressure
    D) Cardiac output
    E) Vena cava hydrostatic pressure

51. Which of the following parts of the circulation has the highest compliance?

    A) Capillaries
    B) Large arteries
    C) Veins
    D) Aorta
    E) Small arteries

52. Using the following data, calculate the filtration coefficient for the capillary bed:

    Plasma colloid osmotic pressure = 30 mm Hg
    Capillary hydrostatic pressure = 40 mm Hg
    Interstitial hydrostatic pressure = 5 mm Hg
    Interstitial colloid osmotic pressure = 5 mm Hg
    Filtration rate = 150 ml/min
    Venous hydrostatic pressure = 10 mm Hg

    A) 10 ml/min/mm Hg
    B) 15 ml/min/mm Hg
    C) 20 ml/min/mm Hg
    D) 25 ml/min/mm Hg
    E) 30 ml/min/mm Hg

53. Which of the following sets of physiological changes would be expected to occur in a person who stands up from a supine position?

	Venous hydrostatic pressure in legs	Heart rate	Renal blood flow
A)	↑	↑	↑
B)	↑	↑	↓
C)	↑	↓	↓
D)	↓	↓	↓
E)	↓	↓	↑
F)	↓	↑	↑

54. Blood flow to a tissue remains relatively constant despite a reduction in arterial pressure (autoregulation). Which of the following would be expected to occur in response to the reduction in arterial pressure?

    A) Decreased conductance
    B) Decreased tissue carbon dioxide concentration
    C) Increased tissue oxygen concentration
    D) Decreased vascular resistance
    E) Decreased arteriolar diameter

55. The tendency for turbulent flow is greatest in which of the following?

    A) Arterioles
    B) Capillaries
    C) Small arterioles
    D) Aorta

56. Autoregulation of tissue blood flow in response to an increase in arterial pressure occurs as a result of which of the following?

    A) Decrease in vascular resistance
    B) Initial decrease in vascular wall tension
    C) Excess delivery of nutrients such as oxygen to the tissues
    D) Decrease in tissue metabolism

57. Which of the following pressures is normally negative in a muscle capillary bed in the lower extremities?

    A) Plasma colloid osmotic pressure
    B) Capillary hydrostatic pressure
    C) Interstitial hydrostatic pressure
    D) Interstitial colloid osmotic pressure
    E) Venous hydrostatic pressure

58. Which of the following would decrease venous hydrostatic pressure in the legs?

    A) Increase in right atrial pressure
    B) Pregnancy
    C) Movement of leg muscles
    D) Presence of ascitic fluid in the abdomen

59. Movement of solutes such as Na^+ across the capillary walls occurs primarily by which of the following processes?

    A) Filtration
    B) Active transport
    C) Vesicular transport
    D) Diffusion

60. Which of the following has the fastest rate of movement across the capillary wall?

    A) Sodium
    B) Albumin
    C) Glucose
    D) Oxygen

61. A decrease in which of the following would be expected to occur in response to a direct increase in renal arterial pressure?

    A) Water excretion
    B) Sodium excretion
    C) Extracellular fluid volume
    D) Glomerular filtration rate
    E) Inrushing of blood into the ventricles in the early to middle part of diastole

62. Excess production of which of the following would most likely result in chronic hypertension?

    A) Atrial natriuretic peptide
    B) Prostacyclin
    C) Angiotensin II
    D) Nitric oxide

63. A decrease in which of the following would be expected to occur in response to an increase in sodium intake?

    A) Angiotensin II
    B) Nitric oxide
    C) Sodium excretion
    D) Atrial natriuretic peptide

64. Which of the following would be expected to occur in response to constriction of the renal artery?

    A) Increase in sodium excretion
    B) Decrease in arterial pressure
    C) Decrease in renin release
    D) Increase angiotensin II

65. An increase in atrial pressure results in which of the following?

    A) Decrease in plasma atrial natriuretic peptide
    B) Increase in plasma angiotensin II concentration
    C) Increase in plasma aldosterone concentration
    D) Increase in heart rate

66. Which of the following would be expected to occur during a Cushing reaction caused by brain ischemia?

    A) Increase in parasympathetic activity
    B) Decrease in arterial pressure
    C) Decrease in heart rate
    D) Increase in sympathetic activity

67. Which of the following often occurs in decompensated heart failure?

    A) Increased renal loss of sodium and water
    B) Decreased mean systemic filling pressure
    C) Increased norepinephrine in cardiac sympathetic nerves
    D) Orthopnea
    E) Weight loss

68. An angiotensin-converting enzyme inhibitor is administered to a 65-year-old man with a 20-year history of hypertension. The drug lowers arterial pressure and increases plasma levels of renin and bradykinin. Which of the following would best explain the elevation in plasma bradykinin?

    A) Inhibition of preprobradykinin
    B) Decreased conversion of angiotensin I to angiotensin II
    C) Increased formation of angiotensin II
    D) Increased formation of kallikrein
    E) Inhibition of kininases

69. A 60-year-old man has a mean arterial blood pressure of 130 mm Hg, a heart rate of 78 beats/min, a right atrial pressure of 0 mm Hg, and a cardiac output of 3.5 L/min. He also has a pulse pressure of 35 mm Hg and a hematocrit of 40. What is the approximate total peripheral vascular resistance in this man?

    A) 17 mm Hg/L/min
    B) 1.3 mm Hg/L/min
    C) 13 mm Hg/L/min
    D) 27 mm Hg/L/min
    E) 37 mm Hg/L/min

70. In the following graph, for the cardiac output and venous return curves defined by the solid red lines (with the equilibrium at A), which of the following is true?

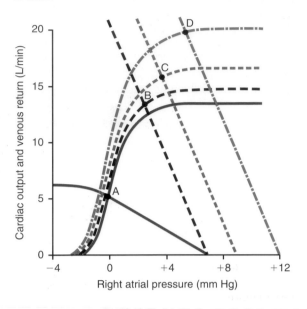

A) Mean systemic filling pressure is 12 mm Hg
B) Right atrial pressure is 2 mm Hg
C) Resistance to venous return is 1.4 mm Hg/L/min
D) Pulmonary arterial flow is approximately 7 L/min
E) Resistance to venous return is 0.71 mm Hg/L/min

71. A 30-year-old male is resting, and his sympathetic output increases to maximal values. Which of the following sets of changes would be expected in response to this increased sympathetic output?

	Resistance to venous return	Mean systemic filling pressure	Venous return
A)	↑	↑	↑
B)	↑	↓	↑
C)	↑	↓	↓
D)	↑	↑	↓
E)	↓	↓	↓
F)	↓	↑	↓
G)	↓	↑	↑
H)	↓	↓	↑

72. If a patient has an oxygen consumption of 240 ml/min, a pulmonary vein oxygen concentration of 180 ml/L of blood and a pulmonary artery oxygen concentration of 160 ml/L of blood units, what is cardiac output in liters per minute?

A) 8
B) 10
C) 12
D) 16
E) 20

73. If the thorax of a normal person is surgically opened, what will happen to the cardiac output curve?

A) It shifts to the left 2 mm Hg
B) It shifts to the left 4 mm Hg
C) It shifts to the right 2 mm Hg
D) It shifts to the right 4 mm Hg
E) It does not shift

74. Which of the following normally cause the cardiac output curve to shift to the left along the right atrial pressure axis?

A) Surgically opening the chest
B) Severe cardiac tamponade
C) Breathing against a negative pressure
D) Playing a trumpet
E) Positive pressure breathing

75. Which of the following will elevate the plateau of the cardiac output curve?

A) Surgically opening the thoracic cage
B) Placing a patient on a mechanical ventilator
C) Cardiac tamponade
D) Increasing parasympathetic stimulation of the heart
E) Increasing sympathetic stimulation of the heart

76. Which of the following normally cause the cardiac output curve to shift to the right along the right atrial pressure axis?

A) Decreasing intrapleural pressure to -6 mm Hg
B) Increasing mean systemic filling pressure
C) Taking a patient off a mechanical ventilator and allowing normal respiration
D) Surgically opening the chest
E) Breathing against a negative pressure

77. Which of the following conditions would be expected to decrease mean systemic filling pressure?

A) Norepinephrine administration
B) Increased blood volume
C) Increased sympathetic stimulation
D) Increased venous compliance
E) Skeletal muscle contraction

78. Which of the following is normally associated with an increased venous return of blood to the heart?

A) Decreased mean systemic filling pressure
B) Acute large vein dilation
C) Decreased sympathetic tone
D) Increased venous compliance
E) Increased blood volume

79. Which of the curves in the following graph (redrawn from Guyton AC, Jones CE, Coleman TB: *Circulatory Physiology: Cardiac Output and Its Regulation*, 2nd ed., Philadelphia: WB Saunders, 1973) has the highest resistance to venous return?

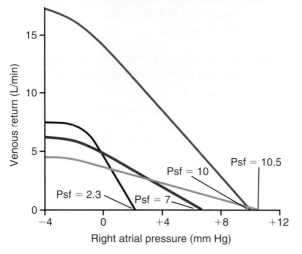

A) Blue line with mean systemic pressure (Psf) = 10
B) Green line with Psf = 10.5
C) Black line with Psf = 2.3
D) Red line with Psf = 7

80. Which of the following is normally associated with an increased cardiac output?

A) Increased venous compliance
B) Cardiac tamponade
C) Surgically opening the chest
D) Moderate anemia
E) Severe aortic stenosis

81. In which of the following conditions would you normally expect to find a decreased cardiac output?

A) Hyperthyroidism
B) Beriberi
C) A-V fistula
D) Anemia
E) Acute myocardial infarction

82. At the onset of exercise, which of the following normally occur?

A) Decreased cerebral blood flow
B) Increased venous constriction
C) Decreased coronary blood flow
D) Decreased mean systemic filling pressure
E) Increased parasympathetic impulses to the heart

83. Which of the following will usually increase the plateau level of the cardiac output curve?

A) Myocarditis
B) Severe cardiac tamponade
C) Decreased parasympathetic stimulation of the heart
D) Myocardial infarction
E) Mitral stenosis

84. If a person has been exercising for 1 hr, which of the following organs will experience the smallest decrease in blood flow?

A) Brain
B) Intestines
C) Kidneys
D) Non-exercising skeletal muscle
E) Pancreas

85. Which of the following increase the risk of adverse cardiac events?

A) Decreased blood levels of LDL
B) Decreased blood levels of HDL
C) Female gender
D) Moderate hypotension
E) Decreased blood triglycerides

86. Which of the following vasoactive agents is usually the most important controller of coronary blood flow?

A) Adenosine
B) Bradykinin
C) Prostaglandins
D) Carbon dioxide
E) Potassium ions

87. During mild exertion, a 70-year-old man experiences an ischemia-induced myocardial infarction and dies from ventricular fibrillation. In this patient, what factor was most likely to increase the tendency of the heart to fibrillate after the infarction?

A) Increased parasympathetic stimulation of the heart
B) A decrease in ventricular diameter
C) Low potassium concentration in the heart extracellular fluid
D) A more negative ventricular membrane potential
E) Current of injury from the damaged area

88. Which of the following statements about coronary blood flow is most accurate?

A) Normal resting coronary blood flow is 500 ml/min
B) The majority of flow occurs during systole
C) During systole the percentage decrease in subendocardial flow is greater than the percentage decrease in epicardial flow
D) Adenosine release will normally decrease coronary flow

89. Which of the following conditions normally cause arteriolar vasodilation during exercise?

A) Decreased plasma potassium ion concentration
B) Increased histamine release
C) Decreased plasma nitric oxide concentration
D) Increased plasma adenosine concentration
E) Decreased plasma osmolality

90. Which of the following vascular beds experiences the most vasoconstriction in a person near the end of a 10-km run?

A) Cerebral
B) Coronary
C) Exercising muscle
D) Intestinal
E) Skin

91. Which of the following blood vessels is responsible for transporting the majority of venous blood flow that leaves the ventricular heart muscle?

A) Anterior cardiac veins
B) Coronary sinus
C) Bronchial veins
D) Azygos vein
E) Thebesian veins

92. A 70-year-old man with a weight of 100 kg and a blood pressure of 160/90 has been told by his doctor that he has angina pain caused by myocardial ischemia. Which of the following treatments would be beneficial to this man?

A) Increased dietary calcium
B) Isometric exercise
C) Give a beta-1 receptor stimulator
D) Angiotensin II infusion
E) Nitroglycerin

93. Which of the following events normally occur during exercise?

A) Arteriolar dilation in non-exercising muscle
B) Decreased sympathetic output
C) Venoconstriction
D) Decreased release of epinephrine by the adrenals
E) Decreased release of norepinephrine by the adrenals

94. Which of the following is the most frequent cause of decreased coronary blood flow in patients with ischemic heart disease?

A) Increased adenosine release
B) Atherosclerosis
C) Coronary artery spasm
D) Increased sympathetic tone of the coronary arteries
E) Occlusion of the coronary sinus

95. Which of the following is an acceptable treatment for patients with an acute myocardial infarction?

A) Daily exercise
B) Beta receptor stimulation
C) Discontinue nitroglycerin intake
D) Discontinue aspirin intake
E) Coronary angioplasty

96. Which of the following would be recommended for a patient with myocardial ischemia?

A) Use of alpha receptor stimulation
B) Discontinue high blood pressure medication
C) Lose excess body weight
D) Angiotensin II infusion
E) Isometric exercise

97. Which of the following is one of the major causes of death after myocardial infarction?

A) Increased cardiac output
B) A decrease in pulmonary interstitial volume
C) Fibrillation of the heart
D) Increased cardiac contractility

98. Which of the following statements about the results of sympathetic stimulation is most accurate?

A) Epicardial flow increases
B) Venous resistance decreases
C) Arteriolar resistance decreases
D) Heart rate decreases
E) Venous reservoirs vasoconstrict

99. Which of the following is normally associated with the chronic stages of compensated heart failure? Assume that the patient is resting.

A) Dyspnea
B) Decreased right atrial pressure
C) Decreased heart rate
D) Sweating
E) Increased mean systemic filling pressure

100. Which of the following normally occur in unilateral right heart failure?

A) Increased pulmonary artery pressure
B) Increased left atrial pressure
C) Increased right atrial pressure
D) Pulmonary edema
E) Increased mean pulmonary filling pressure

101. Which of the following normally causes either renal sodium or water retention during compensated heart failure?

A) Decreased angiotensin II formation
B) Decreased aldosterone formation
C) Sympathetic vasodilation of the afferent arterioles
D) Increased glomerular filtration rate
E) Increased ADH formation

102. Which of the following would normally be beneficial to a patient with acute pulmonary edema?

A) Infuse a vasoconstrictor drug
B) Infuse a balance electrolyte solution
C) Give furosemide
D) Give a bronchoconstrictor
E) Infuse whole blood

103. A 60-year-old man had a heart attack 2 days ago, and his blood pressure has continued to decrease. He is now in cardiogenic shock. Which of the following therapies is most beneficial?

    A) Place tourniquets on all four limbs
    B) Give a sympathetic inhibitor
    C) Give furosemide
    D) Give a blood volume expander
    E) Increase dietary sodium

104. If a 21-year-old male patient has a cardiac reserve of 300% and a maximum cardiac output of 16 L/min, what is his resting cardiac output?

    A) 3 L/min
    B) 4 L/min
    C) 5.33 L/min
    D) 6 L/min
    E) 8 L/min

105. Which of the following occurs during heart failure and causes an increase in renal sodium excretion?

    A) Increased aldosterone release
    B) Increased atrial natriuretic factor release
    C) Decreased glomerular filtration rate
    D) Increased angiotensin II release
    E) Decreased mean arterial pressure

106. Which of the following would be appropriate therapy for a patient in cardiogenic shock?

    A) Place tourniquets on the four limbs
    B) Bleed the patient moderately
    C) Give furosemide
    D) Infuse a vasoconstrictor drug

107. Which of the following conditions normally accompanies acute unilateral right heart failure?

    A) Increased right atrial pressure
    B) Increased left atrial pressure
    C) Increased urinary output
    D) Increased cardiac output
    E) Increased arterial pressure

108. Which of the following often occur in decompensated heart failure?

    A) Edema of the heart muscle
    B) Increased norepinephrine in cardiac sympathetic nerves
    C) Increased calcium in the sarcoplasmic reticulum of cardiac muscle cells
    D) Decreased right atrial pressure
    E) Increased arterial pressure

109. Which of the following would be normally beneficial for patients with acute pulmonary edema?

    A) Place tourniquets on all four limbs
    B) Infuse plasma
    C) Infuse dextran
    D) Infuse norepinephrine
    E) Infuse angiotensin II

110. Which of the following is associated with compensated heart failure?

    A) Increased cardiac output
    B) Increased blood volume
    C) Decreased mean systemic filling pressure
    D) Normal right atrial pressure

111. Which of the following conditions is normally associated with an increase in mean systemic filling pressure?

    A) Decreased blood volume
    B) Congestive heart failure
    C) Sympathetic inhibition
    D) Venous dilation

112. Which of the following conditions normally occurs during the early stages of compensated heart failure?

    A) Increased right atrial pressure
    B) Normal heart rate
    C) Decreased angiotensin II release
    D) Decreased aldosterone release
    E) Increased urinary output of sodium and water

113. Which of the following often occur during decompensated heart failure?

    A) Hypertension
    B) Increased mean pulmonary filling pressure
    C) Decreased pulmonary capillary pressure
    D) Increased cardiac output
    E) Increased norepinephrine in the endings of the cardiac sympathetic nerves

114. Which of the following often occur in decompensated heart failure?

    A) Increased renal loss of sodium and water
    B) Decreased mean systemic filling pressure
    C) Increased norepinephrine in cardiac sympathetic nerves
    D) Orthopnea
    E) Weight loss

115. An 80-year-old male patient at UMC has been diagnosed with a heart murmur. Chest x-ray shows an enlarged heart but no edema fluid in the lungs. The mean QRS axis of his EKG is 170°. Pulmonary wedge pressure is normal. What is the diagnosis?

    A) Mitral stenosis
    B) Aortic stenosis
    C) Pulmonary valve stenosis
    D) Tricuspid stenosis
    E) Mitral regurgitation

116. Which of the following is associated with the second heart sound?

   A) In-rushing of blood into the ventricles due to atrial contraction
   B) Closing of the A-V valves
   C) Closing of the pulmonary valve
   D) Opening of the A-V valves
   E) In-rushing of blood into the ventricles in the early to middle part of diastole

117. A 40-year-old woman has been diagnosed with a heart murmur. A "blowing" murmur of relatively high pitch is heard maximally over the left ventricle. The chest x-ray shows an enlarged heart. Arterial pressure in the aorta is 140/40 mm Hg. What is the diagnosis?

   A) Aortic valve stenosis
   B) Aortic valve regurgitation
   C) Pulmonary valve stenosis
   D) Mitral valve stenosis
   E) Tricuspid valve regurgitation

118. In which of the following disorders would left ventricular hypertrophy normally occur?

   A) Pulmonary valve regurgitation
   B) Tricuspid regurgitation
   C) Mitral stenosis
   D) Tricuspid stenosis
   E) Aortic stenosis

119. Which of the following heart murmurs is heard during systole?

   A) Aortic valve regurgitation
   B) Pulmonary valve regurgitation
   C) Tricuspid valve stenosis
   D) Mitral valve stenosis
   E) Patent ductus arteriosus

120. An increase in left atrial pressure is most likely to occur in which of the following heart murmurs?

   A) Tricuspid stenosis
   B) Pulmonary valve regurgitation
   C) Mitral regurgitation
   D) Tricuspid regurgitation

121. A 50-year-old female patient at UMC has been diagnosed with a heart murmur. A murmur of relatively low pitch is heard maximally over the second intercostal space to the right of the sternum. The chest x-ray shows an enlarged heart. The mean QRS axis of the EKG is −45°. The diagnosis is

   A) Mitral valve stenosis
   B) Aortic valve stenosis
   C) Pulmonary valve stenosis
   D) Tricuspid valve stenosis
   E) Tricuspid valve regurgitation

122. A 29-year-old male patient has been diagnosed with a heart murmur. The mean QRS axis of his EKG is 165°. The arterial blood oxygen content is normal. Which of the following is the likely diagnosis?

   A) Aortic stenosis
   B) Aortic regurgitation
   C) Pulmonary valve stenosis
   D) Mitral stenosis
   E) Tetralogy of Fallot

123. In which of the following will right ventricular hypertrophy normally occur?

   A) Tetralogy of Fallot
   B) Mild aortic stenosis
   C) Mild aortic insufficiency
   D) Mitral stenosis
   E) Tricuspid stenosis

124. Which of the following heart murmurs are only heard during systole?

   A) Patent ductus arteriosus
   B) Mitral stenosis
   C) Tricuspid valve stenosis
   D) Interventricular septal defect
   E) Aortic regurgitation

125. Which of the following is most likely to have low arterial oxygen content?

   A) Tetralogy of Fallot
   B) Pulmonary artery stenosis
   C) Tricuspid insufficiency
   D) Patent ductus arteriosus
   E) Tricuspid stenosis

126. Which of the following is associated with the first heart sound?

   A) In-rushing of blood into the ventricles due to atrial contraction
   B) Closing of the A-V valves
   C) Closing of the pulmonary valve
   D) Opening of the A-V valves
   E) In-rushing of blood into the ventricles in the early to middle part of diastole

127. An echocardiogram was performed on a 50-year-old female patient. The results indicated a thickened right ventricle. Other data indicated that the patient had severely decreased arterial oxygen content and equal systolic pressures in both cardiac ventricles. What condition is present?

   A) Interventricular septal defect
   B) Tetralogy of Fallot
   C) Pulmonary valve stenosis
   D) Pulmonary valve regurgitation
   E) Patent ductus arteriosus

128. Which of the following heart murmurs is only heard during diastole?

 A) Patent ductus arteriosus
 B) Mitral regurgitation
 C) Tricuspid valve stenosis
 D) Interventricular septal defect
 E) Aortic stenosis

129. Which of the following is associated with the third heart sound?

 A) In-rushing of blood into the ventricles due to atrial contraction
 B) Closing of the A-V valves
 C) Closing of the pulmonary valve
 D) Opening of the A-V valves
 E) In-rushing of blood into the ventricles in the early to middle part of diastole

130. Which of the following conditions often occurs in progressive hemorrhagic shock?

 A) Increased capillary permeability
 B) Stress relaxation of veins
 C) Tissue alkalosis
 D) Increased urine output
 E) Increased mean systemic filling pressure

131. In which of the following conditions will administration of a sympathomimetic drug be the therapy of choice to prevent shock?

 A) Spinal cord injury
 B) Shock due to excessive vomiting
 C) Hemorrhagic shock
 D) Shock caused by excess diuretics

132. A 30-year-old female enters the UMC emergency room and has been experiencing severe vomiting. She has pale skin, tachycardia, and arterial pressure of 80/50, and has trouble walking. What therapy do you recommend to prevent shock?

 A) Packed red cell infusion
 B) Administration of an antihistamine
 C) Infusion of a balanced electrolyte solution
 D) Infusion of a sympathomimetic drug
 E) Administration of a glucocorticoid

133. A 65-year-old man enters a local emergency room a few minutes after receiving an influenza inoculation. He has pallor, tachycardia, and arterial pressure of 80/50, and has trouble walking. What therapy do you recommend to prevent shock?

 A) Blood infusion
 B) Administration of an antihistamine
 C) Infusion of a balanced electrolyte solution such as saline
 D) Infusion of a sympathomimetic drug
 E) Administration of tissue plasminogen activator

134. Which of the following conditions often occurs in compensated hemorrhagic shock? Assume systolic pressure is 48 mm Hg.

 A) Decreased heart rate
 B) Stress relaxation of veins
 C) Decreased ADH release
 D) Decreased absorption of interstitial fluid through the capillaries
 E) CNS ischemic response

135. If a patient undergoing spinal anesthesia experiences a large decrease in arterial pressure and goes into shock, which of the following would be the therapy of choice?

 A) Plasma infusion
 B) Blood infusion
 C) Saline infusion
 D) Glucocorticoid infusion
 E) Infusion of sympathomimetic drug

136. A 25-year-old man enters the emergency department and has been in a motorcycle wreck. His clothes are very bloody and arterial pressure is decreased to 70/40. Heart rate is 120 and the respiratory rate is 30/min. Which of the following therapies would the physician recommend?

 A) Blood infusion
 B) Plasma infusion
 C) Infusion of a balanced electrolyte solution
 D) Infusion of a sympathomimetic drug
 E) Administration of a glucocorticoid

137. In which type of shock does cardiac output often increase?

 A) Hemorrhagic shock
 B) Anaphylactic shock
 C) Septic shock
 D) Neurogenic shock

138. A 20-year-old man enters a local emergency room and has been hemorrhaging due to a gunshot wound. He has pale skin, tachycardia, and arterial pressure of 80/50, and has trouble walking. Unfortunately, the blood bank is out of whole blood. Which of the following therapies would the physician recommend to prevent shock?

 A) Administration of a glucocorticoid
 B) Administration of an antihistamine
 C) Infusion of a balanced electrolyte solution
 D) Infusion of a sympathomimetic drug
 E) Plasma infusion

139. A 10-year-old girl in the hospital had an intestinal obstruction and arterial pressure decreased to 70/40. Heart rate is 120 and the respiratory rate is 30/min. Which of the following therapies would the physician recommend?

    A) Blood infusion
    B) Plasma infusion
    C) Infusion of a balanced electrolyte solution
    D) Infusion of a sympathomimetic drug
    E) Administration of a glucocorticoid

140. Which of the following often occur during progressive shock?

    A) Patchy areas of necrosis in the liver
    B) Decreased tendency for blood to clot
    C) Increased glucose metabolism
    D) Decreased release of hydrolases by lysosomes
    E) Decreased capillary permeability

141. Release of which of the following substances causes vasodilation and increased capillary permeability during anaphylactic shock?

    A) Histamine
    B) Bradykinin
    C) Nitric oxide
    D) Atrial natriuretic factor
    E) Adenosine

142. Which of the following is a characteristic of progressive hemorrhagic shock?

    A) Blood clots in small blood vessels
    B) Increased mitochondrial activity in the liver
    C) Decreased lysosomal activity
    D) Decreased active transport of sodium
    E) Tissue alkalosis

143. A 70-year-old man enters the hospital emergency department and has been experiencing severe diarrhea. He has pallor, tachycardia, and an arterial pressure of 80/50, and has trouble walking. Which of the following therapies would the physician recommend to prevent shock?

    A) Blood infusion
    B) Administration of an antihistamine
    C) Infusion of a balanced electrolyte solution
    D) Infusion of a sympathomimetic drug
    E) Administration of a glucocorticoid

144. A 60-year-old woman has been severely burned and has an arterial pressure of 70/40 with a heart rate of 130 bpm. Which of the following therapies would the physician recommend as initial therapy?

    A) Blood infusion
    B) Plasma infusion
    C) Infusion of a balanced electrolyte solution
    D) Infusion of a sympathomimetic drug
    E) Administration of a glucocorticoid

1. **B)** Moving from a supine to a standing position causes an acute fall in arterial pressure that is sensed by arterial baroreceptors located in the carotid bifurcation and aortic arch. Activation of the arterial baroreceptors leads to an increase in sympathetic outflow to the heart, peripheral vasculature, and the kidneys and a decrease in parasympathetic outflow to the heart. The increase in sympathetic activity to peripheral vessels results in an increase in total peripheral resistance. The increase in sympathetic activity and decrease in parasympathetic outflow to the heart result in an increase in heart rate. The increase in renal sympathetic nerve activity results in a decrease in renal blood flow.
   TMP12 205–207

2. **G)** The increase in local metabolism during exercise causes cells to release vasodilator substances such as adenosine. The increase in tissue adenosine concentration decreases arteriolar resistance and increases vascular conductance and blood flow to skeletal muscles.
   TMP12 191–195

3. **G)** Moving from a supine to a standing position causes an acute fall in arterial pressure that is sensed by arterial baroreceptors located in the carotid sinuses and aortic arch. Activation of the baroreceptors results in a decrease in parasympathetic activity (or vagal tone) and an increase in sympathetic activity, which leads to an increase in plasma renin activity (or renin release).
   TMP12 205–207

4. **H)** Atrial natriuretic peptide (ANP) inhibits renin release (and angiotensin II formation). ANP also inhibits aldosterone production, which leads to an increase in sodium excretion.
   TMP12 208

5. **D)** The rate of net fluid movement across a capillary wall is calculated as capillary filtration coefficient × net filtration pressure. Net filtration pressure = capillary hydrostatic pressure − plasma colloid osmotic pressure + interstitial colloid osmotic pressure − interstitial hydrostatic pressure. Thus, the rate of net fluid movement across the capillary wall is 150 ml/min.
   Filtration rate = Capillary filtration coefficient (K_f) × Net filtration pressure
   Filtration rate = $K_f \times [Pc - \Pi c + \Pi i - P_I]$
   Filtration rate = 10 ml/min/mm Hg × [25 − 25 + 10 − (−5)]
   Filtration rate = 10 × 15 = 150 ml/min
   TMP12 181–182

6. **C)** Filtration rate (FR) is the product of the filtration coefficient (Kf) and the net pressure (NP) across the capillary wall. Thus, the filtration coefficient is equal to filtration rate divided by the net pressure. The net pressure for fluid movement across a capillary wall = capillary hydrostatic pressure − plasma colloid osmotic pressure + interstitial colloid osmotic pressure − interstitial hydrostatic pressure. The net pressure in this question calculates to be 15 mm Hg and the filtration is 150. Thus, the Kf is 150/15 or 10 ml/min/mm Hg.
   NP = $[Pc - \Pi p + \Pi_I - P_I]$
   NP = [25 − 25 + 10 − (−5)]
   NP = 15
   Kf = 150/15 = 10 ml/min/mm Hg
   TMP12 181–182

7. **E)** Administration of a drug that decreases the diameter of arterioles in a muscle bed increases the vascular resistance. The increased vascular resistance decreases vascular conductance and blood flow. The reduction in arteriolar diameter also leads to a decrease in capillary hydrostatic pressure and capillary filtration rate.
   TMP12 163–164, 181–182

8. **A)** The difference between systolic pressure and diastolic pressure is the pulse pressure. The two major factors that affect pulse pressure are the stroke volume output of the heart and the compliance of the arterial tree. In patients with moderate aortic regurgitation (due to incomplete closure of aortic valve), the blood that is pumped into the aorta immediately flows back into the left ventricle. The backflow of blood into the left ventricle increases stroke volume and systolic pressure. The rapid backflow of blood also results in a decrease in diastolic pressure. Thus, patients with moderate aortic regurgitation have high systolic pressure, low diastolic pressure, and high pulse pressure.
   TMP12 168–169

9. **E)** Angiotensin II is a powerful vasoconstrictor. Angiotensin I is formed by an enzyme (renin) acting on a substrate called angiotensinogen. Angiotensin I is converted to angiotensin II by a converting enzyme. Angiotensin II is a powerful vasoconstrictor and sodium-retaining hormone that increases arterial pressure. Administration of an ACE inhibitor would be expected to decrease angiotensin II formation, total peripheral resistance, and arterial pressure.
   TMP12 220–223

10. **B)** Cognitive stimuli increase cerebral blood flow by decreasing cerebral vascular resistance. The diameter of cerebral vessels is decreased by various metabolic factors in response to cognitive stimuli. Metabolic factors that enhance cerebral blood flow include increases in carbon dioxide, hydrogen ion (decreased pH), and adenosine.
TMP12 191–194

11. **A)** Stenosis of one kidney results in the release of renin and the formation of angiotensin II from the affected kidney. Angiotensin II stimulates aldosterone production and increases total peripheral resistance by constricting most of the blood vessels in the body.
TMP12 222–224

12. **A)** Histamine is a vasodilator that is typically released by mast cells and basophils. Infusion of histamine into a brachial artery would decrease arteriolar resistance and increase water permeability of the capillary wall. The decrease in arteriolar resistance would also increase capillary hydrostatic pressure. The increase in capillary hydrostatic pressure and water permeability leads to an increase in capillary filtration rate.
TMP12 163–164, 181–182

13. **A)** Bradykinin is a vasodilator that is believed to play a role in regulating blood flow and capillary leakage in inflamed tissue. Infusion of bradykinin into the brachial artery would increase arteriolar diameter and decrease arteriolar resistance. The decrease in arteriolar resistance would also result in an increase in capillary hydrostatic pressure and filtration rate. The increase in filtration rate leads to an increase in interstitial hydrostatic pressure and lymph flow.
TMP12 163–164, 181–182, 187–188

14. **C)** An increase in shear stress in blood vessels is one of the major stimuli for the release of nitric oxide by endothelial cells. Nitric oxide increases blood flow by increasing cyclic guanosine monophosphate.
TMP12 195–196

15. **E)** Solid tumors are metabolically active tissues that need increased quantities of oxygen and other nutrients. When metabolism in a tissue is increased for a prolonged period, the vascularity of the tissue also increases. One of the important factors that increase growth of new blood vessels is vascular endothelial growth factor (VEGF). Presumably, a deficiency of tissue oxygen or other nutrients, or both, leads to the formation of VEGF.
TMP12 198

16. **E)** An increase in the diameter of a precapillary arteriole would decrease arteriolar resistance. The decrease in arteriolar resistance would lead to an increase in vascular conductance and capillary blood flow, hydrostatic pressure, and filtration rate.
TMP12 163–164, 181–182

17. **D)** Blood flow in a vessel is directly proportional to the fourth power of the vessel radius. Increasing vessel diameter by 50% (1.5 times control) would increase blood flow 1.5 to the fourth power × normal blood flow (100 ml/min). Thus, blood flow would increase to 100 ml/min × 5.06, or approximately 500 ml/min.
TMP12 163–164

18. **A)** In patent ductus arteriosus, a large quantity of the blood pumped into the aorta by the left ventricle immediately flows backward into the pulmonary artery and then into the lung and left atrium. The shunting of blood from the aorta results in a low diastolic pressure, while the increased inflow of blood into the left atrium and ventricle increases stroke volume and systolic pressure. The combined increase in systolic pressure and decrease in diastolic pressure results in an increase in pulse pressure.
TMP12 169

19. **A)** The net movement of sodium across a capillary wall is directly proportional to the wall permeability to sodium, wall surface area, and concentration gradient across the capillary wall. Thus, increases in permeability to sodium, surface area, and sodium concentration gradient wall would all increase the net movement of sodium across the capillary wall.
TMP12 178–180

20. **B)** A person with atherosclerosis would be expected to have decreased arterial compliance. The decrease in arterial compliance would lead to an increase in systolic pressure and pulse pressure.
TMP12 168–169

21. **B)** Constriction of the carotid artery reduces blood pressure at the carotid bifurcation where the arterial baroreceptors are located. The decrease in arterial pressure activates baroreceptors, which in turn leads to an increase in sympathetic activity and a decrease in parasympathetic activity (or vagal tone). The enhanced sympathetic activity results in constriction of peripheral blood vessels including the kidneys. The enhanced sympathetic activity leads to an increase in total peripheral resistance and decrease in renal blood flow. The combination of enhanced sympathetic activity and decreased vagal tone also leads to an increase in heart rate.
TMP12 205–207

22. **A)** Atrial natriuretic peptide is released from myocytes in the atria in response to increases in atrial pressure.
TMP12 208

23. **A)** A decrease in the diameter of a precapillary arteriole increases arteriolar resistance while decreasing vascular conductance and capillary blood flow, hydrostatic pressure, filtration rate, interstitial volume, and interstitial hydrostatic pressure.
TMP12 163–164, 181–182

24. C) Excess secretion of aldosterone results in enhanced tubular reabsorption of sodium and secretion of potassium. The increased reabsorption of sodium and water leads to an increase in extracellular fluid volume, which in turn suppresses renin release by the kidney. The increase in potassium secretion leads to a decrease in plasma potassium concentration, or hypokalemia.
TMP12 221–222

25. E) A decrease in tissue oxygen tension is thought to be an important stimulus for vascular endothelial growth factor and the growth of blood vessels in solid tumors.
TMP12 198

26. E) According to Poiseuille's law, flow through a vessel increases in proportion to the fourth power of the radius. A fourfold increase in vessel diameter (or radius) would increase 4 to the fourth power, or 256 times normal. Thus, flow through the vessel after increasing the vessel four times normal would increase from 100 to 25,600 ml/min.
TMP11 163–164

27. H) Constriction of the carotid artery decreases blood pressure at the level of the carotid sinus. A decrease in carotid sinus pressure leads to a decrease in carotid sinus nerve impulses to the vasomotor center, which in turn leads to enhanced sympathetic nervous activity and decreased parasympathetic nerve activity. The increase in sympathetic nerve activity results in peripheral vasoconstriction and an increase in total peripheral resistance.
TMP12 205–208

28. A) The arterial baroreceptors are activated in response to a fall in arterial pressure. During hemorrhage, the fall in arterial pressure at the level of the baroreceptors results in enhanced sympathetic outflow from the vasomotor center and a decrease in parasympathetic nerve activity. The increase in sympathetic nerve activity leads to constriction of peripheral blood vessels, increased total peripheral resistance, and a return of blood pressure toward normal. The decrease in parasympathetic nerve activity and sympathetic outflow would result in an increase in heart rate.
TMP12 205–208

29. C) Vascular resistance = arterial pressure − venous pressure ÷ blood flow. In this example, arterial pressure is 130 mm Hg, venous pressure is 5 mm Hg, and blood flow is 250 ml/min. Thus, vascular resistance = 125 ÷ 250, or 0.50 mm Hg/ml/min.
TMP12 162–163

30. A) Activation of the baroreceptors leads to an increase in sympathetic activity, which in turn increases heart rate, strength of cardiac contraction, and constriction of arterioles and veins. The increase in

venous constriction results in an increase in mean circulatory filling pressure, venous return, and cardiac output.
TMP12 205–208

31. E) Pulse pressure is the difference between systolic pressure and diastolic pressure. The two major factors that affect pulse pressure are the stroke volume output of the heart and the compliance of the arterial tree. An increase in stroke volume increases systolic and pulse pressure, while an increase in compliance of the arterial tree decreases pulse pressure. Moderate aortic valve stenosis results in a decrease in stroke volume, which leads to a decrease in systolic pressure and pulse pressure.
TMP12 168–169

32. G) When blood pressure falls below 80 mm Hg, carotid and aortic chemoreceptors are activated to elicit a neural reflex to minimize the fall in blood pressure. The chemoreceptors are chemosensitive cells that are sensitive to oxygen lack, carbon dioxide excess, or hydrogen ion excess (or fall in pH). The signals transmitted from the chemoreceptors into the vasomotor center excite the vasomotor center to increase arterial pressure.
TMP12 208

33. E) The two main factors that increase lymph flow are an increase in capillary filtration rate and an increase in lymphatic pump activity. An increase in plasma colloid osmotic pressure decreases capillary filtration rate, interstitial volume and hydrostatic pressure, and lymph flow. In contrast, an increase in hydraulic conductivity of the capillary wall and capillary hydrostatic pressure increase capillary filtration rate, interstitial volume and pressure, and lymph flow. An increase arteriole resistance would decrease capillary hydrostatic pressure, capillary filtration rate, interstitial volume and pressure, and lymph flow.
TMP12 181–187

34. D) Although sympathetic nerves, angiotensin II, and vasopressin are powerful vasoconstrictors, blood flow to skeletal muscles under normal physiological conditions is mainly determined by local metabolic needs.
TMP12 194–196

35. C) Those molecules or ions that fail to pass through the pores of the capillary wall exert osmotic pressure. The capillary wall is highly permeable to sodium chloride, glucose, cholesterol, and potassium but relatively impermeable to albumin. Thus, albumin in the plasma is the major contributor to plasma colloid osmotic pressure.
TMP12 184

36. E) During exercise, tissue levels of carbon dioxide and lactic acid increase. These metabolites dilate blood vessels, decrease arteriolar resistance, and enhance vascular conductance and blood flow.
TMP12 194–195

37. **D)** The flow in a vessel is directly proportional to the pressure gradient across the vessel and to the fourth power of the radius of the vessel. In contrast, blood flow is inversely proportional to the viscosity of the blood. Because blood flow is proportional to the fourth power of the vessel radius, the vessel with the largest radius (vessel D) would have the greatest flow.
TMP12 163

38. **A)** Resistance of a vessel = pressure gradient ÷ blood flow of the vessel. In this example, vessel A has the highest vascular resistance (100 mm Hg/1000 ml/min, or 0.1 mm Hg/ml/min).
TMP12 162–163

39. **C)** The transport of oxygen across a capillary wall is proportional to the capillary surface area, capillary wall permeability to oxygen, and oxygen gradient across the capillary wall. Thus, a twofold increase in the oxygen concentration gradient would result in the greatest increase in the transport of oxygen across the capillary wall. A twofold increase in intercellular clefts in the capillary wall would not significantly impact oxygen transport, because oxygen can permeate the endothelial cell wall.
TMP12 179–180

40. **C)** The capillaries have the largest total cross-sectional area of all vessels of the circulatory system. The venules also have a relatively large total cross-sectional area, but not as great as the capillaries, which explains the large storage of blood in the venous system compared with that in the arterial system.
TMP12 160–161

41. **C)** The percentage of total blood volume in the veins is approximately 64%.
TMP12 157

42. **D)** The rate of blood flow is directly proportional to the fourth power of the vessel radius and to the pressure gradient across the vessel. In contrast, the rate of blood flow is inversely proportional to the viscosity of the blood. Thus, an increase in blood viscosity would decrease blood flow in a vessel.
TMP12 163–164

43. **A)** The velocity of blood flow within each segment of the circulatory system is inversely proportional to the total cross-sectional area of the segment. Because the aorta has the smallest total cross-sectional area of all circulatory segments, it has the highest velocity of blood flow.
TMP12 161–162

44. **C)** The difference between systolic pressure and diastolic pressure is called the pulse pressure. The two main factors that affect pulse pressure are stroke volume and arterial compliance. Pulse pressure is directly proportional to the stroke volume and inversely proportional to the arterial compliance. Thus, a decrease in arterial compliance would tend to increase pulse pressure.
TMP11 168–169

45. **B)** An increase in plasma colloid osmotic pressure would reduce net filtration pressure and capillary filtration rate. Increases in capillary hydrostatic pressure and interstitial colloid osmotic pressure would also favor capillary filtration. An increase in venous hydrostatic pressure and arteriolar diameter would tend to increase capillary hydrostatic pressure and capillary filtration rate.
TMP12 181–185

46. **A)** An increase in capillary wall permeability to water would increase capillary filtration rate, whereas increases in arteriolar resistance, plasma colloid osmotic pressure, and interstitial hydrostatic pressure would all decrease filtration rate. Plasma sodium concentration would have no effect on filtration.
TMP12 181–186

47. **C)** The rate of lymph flow increases in proportion to the interstitial hydrostatic pressure and the lymphatic pump activity. A decrease in plasma colloid osmotic pressure would increase filtration rate, interstitial volume, interstitial hydrostatic pressure, and lymph flow. A decrease in arteriolar diameter would decrease capillary hydrostatic pressure, capillary filtration, and lymph flow.
TMP12 181–188

48. **E)** The brain has tight junctions between capillary endothelial cells that allow only extremely small molecules such as water, oxygen, and carbon dioxide to pass in or out of the brain tissues.
TMP12 178

49. **B)** The factors that determine the net movement of glucose across a capillary wall include the wall permeability to glucose, the glucose concentration gradient across the wall, and the capillary wall surface area. Thus, an increase in the concentration difference of glucose across the wall would enhance the net movement of glucose.
TMP12 179–180

50. **E)** An increase in atrial pressure of 10 mm Hg would tend to decrease venous return to the heart and increase vena cava hydrostatic pressure. Plasma colloid osmotic pressure, interstitial colloid osmotic pressure, arterial pressure, and cardiac output would generally be low to normal in this patient.
TMP12 172–173

51. **C)** The vascular compliance is proportional to the vascular distensibility and vascular volume of any given segment of the circulation. The compliance of a

systemic vein is 24 times that of its corresponding artery because it is about 8 times as distensible and it has a volume about 3 times as great.
   TMP12 167

52. **B)** Filtration coefficient (K_f) = filtration rate ÷ net filtration pressure. Net filtration pressure = capillary hydrostatic pressure − plasma colloid osmotic pressure + interstitial colloid osmotic pressure − interstitial hydrostatic pressure. The net filtration pressure in this example is 10 mm Hg. Thus, K_f = 150 ml/min ÷ 10 mm Hg, or 15 ml/min/mm Hg.
   TMP12 181–186

53. **B)** Moving from a supine to a standing position results in pooling of blood in the lower extremities and a fall in blood pressure. The pooling of blood in the legs increases venous hydrostatic pressure. The fall in arterial pressure activates the arterial baroreceptors, which in turn increases sympathetic nerve activity and decreases parasympathetic nerve activity. The increase in sympathetic activity constricts renal vessels and reduces renal blood flow. The heart rate also increases.
   TMP12 205–207

54. **D)** Reduction in perfusion pressure to a tissue leads to a decrease in tissue oxygen concentration and an increase in tissue carbon dioxide concentration. Both events lead to an increase in arteriolar diameter, decreased vascular resistance, and increased vascular conductance.
   TMP12 194–196

55. **D)** The largest portion of the arterial pressure is at the site of greatest vascular resistance, which is the arteriolar–capillary juncture.
   TMP12 158

56. **D)** The tendency for turbulent flow occurs at vascular sites where the velocity of blood flow is high. The aorta has the highest velocity of blood flow.
   TMP12 161–162

57. **C)** An increase in perfusion pressure to a tissue results in excessive delivery of nutrients such as oxygen to a tissue. The increase in tissue oxygen concentration constricts arterioles and returns blood flow and nutrient delivery toward normal levels.
   TMP12 194–195

58. **C)** Interstitial hydrostatic pressure in a muscle capillary bed is normally negative (−3 mm Hg). Pumping by the lymphatic system is the basic cause of the negative pressure.
   TMP12 183–184

59. **C)** Movement of the leg muscles causes blood to flow toward the vena cava, which reduces venous hydrostatic pressure. An increase in right atrial pressure would decrease venous return and increase venous

hydrostatic pressure. Pregnancy and the presence of ascitic fluid in the abdomen would tend to compress the vena cava and increase venous hydrostatic pressure in the legs.
   TMP12 172–173

60. **D)** The primary mechanism whereby solutes move across a capillary wall is simple diffusion.
   TMP12 179

61. **D)** Because oxygen is lipid soluble and can cross the capillary wall with ease, it has the fastest rate of movement across the capillary wall.
   TMP12 179

62. **C)** An increase in renal arterial pressure results in pressure natriuresis and diuresis. The loss of sodium and water tends to decrease extracellular fluid volume. Glomerular filtration rate would be normal or slightly increased in response to an increase in renal artery pressure.
   TMP12 213–215

63. **C)** Nitric oxide and prostacyclin are potent vasodilator and natriuretic substances. In addition, atrial natriuretic peptide is natriuretic and antihypertensive. In contrast, angiotensin II is a powerful vasoconstrictor, antinatriuretic, and hypertensive hormone.
   TMP12 195–196

64. **A)** An increase in sodium intake would result in an increase in sodium excretion to maintain sodium balance. Angiotensin II decreases in response to a chronic elevation in sodium intake while nitric oxide and atrial natriuretic peptide increase.
   TMP12 217–222

65. **D)** Constriction of the renal artery increases renin release, angiotensin II formation, and arterial pressure. Sodium excretion decreases, but only transiently, because as arterial pressure increases, sodium excretion returns to normal levels via a pressure natriuresis mechanism.
   TMP12 223–225

66. **D)** An increase in atrial pressure causes an increase in heart rate by a nervous reflex called the Bainbridge reflex. The stretch receptors of the atria that elicit the Bainbridge reflex transmit their afferent signals through the vagus nerves to the medulla of the brain. The efferent signals are transmitted back via vagal and sympathetic nerves to increase the heart rate. An increase in atrial pressure would also increase plasma levels of atrial natriuretic peptide, which in turn would decrease plasma levels of angiotensin II and aldosterone.
   TMP12 208–209

67. **D)** The Cushing reaction is a special type of central nervous system (CNS) ischemic response that results from increased pressure of the cerebrospinal fluid

around the brain in the cranial vault. When the cerebrospinal fluid pressure rises, it decreases the blood supply to the brain and elicits a CNS ischemic response. The CNS ischemic response includes enhanced sympathetic activity; decreased parasympathetic activity; and increased heart rate, arterial pressure, and total peripheral resistance.
TMP12 209–210

68. **E)** The conversion of angiotensin I to angiotensin II is catalyzed by a converting enzyme that is present in the endothelium of the lung vessels and in the kidneys. The converting enzyme also serves as a kininase that degrades bradykinin. Thus, a converting enzyme inhibitor not only decreases the formation of angiotensin II but also inhibits kininases and the breakdown of bradykinin.
TMP12 220

69. **E)** Total peripheral vascular resistance = arterial pressure − right atrial pressure ÷ cardiac output. In this example, total peripheral vascular resistance = 130 mm Hg ÷ 3.5 L/min, or approximately 37 mm Hg/L/min.
TMP12 162-163

70. **C)** The formula for resistance to venous return is mean systemic filling pressure − right atrial pressure/cardiac output. In this example the mean systemic filling pressure is 7 mm Hg and the right atrial pressure is 0 mm Hg. The cardiac output is 5 L/min. Using these values in the previous formula indicates that the resistance to venous return is 1.4 mm Hg/L/min. Note that this formula only applies to the linear portion of the venous return curve.
TMP12 238–239

71. **A)** During increases in sympathetic output to maximal values, several changes occur. First, the mean systemic filling pressure increases markedly, but at the same time the resistance to venous return increases. Venous return is determined by the formula: mean systemic filling pressure − right atrial pressure/resistance to venous return. During maximal sympathetic output, the increase in systemic filling pressure is greater than the increase in resistance to venous return. Therefore, in this formula the numerator has a much greater increase than the denominator. This results in an increase in the venous return.
TMP12 238–239

72. **C)** This problem concerns the Fick principle for determining cardiac output. The formula for cardiac output is oxygen absorbed per minute by the lungs divided by the arterial-venous oxygen difference. In this problem, oxygen consumption of the body is 240 ml/min, and in a steady-state condition this would exactly equal the oxygen absorbed by the lungs. Therefore, by inserting these values into the equation we see that the cardiac output will equal 12 L/min.
TMP12 240

73. **D)** The normal intrapleural pressure is -4 mm Hg. When the thorax is surgically opened, all pressures inside the chest will immediately have a value of 0 mm Hg, which is the atmospheric pressure. This increased pressure in the chest tends to collapse the atria and decreases the transmural pressure across each of the atria. In particular, the right atrial transmural pressure gradient decreases about 4 mm Hg. Therefore, the cardiac output curve will shift to the right by 4 mm Hg.
TMP12 234

74. **C)** Several factors can cause the cardiac output to shift to the right or to the left. These factors include surgically opening the chest, which makes the cardiac output curve shift 4 mm Hg to the right, and severe cardiac tamponade, which increases the pressure inside the pericardium, thus tending to collapse the heart, particularly the atria. Playing a trumpet or positive pressure breathing tremendously increases the interpleural pressure, thus collapsing the atria and shifting the cardiac output curve to the right. Breathing against a negative pressure will shift the cardiac output curve to the left.
TMP12 234

75. **E)** The plateau level of the cardiac output curve, which is one measure of cardiac contractility, decreases in several circumstances. Some of these include severe cardiac tamponade that increases the pressure in the pericardial space and increasing parasympathetic stimulation of the heart. Increased sympathetic stimulation of the heart increases the level of the cardiac output curve by increasing heart rate and contractility.
TMP12 231

76. **D)** Several factors can cause the cardiac output to shift to the right or to the left. These factors include surgically opening the chest, which makes the cardiac output curve shift 4 mm Hg to the right, and severe cardiac tamponade, which increases the pressure inside the pericardium, thus tending to collapse the heart, particularly the atria. Playing a trumpet or positive pressure breathing including being on a mechanical ventilator tremendously increases the interpleural pressure, thus collapsing the atria and shifting the cardiac output curve to the right.
TMP12 234

77. **D)** Mean systemic filling pressure is a measure of the tightness of fit of the blood in the circulation. Mean systemic filling pressure is increased by factors which increase blood volume and by factors that decrease the vascular compliance. Therefore, a decreased venous compliance, not an increased compliance, would cause an increase in mean systemic filling pressure. Norepinephrine administration and sympathetic stimulation cause arteriolar vasoconstriction and decreased vascular compliance resulting in an increase in mean

systemic filling pressure. Increased blood volume and skeletal muscle contraction, which cause a contraction of the vasculature, also increase this filling pressure.
TMP12 236

78. **E)** Venous return of the heart is equal to the mean systemic filling pressure minus the right atrial pressure divided by the resistance to venous return. Therefore, decreased mean systemic filling pressure will decrease the venous return to the heart. Factors that will decrease the systemic filling pressure include large vein dilation, decreased sympathetic tone, increased venous compliance and increased blood volume.
TMP12 236–237

79. **B)** The resistance to venous return is the inverse of the slope of the linear portion of the venous return curve. Therefore, the curve with the lowest slope will have the highest resistance to venous return.
TMP12 238

80. **D)** Decreased cardiac output can result from a weakened heart or from a decrease in venous return. Increased venous compliance decreases the venous return of blood to the heart. Cardiac tamponade, surgically opening the chest and severe aortic stenosis will effectively weaken the heart and thus decrease cardiac output. Moderate anemia will cause an arteriolar vasodilation, which increases venous return of blood back to the heart thus increasing cardiac output.
TMP12 239

81. **E)** Cardiac output increases in several conditions because of increased venous return. Cardiac output increases in hyperthyroidism because of the increased oxygen use by the peripheral tissues resulting in arteriolar vasodilation and thus increased venous return. Beriberi causes increased cardiac output because a lack of the vitamin thiamine results in peripheral vasodilation. A-V fistulae also cause a decreased resistance to venous return thus increasing cardiac output. Anemia, because of the decreased oxygen delivery to the tissues, causes an increase in venous return to the heart and thus an increase in cardiac output. Cardiac output decreases in patients with myocardial infarction.
TMP12 232–233

82. **B)** During exercise there is very little change in cerebral blood flow and coronary blood flow increases. Because of the increased sympathetic output, mean systemic filling pressure increases and the veins constrict. During exercise there is also a decrease in parasympathetic impulses to the heart.
TMP12 238–239

83. **C)** The plateau level of the cardiac output curve, which is one measure of cardiac contractility, decreases in several circumstances. Some of these include myocarditis, severe cardiac tamponade that increases the pressure in the pericardial space, myocardial infarction and various valvular diseases such as mitral stenosis. Decreased parasympathetic stimulation of the heart actually moderately increases the level of the cardiac output curve by increasing heart rate.
TMP12 231

84. **A)** During increases in sympathetic output the main two organs to maintain their blood flow are the brain and the heart. During exercise for 1 hour, the intestinal flow decreases significantly as will the renal and pancreatic blood flows. The skeletal muscle blood flow to non-exercising muscles also decreases at this time. Therefore, the cerebral blood flow remains close to its control value.
TMP12 244

85. **B)** There are several factors that decrease the risk of adverse cardiac events, including decreased blood levels of LDL, female gender, moderate hypotension, and decreased blood triglycerides. Decreased blood levels of HDL will increase cardiac risks, since HDL is a protective cholesterol.
TMP12 248–249

86. **A)** Bradykinin, prostaglandins, carbon dioxide, and potassium ions serve as vasodilators for the coronary artery system. However, the major controller of coronary blood flow is adenosine. Adenosine is formed as ATP degrades to adenosine monophosphate. Then, small portions of the adenosine monophosphate are further degraded to release adenosine into the tissue fluids of the heart muscle, and this adenosine vasodilates the coronary arteries.
TMP12 247

87. **E)** An acute loss of blood supply to a cardiac muscle causes depletion of potassium from the cardiac myocytes. This locally increases the extracellular potassium concentration. In turn, this increases the irritability of the cardiac musculature and therefore its likelihood for fibrillating. Therefore, a decreased potassium ion concentration in the extracellular fluids of the heart does not lead to fibrillation. Powerful sympathetic and not parasympathetic reflexes also increase the irritability of the cardiac muscle and predispose it to fibrillation. A more negative membrane potential protects the heart from fibrillation, and a current of injury allows electrical current flow from an ischemic area of the heart to a normal area and can elicit fibrillation.
TMP12 250–251

88. **C)** The normal resting coronary blood flow is approximately 225 ml/min. Infusion of adenosine or local release of adenosine normally increases the coronary blood flow. The contraction of the cardiac muscle around the vasculature, particularly in the subendocardial vessels, causes a decrease in blood flow. Therefore, during the systolic phase of the cardiac cycle the

subendocardial flow clearly decreases while the decrease in epicardial flow is relatively minor.
TMP12 247

89. **D)** There are several factors that cause arteriolar vasodilation during exercise including increases in potassium ion concentration, plasma nitric oxide concentration, plasma adenosine concentration and plasma osmolality. Although histamine causes arteriolar vasodilation, histamine release does not normally occur during exercise.
TMP12 243

90. **D)** The vascular beds that are spared from vasoconstriction due to increased sympathetic output during exercise include the cerebral and coronary vascular beds. In exercising muscle the metabolic vasodilatory response overcomes the sympathetic nervous system resulting in vasodilation. In the skin vasculature, vasoconstriction occurs only at the beginning of exercise, and when the body heats up, the skin arterioles dilate. The intestinal vasculature significantly constricts during long-term exercise.
TMP12 244

91. **B)** The anterior cardiac veins and the thebesian veins both drain venous blood from the heart. However, 75% of the total coronary flow drains from the heart by the coronary sinus.
TMP12 246

92. **E)** Several drugs have proven to be helpful to patients with myocardial ischemia. Beta receptor blockers (not stimulators) inhibit the sympathetic effects on the heart and are very helpful. Angiotensin converting enzyme inhibition prevents the production of angiotensin II and thus decreases the afterload effect on the heart. Nitroglycerin causes nitric oxide release resulting in coronary vasodilation. Isometric exercise increases blood pressure markedly and can be harmful, and increased dietary calcium would be of little benefit.
TMP12 252

93. **C)** During exercise the sympathetic output increases markedly which causes arteriolar constriction in many places of the body including non-exercising muscle. The increased sympathetic output also causes venoconstriction throughout the body. During exercise there also is an increased release of norepinephrine and epinephrine by the adrenal glands.
TMP12 244–245

94. **B)** Several factors contribute to decreased coronary flow in patients with ischemic heart disease. Some patients will have spasm of the coronary arteries which acutely decreases coronary flow. However, the major cause of decreased coronary flow is an atherosclerotic narrowing of the lumen of the coronary arteries.
TMP12 248

95. **E)** There are a several acceptable treatments for patients with myocardial ischemia. Many patients take a daily dose of aspirin to prevent coronary thrombosis. Angioplasty with placement of stents or coronary by-pass surgery effectively increases the coronary blood flow. Lowering of blood pressure, angiotensin converting enzyme inhibitors, or beta receptor blockade are also effective treatments. However, beta receptor stimulation or exercise would be detrimental to a patient with ischemia.
TMP12 252–253

96. **C)** In a patient with myocardial ischemia, factors which increase stress on the heart must be minimized. This can be done with the use of beta sympathetic blockers, which inhibit the effects of excess sympathetic output on the heart. It is also important to maintain a normal body weight and a normal arterial pressure, which prevent excess stress on the heart. And in conditions of acute myocardial ischemia, nitroglycerin can be taken. Isometric exercise should be avoided because of the large increase in arterial pressure that occurs.
TMP12 252

97. **C)** The major causes of death after myocardial infarction include a decrease in cardiac output that prevents tissues of the body from receiving adequate nutrition and oxygen delivery and prevents removal of waste materials. Other causes of death are pulmonary edema, which reduces the oxygenation of the blood, fibrillation of the heart, and rupture of the heart. Cardiac contractility decreases after a myocardial infarction.
TMP12 250

98. **E)** During sympathetic stimulation venous reservoirs constrict, venous vascular resistance also increases, arterioles constrict which increases their resistance, and heart rate increases. The epicardial coronary vessels have a large number of alpha receptors but the subendocardial vessels have more beta receptors. Therefore, sympathetic stimulation causes at least a slight constriction of the epicardial vessels. This results in a slight decrease in epicardial flow.
TMP12 244–245, 247

99. **E)** Several factors change during compensated heart failure to stabilize the circulatory system. Because of increased sympathetic output the heart rate increases during compensated heart failure. The kidneys retain sodium and water which increases blood volume and thus right atrial pressure. The increased blood volume that results causes an increase in mean systemic filling pressure, which will help to increase the cardiac output. Dyspnea usually will occur only in the early stages of compensated failure.
TMP12 255–256

100. **C)** In acute right heart failure the kidneys retain sodium and water, and the systemic but not the pulmonary veins become congested. Therefore, mean pulmonary filling pressure and left atrial pressure do not increase, but right atrial pressure increases and edema of the lower extremities including the feet and ankles occurs.
    TMP12 259

101. **E)** In compensated heart failure the sympathetic output increases. One of the results is a sympathetic vasoconstriction of the afferent arterioles of the kidney. This decreases the glomerular hydrostatic pressure and thus the glomerular filtration rate, resulting in an increase in sodium and water retention in the body. An increased release of angiotensin II also occurs which causes direct renal sodium retention and also stimulates aldosterone secretion which will, in turn, cause further increases in sodium retention in the kidney. The excess sodium in the body will increase osmolality and this increases the release of antidiuretic hormone which causes renal water retention.
    TMP12 260

102. **C)** During acute pulmonary edema, the increased fluid in the lungs diminishes the O_2 content in the blood. This decreased oxygen weakens the heart even further and also causes arteriolar dilation in the body. This results in increases in venous return of blood to the heart which cause further leakage of the fluid in the lungs and further decreases in oxygen content in the blood. It is important to interrupt this vicious circle to save a patient's life. This can be done by placing tourniquets on all four limbs which effectively removes blood volume from the chest. The patient can also breathe oxygen and you can give a bronchodilator. Furosemide can be given to reduce some of the fluid volume in the body and especially in the lungs. One thing that you do not want to do is infuse whole blood or an electrolyte solution in this patient as it may exacerbate the pulmonary edema that is already present.
    TMP12 261

103. **D)** Cardiogenic shock results from a weakening of the cardiac muscle many times following coronary thrombosis. This can result in a vicious circle because of low cardiac output resulting in a low diastolic pressure. This causes a decrease in coronary flow which decreases the cardiac strength even more. Therefore, arterial pressure, particularly diastolic pressure, must be increased in patients with cardiogenic shock by either vasoconstrictors or volume expanders. In this patient the best answer is to infuse plasma. Placing tourniquets on all four limbs decreases the central blood volume, which would worsen the condition of the patient in shock.
    TMP12 259

104. **B)** This patient has a resting cardiac output of 4 L/min, and his cardiac reserve is 300% of this resting cardiac output or 12 L/min. This gives a total maximum cardiac output of 16 L/min. Therefore, the cardiac reserve is the percentage increase that the cardiac output can be elevated over the resting cardiac output.
    TMP12 261

105. **B)** Several factors cause sodium retention during heart failure including aldosterone release, decreased glomerular filtration rate, and an increased angiotensin II release. A decrease in mean arterial pressure also results in decreases in glomerular hydrostatic pressure and causes a decrease in renal sodium excretion. During heart failure blood volume increases, resulting in an increased cardiac stretch. In particular, the atrial pressure increases causing a release of atrial natriuretic factor resulting in an increase in renal sodium excretion.
    TMP12 260

106. **D)** There is a vicious circle of cardiac deterioration in cardiogenic shock. A weakened heart causes a decreased cardiac output, which decreases arterial pressure. The decreased arterial pressure, particularly the decrease in diastolic pressure, decreases the coronary blood flow and further weakens the heart and thus further decreases cardiac output. The therapy of choice for a patient in cardiogenic shock is to increase the arterial pressure either with a vasoconstrictor drug or with a volume-expanding drug. Placing tourniquets on the four limbs, bleeding the patient moderately, or giving furosemide decreases the thoracic blood volume and thus worsens the condition of the patient in cardiogenic shock.
    TMP12 259

107. **A)** In unilateral right heart failure, the right atrial pressure decreases and the overall cardiac output decreases. This results in a decrease in arterial pressure and urinary output. However, left atrial pressure does not increase but in fact decreases.
    TMP12 259

108. **A)** During decompensated heart failure the kidneys decrease their urinary output of sodium and water in order to increase the blood volume. This increases the mean systemic filling pressure and the venous return of blood back toward the heart thus increasing right atrial pressure. Unfortunately, if the heart is very weak, the end diastolic volume increases, which overstretches the cardiac sarcomeres, and the heart muscle becomes very edematous. At the same time, there is a decreased accumulation of calcium ions in the longitudinal tubules of the sarcoplasmic reticulum. Therefore, there is less calcium available for the cardiac muscle resulting in a further weakened heart.
    TMP12 257–258

109. A) Patients with acute pulmonary edema rapidly deteriorate unless the proper therapy is given. The thoracic blood volume must be decreased and several techniques are available. Tourniquets can be placed on all four limbs and then the constriction rotated to increase the blood volume of the limbs and thus decrease the volume of the blood in the chest. They can also be given rapidly acting diuretics such as furosemide, which reduces plasma volume. Blood can be actually removed in moderate quantities from the patient to decrease the volume of blood in the chest. Patients should also breathe oxygen to increase the oxygen levels in the blood. But they should never be given a volume expander such as plasma or dextran, since it could worsen the pulmonary edema.
TMP12 261

110. B) In compensated heart failure, mean systemic filling pressure increases because of hypervolemia, and cardiac output is often at normal values. There is air hunger, called dyspnea, and excess sweating occurs in the early phases of compensated heart failure. However, right atrial pressure elevates to very high values in these patients and is a hallmark of this disease.
TMP12 256–257

111. B) Mean systemic pressure is increased by factors which increase blood volume or decrease vascular capacity. Sympathetic inhibition and venous dilation both decrease the mean systemic filling pressure. In congestive heart failure, the kidneys retain great quantities of sodium and water resulting in an increase in blood volume, which causes large increases in mean systemic filling pressure.
TMP12 256

112. A) During compensated heart failure angiotensin II and aldosterone release increase causing the kidneys to retain sodium and water which increases the blood volume in the body and increases the venous return of blood to the heart. This results in an increase in right atrial pressure. Increased sympathetic output during compensated heart failure will increase heart rate. There is also an air hunger, called dyspnea, during any type of exertion. There is orthopnea, which is the air hunger that occurs when one lies in a recumbent position.
TMP12 256–257

113. B) During decompensated heart failure cardiac output decreases because of weakness of the heart and edema of the cardiac muscle. Pressures in the pulmonary capillary system increase including the pulmonary capillary pressure and the mean pulmonary filling pressure. Depletion of norepinephrine in the endings of the cardiac sympathetic nerves is another factor which causes weakness of the heart.
TMP12 257–258

114. D) In decompensated heart failure the kidneys retain sodium and water which causes a weight gain and an increase in blood volume. This increases the mean systemic filling pressure which also stretches the heart. Therefore, a decreased mean systemic filling pressure does not occur in decompensated heart failure. The excess blood volume will many times over-stretch the sarcomeres of the heart, which will prevent them from achieving their maximal tension. An excess central fluid volume also results in orthopnea which is the inability to breathe properly except in the upright position.
TMP12 257–258

115. C) The mean electrical axis of the QRS of this patient is shifted rightward to 170°. This indicates that the right side of the heart is involved. Both aortic stenosis and mitral regurgitation will cause a leftward shift of the QRS axis. Mitral stenosis will not affect the left ventricle but in severe enough circumstances could cause an increase in pulmonary artery pressure. This would cause an increase in pulmonary capillary pressure at the same time. Tricuspid stenosis will not affect the right ventricle. Therefore, pulmonary valve stenosis is the only condition that fits this set of symptoms.
TMP12 265–266

116. C) The second heart sound is caused by the closing of the aortic and pulmonary valves at the end of systole. This initiates a vibration similar throughout the ventricles, aorta, and pulmonary artery. By comparison the first heart sound is caused by closing of the A-V valves.
TMP12 267

117. B) The blowing murmurs of relatively high pitch are usually the murmurs associated with valvular insufficiency. The key pieces of data to identify this murmur are the systolic and diastolic pressures. Aortic valve regurgitation typically has a high pulse pressure, which is the systolic − the diastolic pressure, and in this case is 100 mm Hg. Also note that the diastolic pressure decreases to very low values of 40 mm Hg as the blood leaks back into the left ventricle.
TMP12 267–268

118. E) Left ventricular hypertrophy occurs when the left ventricle either has to produce high pressure or when it pumps extra volume with each stroke. During aortic regurgitation extra blood leaks back into the ventricle during the diastolic period. This extra volume must be expelled during the next heartbeat. During mitral regurgitation some blood gets pumped out into the aorta, while at the same time blood leaks back into the left atrium. Therefore, the left ventricle is pumping extra volume with each heartbeat. During aortic stenosis the left ventricle must contract

very strongly producing high wall tension in order to increase the aortic pressure to the high enough values necessary to expel blood into the aorta. During mitral stenosis the ventricle is normal, because the atrium produces the extra pressure to get blood through the stenotic mitral valve.
TMP12 267–268

119. **E)** There are several diastolic murmurs that can be easily heard with a stethoscope. During diastole aortic and pulmonary valve regurgitation occurs through the insufficient valves causing the heart murmur at this time. Tricuspid and mitral stenosis are diastolic murmurs because blood flows through the restricted valves during the diastolic period. Patent ductus arteriosus is heard in both systole and diastole.
TMP12 265–266

120. **C)** Mitral regurgitation causes large increases in left atrial pressure. However, tricuspid stenosis and regurgitation and pulmonary valve regurgitation only increase the right atrial pressure and should not affect pressure in the left atrium.
TMP12 267–268

121. **B)** This patient has a QRS axis of −45°, indicating a leftward axis shift. In other words, the left side of the heart is enlarged. In aortic valve stenosis the left side of the heart is enlarged because of the extra tension the left ventricular walls must exert to expel blood out the aorta. Therefore, these symptoms fit with a patient with aortic stenosis. In pulmonary valve stenosis, the right side of the heart hypertrophies, and in mitral valve stenosis there is no left ventricular hypertrophy. In tricuspid valve regurgitation the right side of the heart enlarges, and in tricuspid valve stenosis no ventricular hypertrophy occurs.
TMP12 267–268

122. **C)** This patient has a rightward axis shift which indicates that the right side of the heart has hypertrophied. The two choices that have a rightward axis shift are pulmonary valve stenosis and tetralogy of Fallot. In tetralogy of Fallot, the arterial blood oxygen content is low, which is not the case with this patient. Therefore, pulmonary valve stenosis is the correct answer.
TMP12 267–268

123. **A)** Right ventricular hypertrophy occurs when the right heart has to pump a higher volume of blood or pump it against a higher pressure. Tetralogy of Fallot is associated with right ventricular hypertrophy because of the increased pulmonary valvular resistance, and this also occurs during pulmonary artery stenosis. Tricuspid insufficiency causes an increased stroke volume by the right heart which causes hypertrophy. However, tricuspid stenosis does not affect the right ventricle.
TMP12 271

124. **D)** During systole the murmurs from an interventricular septal effect and patent ductus arteriosis are clearly heard. However, patent ductus arteriosis also is heard during diastole. Mitral stenosis, tricuspid valve stenosis, and aortic regurgitation are diastolic murmurs.
TMP12 267

125. **A)** In tetralogy of Fallot, there is an interventricular septal defect as well as stenosis of either the pulmonary artery or the pulmonary valve. Therefore, it is very difficult for blood to pass into the pulmonary artery and into the lungs to be oxygenated. Instead, the blood partially shunts to the left side of the heart thus bypassing the lungs. This results in low arterial oxygen content.
TMP12 271

126. **B)** The first heart sound by definition is always associated with the closing of the A-V valves. The heart sounds are never associated with opening of any of the valves but always with the closing of the valves and the associated vibration of the blood and the walls of the heart.
TMP12 265–266

127. **B)** In tetralogy of Fallot there is an interventricular septal defect and increased resistance in the pulmonary valve or pulmonary artery. This causes partial blood shunting toward the left side of the heart without going through the lungs. This results in severely decreased arterial oxygen content. The interventricular septal defect causes equal systolic pressures in both cardiac ventricles. This causes right ventricular hypertrophy and a wall thickness very similar to that of the left ventricle.
TMP12 271

128. **C)** Mitral regurgitation and aortic stenosis are murmurs heard during the systolic period. A ventricular septal defect murmur is normally heard only during the systolic phase. Tricuspid valve stenosis and patent ductus arteriosus murmurs are heard during diastole. However, a patent ductus arteriosus murmur is also heard during systole.
TMP12 267

129. **E)** The third heart sound is associated with inrushing of blood into the ventricles in the early to middle part of diastole. The next heart sound, the fourth heart sound, is caused by inrushing of blood in the ventricles caused by atrial contraction. The first heart sound is caused by the closing of the A-V valves and the second heart sound by the closing of the pulmonary and aortic valves.
TMP12 265–266

130. **A)** A number of things occur in progressive shock, including increased capillary permeability, which allows fluid to leak out of the vasculature thus

decreasing the blood volume. Other deteriorating factors include vasomotor center failure, peripheral circulatory failure, decreased cellular mitochondrial activity, and acidosis throughout the body. Usually urine output strikingly decreases; therefore, the increased urinary output answer is incorrect. Tissue pH decreases and reverse stress relaxation of the veins occurs.

TMP12 276

131. **A)** Sympathomimetic drugs are given to counteract hypotension during a number of conditions. These include spinal cord injury in which the sympathetic output is interrupted. Sympathomimetic drugs are also given during very deep anesthesia which decreases the sympathetic output, and in anaphylactic shock that results from histamine release and the accompanying vasodilatation. Sympathomimetic drugs, such as norepinephrine, increase blood pressure by causing a vasoconstriction. Shock caused by excess vomiting, hemorrhage or excessive administration of diuretics result in fluid volume depletion resulting in decreased blood volume and decreased mean systemic filling pressure. Giving a balanced electrolyte solution best counteracts this condition.

TMP12 281

132. **C)** Vomiting can cause a large loss of electrolytes which results in a substantial decrease in the plasma volume. Therefore, blood volume decreases, and the arterial pressure reaches very low levels. The appropriate therapy is to replace the volume that was lost by the infusion of a balanced electrolyte solution.

TMP12 280–281

133. **D)** The patient received an influenza inoculation and quickly went into shock, which leads one to believe that he may be in anaphylactic shock. This is in a state of extreme vasodilation because of histamine release. Antihistamines would be somewhat helpful but they are very slow-acting and the patient could die in the meantime. Therefore, a very rapid-acting agent must be used such as a sympathomimetic drug.

TMP12 280–281

134. **E)** In compensated hemorrhagic shock a number of factors prevent the progression of the shock including increased heart rate. Also occurring is reverse stress relaxation in which the vasculature, particularly the veins, constrict around the available blood volume. Increased ADH release also occurs, which causes water retention from the kidney but also vasoconstriction of the arterioles. A CNS ischemic response also occurs if blood pressure drops to very low values. This causes an increase in sympathetic output. Increased absorption of interstitial fluid through the capillaries also occurs which increases the volume in the vasculature.

TMP12 275

135. **E)** Spinal anesthesia especially when the anesthesia extends all the way up the spinal cord can block the sympathetic nervous outflow from the spinal cord. This can be a very potent cause of neurogenic shock. The therapy of choice is to replace the sympathetic tone that was lost in the body. The best way to increase the sympathetic tone is by infusing a sympathomimetic drug.

TMP12 281

136. **A)** This patient has obviously lost a lot of blood because of the motorcycle wreck. The most advantageous therapy is to replace what was lost in the accident. This would be whole blood and is much superior to a plasma infusion, since you are also putting in red blood cells, which have a much superior oxygen carrying capacity than the plasma component of blood. Sympathetic nerves are firing very rapidly in this condition and an infusion of a sympathomimetic agent would be of little advantage.

TMP12 280–281

137. **C)** In hemorrhagic shock, anaphylactic shock and neurogenic shock the venous return of blood to the heart markedly decreases. However, in septic shock the cardiac output increases in many patients because of vasodilation in affected tissues and by a high metabolic rate causing vasodilation in other parts of the body.

TMP12 280

138. **E)** This patient has been hemorrhaging, and the optimal therapy is to replace the blood that he has lost. Unfortunately, there is no blood available; therefore, we must pick next best therapy. Increasing the volume of his blood is the best therapy. Plasma infusion is the next best therapy, because its high colloid osmotic pressure will help the infused fluid stay in the circulation much longer than a balanced electrolyte solution.

TMP12 280–281

139. **B)** Intestinal obstruction often causes severe reduction in plasma volume. Obstruction causes a distention of the intestine and partially blocks the venous blood flow in the intestines. This results in an increased intestinal capillary pressure which causes fluid to leak from the capillary into the walls of the intestines and also into the intestinal lumen. The leaking fluid has a high protein content very similar to that of the plasma, which reduces the total plasma protein and the plasma volume. Therefore, the therapy of choice would be to replace the fluid lost by infusing plasma.

TMP12 280–281

140. **A)** In progressive shock because of the poor blood flow the pH in the tissues throughout the body decreases. Many vessels become blocked because of

local blood agglutination, which is called *sludged blood*. Patchy areas of necrosis also occur in the liver. Mitochondrial activity decreases and capillary permeability increases. There is also an increased release of hydrolases by the lysosomes and a decrease in cellular metabolism of glucose.

TMP12 280–281

141. **A)** Anaphylaxis is an allergic condition which results from an antigen-antibody reaction that takes place after exposure of an individual to an antigenic substance. The basophils and mast cells in the pericapillary tissues release histamine or histamine-like substances. The histamine causes venous dilation, dilation of arterioles and greatly increased capillary permeability with rapid loss of fluid and protein into the tissue spaces. This reduces venous return and often results in anaphylactic shock.

TMP12 280–281

142. **A)** During progressive hemorrhagic shock blood clots begin to occur in many minute blood vessels. Lack of blood flow throughout the body causes acidosis because of lack of removal of carbon dioxide. Active transport of sodium and potassium also decreases. In the liver mitochondrial activity decreases, and lysosomal activity increases in widespread areas.

TMP12 276

143. **C)** With severe diarrhea, there is a large loss of sodium and water from the body resulting in dehydration and sometimes shock. The best therapy is to replace the electrolytes that were lost during diarrhea. Therefore, infusion of a balanced electrolyte solution is the therapy of choice.

TMP12 280–281

144. **B)** In patients with severe burns there is a large loss of plasma-like substances from the burned tissues. Therefore, the plasma protein concentration decreases severely and the therapy of choice would therefore be plasma infusion.

TMP12 279–280

The Body Fluids and Kidneys

Questions 1 and 2

Use the following clinical laboratory test results for questions 1 and 2:

Urine flow rate = 1 ml/min
Urine inulin concentration = 100 mg/ml
Plasma inulin concentration = 2 mg/ml
Urine urea concentration = 50 mg/ml
Plasma urea concentration = 2.5 mg/ml

1. What is the glomerular filtration rate (GFR)?

   A) 25ml/min
   B) 50 ml/min
   C) 100 ml/min
   D) 125ml/min
   E) None of the above

2. What is the net urea reabsorption rate?

   A) 0 mg/min
   B) 25 mg/min
   C) 50 mg/min
   D) 75 mg/min
   E) 100 mg/min

3. Which of the following solutions when infused intravenously would result in an increase in extracellular fluid volume, a decrease in intracellular fluid volume, and an increase in total body water after osmotic equilibrium?

   A) 1 L of 0.9% sodium chloride solution
   B) 1 L of 0.45% sodium chloride solution
   C) 1 L of 3% sodium chloride solution
   D) 1 L of 5% dextrose solution
   E) 1 L of pure water

4. A 65-year-old man has a heart attack and experiences cardiopulmonary arrest while being transported to the emergency room. The following laboratory values are obtained from arterial blood:

   plasma pH = 7.12,
   plasma P_{CO_2} = 60mm Hg, and
   plasma HCO_3^- concentration = 19 mEq/L.
   Which of the following best describes his acid-base disorder?

   A) Respiratory acidosis with partial renal compensation
   B) Metabolic acidosis with partial respiratory compensation
   C) Mixed acidosis: combined metabolic and respiratory acidosis
   D) Mixed alkalosis: combined respiratory and metabolic alkalosis

5. In the patient described in question 4, which of the following laboratory results would be expected, compared with normal?

   A) Increased renal excretion of HCO_3^-
   B) Decreased urinary titratable acid
   C) Increased urine pH
   D) Increased renal excretion of NH_4^+

6. In normal kidneys, which of the following is true of the osmolarity of renal tubular fluid that flows through the early distal tubule in the region of the macula densa?

   A) Usually isotonic compared with plasma
   B) Usually hypotonic compared with plasma
   C) Usually hypertonic compared with plasma
   D) Hypertonic, compared with plasma, in antidiuresis

Questions 7–9

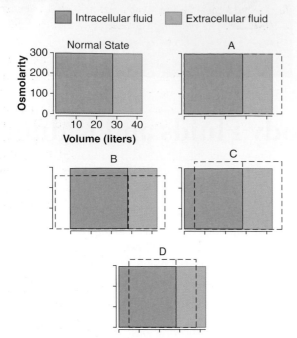

The diagrams represent various states of abnormal hydration. In each diagram, the normal state (orange and lavender) is superimposed on the abnormal state (dashed lines) to illustrate the shifts in the volume (width of rectangles) and total osmolarity (height of rectangles) of the extracellular and intracellular fluid compartments.

7. Which of the diagrams represents the changes (after osmotic equilibrium) in extracellular and intracellular fluid volumes and osmolarities after the infusion of 1% dextrose?

8. Which of the diagrams represents the changes (after osmotic equilibrium) in extracellular and intracellular fluid volumes and osmolarities after the infusion of 3% sodium chloride?

9. Which of the diagrams represents the changes (after osmotic equilibrium) in extracellular and intracellular fluid volumes and osmolarities in a patient with the syndrome of inappropriate antidiuretic hormone (excessive secretion of antidiuretic hormone)?

10. After receiving a renal transplant, a patient develops severe hypertension (170/110 mm Hg). A renal arteriogram indicates severe renal artery stenosis in his single remaining kidney, with a reduction in GFR to 25% of normal. Which of the following changes, compared with normal, would be expected in this patient, assuming steady-state conditions?

    A) Large increase in plasma sodium concentration
    B) Reduction in urinary sodium excretion to 25% of normal
    C) Reduction in urinary creatinine excretion to 25% of normal

D) Increase in serum creatinine to about four times normal
E) Normal renal blood flow in the stenotic kidney due to autoregulation

11. Which of the following tends to decrease potassium secretion by the cortical collecting tubule?

    A) Increased plasma potassium concentration
    B) A diuretic that decreases proximal tubule sodium reabsorption
    C) A diuretic that inhibits the action of aldosterone (e.g., spironolactone)
    D) Acute alkalosis
    E) High sodium intake

12. If a patient has a creatinine clearance of 90 ml/min, a urine flow rate of 1 ml/min, a plasma K^+ concentration of 4 mEq/L, and a urine K^+ concentration of 60 mEq/L, what is the approximate rate of K^+ excretion?

    A) 0.06 mEq/min
    B) 0.30 mEq/min
    C) 0.36 mEq/min
    D) 3.6 mEq/min
    E) 60 mEq/min

13. Which of the following changes would be expected in a patient with diabetes insipidus due to a lack of antidiuretic hormone (ADH) secretion?

	Plasma osmolarity concentration	Plasma sodium concentration	Plasma renin	Urine volume
A)	↔	↔	↓	↑
B)	↔	↔	↑	↑
C)	↑	↑	↑	↑
D)	↑	↑	↔	↔
E)	↓	↓	↓	↔

14. A patient with severe hypertension (blood pressure 185/110 mm Hg) is referred to you. A renal magnetic resonance imaging scan shows a tumor in the kidney, and laboratory findings include a very high plasma renin activity of 12 ng angiotensin 1/ml/hr (normal = 1). The diagnosis is a renin-secreting tumor. Which of the following changes would you expect to find in this patient, under steady-state conditions, compared with normal?

	Plasma aldosterone concentration	Sodium excretion rate	Plasma potassium concentration	Renal blood flow
A)	↔	↓	↓	↑
B)	↔	↔	↓	↑
C)	↑	↔	↓	↓
D)	↑	↓	↔	↓
E)	↑	↓	↓	↔

15. Which of the following changes, compared with normal, would you expect to find 3 weeks after a patient ingested a toxin that caused sustained impairment of proximal tubular sodium chloride (NaCl) reabsorption? Assume that there has been no change in diet or ingestion of electrolytes.

	Glomerular filtration rate	Afferent arteriolar resistance	Sodium excretion
A)	↔	↔	↑
B)	↔	↔	↑
C)	↓	↑	↑
D)	↓	↑	↔
E)	↑	↓	↔

16. A 26-year-old woman recently decided to adopt a healthier diet and eat more fruits and vegetables. As a result, her potassium intake increased from 80 to 160 mmol/day. Which of the following conditions would you expect to find 2 weeks after she increased her potassium intake, compared with before the increase?

	Potassium excretion rate	Sodium excretion rate	Plasma aldosterone concentration	Plasma potassium concentration
A)	↔	↔	↑	Large increase (>1 mmol/L)
B)	↔	↓	↑	Small increase (<1 mmol/L)
C)	↑2×	↔	↑	Small increase (<1 mmol/L)
D)	↑2×	↑	↓	Large increase (>1 mmol/L)
E)	↑2×	↑	↔	Large increase (>1 mmol/L)

17. An 8-year-old boy is brought to your office with extreme swelling of the abdomen. His parents indicate that he had a very sore throat a "month or so" ago and that he has been "swelling up" since that time. He appears to be edematous, and when you check his urine, you find large amounts of protein being excreted. Your diagnosis is nephrotic syndrome subsequent to glomerulonephritis. Which of the following changes would you expect to find, compared with normal?

	Thoracic lymph flow	Interstitial fluid protein concentration	Interstitial fluid hydrostatic pressure	Plasma renin concentration
A)	↑	↓	↑	↑
B)	↑	↓	↑	↔
C)	↑	↓	↔	↑
D)	↓	↑	↔	↔
E)	↓	↓	↓	↓

18. Which of the following changes would you expect to find after administering a vasodilator drug that caused a 50% decrease in afferent arteriolar resistance and no change in arterial pressure?

A) Decreased renal blood flow, decreased GFR, and decreased peritubular capillary hydrostatic pressure
B) Decreased renal blood flow, decreased GFR, and increased peritubular capillary hydrostatic pressure
C) Increased renal blood flow, increased GFR, and increased peritubular capillary hydrostatic pressure
D) Increased renal blood flow, increased GFR, and no change in peritubular capillary hydrostatic pressure
E) Increased renal blood flow, increased GFR, and decreased peritubular capillary hydrostatic pressure

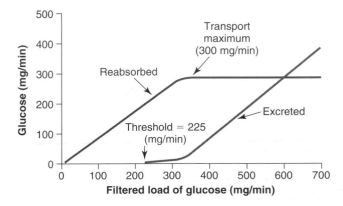

19. A 32-year-old man complains of frequent urination. He is overweight (280 lb, 5 ft 10 in tall), and after measuring the 24-hr creatinine clearance, you estimate his GFR to be 150 ml/min. His plasma glucose is 300 mg/dL. Assuming that his renal transport maximum for glucose is normal, as shown in the figure above, what would be this patient's approximate rate of urinary glucose excretion?

A) 0 mg/min
B) 100 mg/min
C) 150 mg/min
D) 225 mg/min
E) 300 mg/min
F) Information provided is inadequate to estimate the glucose excretion rate

20. The clinical laboratory returned the following values for arterial blood taken from a patient: plasma pH = 7.28, plasma HCO_3^- = 32 mEq/L, and plasma PCO_2 = 70 mm Hg. What is this patient's acid–base disorder?

A) Acute respiratory acidosis without renal compensation
B) Respiratory acidosis with partial renal compensation
C) Acute metabolic acidosis without respiratory compensation
D) Metabolic acidosis with partial respiratory compensation

21. Which of the following changes tends to increase peritubular capillary fluid reabsorption?

    A) Increased blood pressure
    B) Decreased filtration fraction
    C) Increased efferent arteriolar resistance
    D) Decreased angiotensin II
    E) Increased renal blood flow

22. Which of the following would cause the greatest degree of hyperkalemia?

    A) Increase in potassium intake from 60 to 180 mmol/day in a person with normal kidneys and a normal aldosterone system
    B) Chronic treatment with a diuretic that inhibits the action of aldosterone
    C) Decrease in sodium intake from 200 to 100 mmol/day
    D) Chronic treatment with a diuretic that inhibits loop of Henle Na^+-$2Cl^-$-K^+ co-transport
    E) Chronic treatment with a diuretic that inhibits sodium reabsorption in the collecting ducts

23. Which of the following is filtered most readily by the glomerular capillaries?

    A) Albumin in plasma
    B) Neutral dextran with a molecular weight of 25,000
    C) Polycationic dextran with a molecular weight of 25,000
    D) Polyanionic dextran with a molecular weight of 25,000
    E) Red blood cells

24. Under conditions of normal renal function, which of the following is true of the concentration of urea in tubular fluid at the end of the proximal tubule?

    A) It is higher than the concentration of urea in tubular fluid at the tip of the loop of Henle
    B) It is higher than the concentration of urea in the plasma
    C) It is higher than the concentration of urea in the final urine in antidiuresis
    D) It is lower than plasma urea concentration because of active urea reabsorption along the proximal tubule

25. Which of the following changes would be expected in a patient with Liddle's syndrome (excessive activity of amiloride-sensitive sodium channel in the collecting tubule) under steady-state conditions, assuming that intake of electrolytes remained constant?

	Plasma renin concentration	Blood pressure	Sodium excretion concentration	Plasma aldosterone
A)	↔	↑	↓	↔
B)	↑	↑	↔	↑
C)	↑	↑	↓	↓
D)	↓	↑	↔	↓
E)	↓	↑	↓	↓
F)	↓	↓	↑	↑

26. A patient's urine is collected for 2 hr, and the total volume is 600 ml during this time. Her urine osmolarity is 150 mOsm/L, and her plasma osmolarity is 300 mOsm/L. What is her "free water clearance"?

    A) +5.0 ml/min
    B) +2.5 ml/min
    C) 0.0 ml/min
    D) −2.5 ml/min
    E) −5.0 ml/min

27. A patient is referred for treatment of hypertension. After testing, you discover that he has a very high level of plasma aldosterone, and your diagnosis is Conn's syndrome. Assuming no change in electrolyte intake, which of the following changes would you expect to find, compared with normal?

	Plasma pH	Plasma K^+ concentration	Urine K^+ excretion	Urine Na^+ excretion	Plasma renin concentration
A)	↑	↓	↔	↔	↓
B)	↓	↓	↔	↔	↓
C)	↑	↓	↑	↓	↓
D)	↑	↑	↔	↓	↑
E)	↑	↑	↑	↑	↑

28. A patient with renal disease had a plasma creatinine of 2 mg/dL during an examination 6 months ago. You note that his blood pressure has increased about 30 mm Hg since his previous visit, and the lab tests indicate that his plasma creatinine is now 4 mg/dL. Which of the following changes, compared with his previous visit, would you expect to find, assuming steady-state conditions and no changes in electrolyte intake or metabolism?

	Sodium excretion rate	Creatinine excretion rate	Creatinine clearance	Filtered load of creatinine
A)	↔	↔	↓ by 50%	↓
B)	↔	↔	↓ by 50%	↔
C)	↔	↔	↓ by 75%	↓
D)	↓	↓	↔	↔
E)	↓	↓	↓ by 50%	↓

29. Which of the following changes tends to increase GFR?

    A) Increased afferent arteriolar resistance
    B) Decreased efferent arteriolar resistance
    C) Increased glomerular capillary filtration coefficient
    D) Increased Bowman's capsule hydrostatic pressure
    E) Decreased glomerular capillary hydrostatic pressure

30. The maximum clearance rate possible for a substance that is totally cleared from the plasma is equal to which of the following?

    A) GFR
    B) Filtered load of that substance
    C) Urinary excretion rate of that substance
    D) Renal plasma flow
    E) Filtration fraction

31. A patient has the following laboratory values: arterial pH = 7.13, plasma HCO_3^- = 15 mEq/L, plasma chloride concentration = 118 mEq/L, arterial P_{CO_2} = 28 mm Hg, and plasma Na^+ concentration = 141 mEq/L. What is the most likely cause of his acidosis?

    A) Salicylic acid poisoning
    B) Diabetes mellitus
    C) Diarrhea
    D) Emphysema

32. A 26-year-old man develops glomerulonephritis, and his GFR decreases by 50% and remains at that level. For which of the following substances would you expect to find the greatest increase in plasma concentration?

    A) Creatinine
    B) K^+
    C) Glucose
    D) Na^+
    E) Phosphate
    F) H^+

33. A patient with a history of frequent and severe migraine headaches arrives at your office complaining of stomach pain and breathing rapidly. She informs you that she has had a severe migraine for the past 2 days and has taken eight times the recommended dose of aspirin to relieve her headache during that time. Which of the following changes would you expect to find, compared with normal?

	Plasma HCO_3^- concentration	Plasma P_{CO_2}	Urine HCO_3^- excretion	Urine NH_4^+ excretion	Plasma anion gap
A)	↑	↓	↑	↑	↑
B)	↑	↑	↑	↓	↑
C)	↓	↓	↓	↓	↓
D)	↓	↓	↓	↑	↑
E)	↓	↓	↓	↑	↓

Questions 34 and 35

Assume the following initial conditions: intracellular fluid volume = 40% of body weight before fluid administration, extracellular fluid volume = 20% of body weight before fluid administration, molecular weight of NaCl = 58.5g/mol, and no excretion of water or electrolytes.

34. A male patient appears to be dehydrated, and after obtaining a plasma sample, you find that he has hyponatremia, with a plasma sodium concentration of 130 mmol/L and a plasma osmolarity of 260 mOsm/L. You decide to administer 2 L of 3% sodium chloride (NaCl). His body weight was 60 kilograms before giving the fluid. What is his approximate plasma osmolarity after administration of the NaCl solution and after osmotic equilibrium? Assume the initial conditions described above.

    A) 273 mOsm/L
    B) 286 mOsm/L
    C) 300 mOsm/L
    D) 310 mOsm/L
    E) 326 mOsm/L

35. What is the approximate extracellular fluid volume in this patient after administration of the NaCl solution and after osmotic equilibrium?

    A) 15.1 L
    B) 17.2 L
    C) 19.1 L
    D) 19.8 L
    E) 21.2 L

36. The most serious hypokalemia would occur in which of the following conditions?

    A) Decrease in potassium intake from 150 to 60 mEq/day
    B) Increase in sodium intake from 100 to 200 mEq/day
    C) Fourfold increase in aldosterone secretion plus high sodium intake
    D) Fourfold increase in aldosterone secretion plus low sodium intake
    E) Addison's disease

37. If the average hydrostatic pressure in the glomerular capillaries is 50 mm Hg, the hydrostatic pressure in the Bowman's space is 12 mm Hg, the average colloid osmotic pressure in the glomerular capillaries is 30 mm Hg, and there is no protein in the glomerular ultrafiltrate, what is the net pressure driving glomerular filtration?

    A) 8 mm Hg
    B) 32 mm Hg
    C) 48 mm Hg
    D) 60 mm Hg
    E) 92 mm Hg

38. In a patient who has chronic, uncontrolled diabetes mellitus, which of the following sets of conditions would you expect to find, compared with normal?

	Titratable acid excretion	NH$^+$ excretion	HCO$_3^-$ excretion	Plasma Pco$_2$
A)	↔	↑	↓	↔
B)	↓	↑	↔	↓
C)	↑	↑	↔	↑
D)	↑	↑	↓	↓
E)	↓	↓	↓	↓
F)	↔	↑	↓	↔

39. Intravenous infusion of 1 L of 0.45% sodium chloride (NaCl) solution (molecular weight of NaCl = 58.5) would cause which of the following changes, after osmotic equilibrium?

	Intracellular fluid volume	Intracellular fluid osmolarity	Extracellular fluid volume	Extracellular fluid osmolarity
A)	↑	↑	↑	↑
B)	↑	↓	↑	↓
C)	↔	↑	↑	↑
D)	↓	↑	↑	↑
E)	↓	↓	↓	↓

40. The figure above shows the concentration of inulin at different points along the renal tubule, expressed as the tubular fluid/plasma ratio of inulin concentration. If inulin is not reabsorbed, what is the approximate percentage of the filtered water that has been reabsorbed prior to the distal convoluted tubule?

A) 25%
B) 33%
C) 66%
D) 75%
E) 99%
F) 100%

41. Which of the following tends to increase potassium secretion by the cortical collecting tubule?

A) A diuretic that inhibits the action of aldosterone (e.g., spironolactone)
B) A diuretic that decreases loop of Henle sodium reabsorption (e.g., furosemide)
C) Decreased plasma potassium concentration
D) Acute metabolic acidosis
E) Low sodium intake

42. Which of the following changes would you expect to find in a patient with primary aldosteronism (Conn's syndrome) under steady-state conditions, assuming that electrolyte intake remained constant?

	Sodium excretion rate	Potassium excretion rate	Plasma renin concentration	Plasma potassium concentration	Blood pressure
A)	↔	↔	↔	↓	↑
B)	↔	↔	↓	↓	↑
C)	↔	↑	↓	↓	↑
D)	↓	↑	↓	↔	↑
E)	↑	↓	↑	↑	↔

43. A diabetic patient has developed chronic renal disease and is referred to your nephrology clinic. According to his family physician, his creatinine clearance has decreased from 100 ml/min to 40 ml/min over the past 4 years. His glucose has not been well controlled, and his plasma pH is 7.14. Which of the following changes, compared with before the development of renal disease, would you expect to find, assuming steady-state conditions and no change in electrolyte intake?

	Sodium excretion rate	Creatinine excretion rate	Plasma creatinine concentration	Plasma HCO$_3^-$ concentration	NH$_4^+$ excretion rate
A)	↓	↓	↑	↑	↑
B)	↔	↔	↑	↓	↑
C)	↔	↔	↑	↓	↔
D)	↔	↓	↑	↓	↔
E)	↓	↓	↓	↓	↑
F)	↓	↓	↓	↓	↓

44. A 20-year-old woman arrives at your office complaining of rapid weight gain and marked fluid retention. Her blood pressure is 105/65 mm Hg, her plasma protein concentration is 3.6g/dL (normal = 7.0), and she has no detectable protein in her urine. Which of the following changes would you expect to find, compared with normal?

	Thoracic lymph flow	Interstitial fluid protein concentration	Capillary filtration	Interstitial fluid pressure
A)	↓	↓	↓	↓
B)	↓	↑	↔	↔
C)	↑	↓	↑	↑
D)	↑	↓	↑	↔
E)	↑	↑	↑	↑

45. A 48-year-old woman complains of severe polyuria (producing about 0.5 L of urine each hour) and polydipsia (drinking two to three glasses of water every hour). Her urine contains no glucose, and she is placed on overnight water restriction for further evaluation. The next morning, she is weak and confused, her sodium concentration is 160 mEq/L, and her urine osmolarity is 80 mOsm/L. Which of the following is the most likely diagnosis?

A) Diabetes mellitus
B) Diabetes insipidus
C) Primary aldosteronism
D) Renin-secreting tumor
E) Syndrome of inappropriate antidiuretic hormone

46. Furosemide (Lasix) is a diuretic that also produces natriuresis. Which of the following is an undesirable side effect of furosemide due to its site of action on the renal tubule?

A) Edema
B) Hyperkalemia
C) Hypercalcemia
D) Decreased ability to concentrate the urine
E) Heart failure

47. A patient complains of headaches, and an examination reveals that her blood pressure is 175/112 mm Hg. Laboratory tests give the following results: plasma renin activity = 11.5 ng angiotensin I/ml/hr (normal = 1), plasma Na^+ = 144 mmol/L, and plasma K^+ = 3.4 mmol/L. A magnetic resonance imaging procedure suggests that she has a renin-secreting tumor. Which of the following changes would you expect, compared with normal?

	Renal blood flow	Filtration fraction	Glomerular capillary hydrostatic pressure	Peritubular capillary hydrostatic pressure
A)	↓	↑	↑	↓
B)	↓	↑	↑	↑
C)	↓	↓	↑	↓
D)	↓	↑	↓	↑
E)	↓	↓	↓	↓

48. When the dietary intake of K^+ increases, body K^+ balance is maintained by an increase in K^+ excretion primarily by which of the following?

A) Decreased glomerular filtration of K^+
B) Decreased reabsorption of K^+ by the proximal tubule
C) Decreased reabsorption of K^+ by the thick ascending limb of the loop of Henle
D) Increased K^+ secretion by the late distal and collecting tubules
E) Shift of K^+ into the intracellular compartment

49. A female patient has unexplained severe hypernatremia (plasma Na^+ = 167 mmol/L) and complains of frequent urination and large urine volumes. A urine specimen reveals that the Na^+ concentration is 15 mmol/L (very low) and the osmolarity is 155 mOsm/L (very low). Laboratory tests reveal: plasma renin activity = 3 ng angiotensin I/ml/hr (normal = 1.0), plasma antidiuretic hormone (ADH) = 30 pg/ml (normal = 3 pg/ml), and plasma aldosterone = 20 ng/dL (normal = 6 ng/dL). Which of the following is the most likely reason for her hypernatremia?

A) Simple dehydration due to decreased water intake
B) Nephrogenic diabetes insipidus
C) Central diabetes insipidus
D) Syndrome of inappropriate ADH
E) Primary aldosteronism
F) Renin-secreting tumor

50. Juvenile (type I) diabetes mellitus is often diagnosed because of polyuria (high urine flow) and polydipsia (frequent drinking) that occur because of which of the following?

A) Increased delivery of glucose to the collecting duct interferes with the action of antidiuretic hormone
B) Increased glomerular filtration of glucose increases Na^+ reabsorption via the sodium-glucose co-transporter
C) When the filtered load of glucose exceeds the renal threshold, a rising glucose concentration in the proximal tubule decreases the osmotic driving force for water reabsorption
D) High plasma glucose concentration decreases thirst
E) High plasma glucose concentration stimulates antidiuretic hormone release from the posterior pituitary

51. You begin treating a hypertensive patient with a powerful loop diuretic (e.g., furosemide). Which of the following changes would you expect to find, compared with pretreatment values, when he returns for a follow-up examination 2 weeks later?

	Urine sodium excretion	Extracellular fluid volume	Blood pressure	Plasma potassium concentration
A)	↑	↓	↓	↓
B)	↑	↓	↔	↔
C)	↔	↓	↓	↓
D)	↔	↓	↔	↔
E)	↑	↔	↓	↑

52. In acidosis, most of the hydrogen ions secreted by the proximal tubule are associated with which of the following processes?

 A) Excretion of hydrogen ions
 B) Excretion of NH_4^+
 C) Reabsorption of bicarbonate ions
 D) Reabsorption of phosphate ions
 E) Reabsorption of potassium ions

53. Administration of a thiazide diuretic (e.g., chlorothiazide) would be expected to cause which of the following effects as its primary mechanism of action?

 A) Inhibition of NaCl co-transport in the early distal tubules
 B) Inhibition of NaCl co-transport in the proximal tubules
 C) Inhibition of Na^+-$2Cl^-$-K^+ co-transport in the loop of Henle
 D) Inhibition of Na^+-$2Cl^-$-K^+ co-transport in the collecting tubules
 E) Inhibition of the renal tubular actions of aldosterone
 F) Blockade of sodium channels in the collecting tubules

54. Two weeks after constricting the renal artery of a sole remaining kidney to initially reduce renal artery pressure by 20 mm Hg (from 100 to 80 mm Hg), which of the following changes would you expect, compared with before constriction of the artery?

 A) Large decrease in sodium excretion (>20%)
 B) Large increase in renin secretion (more than twofold)
 C) Return of renal artery pressure to nearly 100 mm Hg
 D) Large decrease in GFR (>20%)
 E) Large reduction in renal blood flow (>20%)

55. Because the usual rate of phosphate filtration exceeds the transport maximum for phosphate reabsorption, which of the following is true?

 A) All the phosphate that is filtered is reabsorbed
 B) More phosphate is reabsorbed than is filtered
 C) Phosphate in the tubules can contribute significantly to titratable acid in the urine

 D) The "threshold" for phosphate is usually not exceeded
 E) Parathyroid hormone must be secreted for phosphate reabsorption to occur

56. Which of the following changes, compared with normal, would be expected to occur, under steady-state conditions, in a patient whose severe renal disease has reduced the number of functional nephrons to 25% of normal?

 A) Increased GFR of the surviving nephrons
 B) Decreased urinary creatinine excretion rate
 C) Decreased urine flow rate in the surviving nephrons
 D) Decreased urinary excretion of sodium
 E) Increased urine concentrating ability

57. In a patient with severe syndrome of inappropriate antidiuretic hormone (excessive antidiuretic hormone secretion), which of the following changes, compared with normal, would you expect to find? Assume steady-state conditions and that the intake of water and electrolytes has remained constant.

	Plasma renin concentration	Plasma aldosterone concentration	Urine flow rate	Plasma sodium concentration	Plasma protein concentration
A)	↔	↔	↓	↓	↓
B)	↔	↔	↔	↓	↑
C)	↓	↓	↔	↓	↓
D)	↓	↓	↔	↔	↓
E)	↑	↑	↓	↓	↔

58. Which of the following would likely lead to hyponatremia?

 A) Excessive antidiuretic hormone secretion
 B) Restriction of fluid intake
 C) Excess aldosterone secretion
 D) Administration of 2 L of 3% sodium chloride solution
 E) Administration of 2 L of 0.9% sodium chloride solution

Questions 59–62

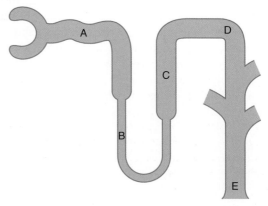

Choose the appropriate nephron site in the diagram above.

59. In a patient with severe central diabetes insipidus caused by a lack of antidiuretic hormone secretion, which part of the tubule would have the lowest tubular fluid osmolarity?

60. In a person on a very low potassium diet, which part of the nephron would be expected to reabsorb the most potassium?

61. Which part of the nephron normally reabsorbs the most water?

62. In a normally functioning kidney, which part of the tubule has the lowest permeability to water during antidiuresis?

63. Which of the following substances are best suited to measure interstitial fluid volume?

    A) Inulin and heavy water
    B) Inulin and ^{22}Na
    C) Heavy water and ^{125}I-albumin
    D) Inulin and ^{125}I-albumin
    E) ^{51}Cr red blood cells and ^{125}I-albumin

64. Which of the following changes would you expect to find in a dehydrated person deprived of water for 24 hours?

    A) Decreased plasma renin activity
    B) Decreased plasma antidiuretic hormone concentration
    C) Increased plasma atrial natriuretic peptide concentration
    D) Increased water permeability of the collecting duct
    E) Increased water permeability in the ascending loop of Henle

65. Which of the following changes would you expect to find after acute administration of a vasodilator drug that caused a 50% decrease in renal efferent arteriolar resistance and no change in afferent arteriolar resistance or arterial pressure?

	Renal blood flow	Glomerular filtration rate	Glomerular capillary hydrostatic pressure	Peritubular capillary hydrostatic pressure
A)	↑	↑	↑	↔
B)	↑	↑	↑	↑
C)	↑	↔	↔	↔
D)	↑	↓	↓	↓
E)	↑	↓	↓	↑

66. Which of the following would be expected to cause a decrease in extracellular fluid potassium concentration (hypokalemia) at least in part by stimulating potassium uptake into the cells?

    A) β-adrenergic blockade
    B) Insulin deficiency

C) Strenuous exercise
D) Aldosterone deficiency (Addison's disease)
E) Metabolic alkalosis

67. Which of the following is true of the tubular fluid that passes through the lumen of the early distal tubule in the region of the macula densa?

    A) It is usually isotonic
    B) It is usually hypotonic
    C) It is usually hypertonic
    D) It is hypertonic in antidiuresis
    E) It is hypertonic when the filtration rate of its own nephron decreases to 50% below normal

68. If a person has a kidney transport maximum for glucose of 350 mg/min, a GFR of 100 ml/min, a plasma glucose of 150 mg/dL, a urine flow rate of 2 ml/min, and no detectable glucose in the urine, what would be the approximate rate of glucose reabsorption, assuming normal kidneys?

    A) Glucose reabsorption cannot be estimated from these data
    B) 0 mg/min
    C) 50 mg/min
    D) 150 mg/min
    E) 350 mg/min

69. A patient complains that he is always thirsty, and his breath has an acetone smell. You suspect that he has diabetes mellitus, and that diagnosis is confirmed by a urine sample that tests very positive for glucose and a blood sample that shows a fasting blood glucose concentration of 400 mg/dL. Compared with normal, you would expect to find which of the following changes in his urine?

	Urine pH	NH_4^+ excretion	Urine volume (ml/24 hr)	Renal HCO_3^- production
A)	↓	↓	↓	↓
B)	↓	↑	↓	↓
C)	↑	↓	↓	↓
D)	↓	↑	↑	↑
E)	↑	↑	↑	↑

70. Which of the following statements is correct?

    A) Urea reabsorption in the medullary collecting tubule is less than in the distal convoluted tubule during antidiuresis
    B) Urea concentration in the interstitial fluid of the renal cortex is greater than in the interstitial fluid of the renal medulla during antidiuresis
    C) The thick ascending limb of the loop of Henle reabsorbs more urea than the inner medullary collecting tubule during antidiuresis
    D) Urea reabsorption in the proximal tubule is greater than in the cortical collecting tubule

71. A healthy 29-year-old man runs a 10-km race on a hot day and becomes very dehydrated. Assuming that his antidiuretic hormone levels are very high, in which part of the renal tubule is the most water reabsorbed?

    A) Proximal tubule
    B) Loop of Henle
    C) Distal tubule
    D) Cortical collecting tubule
    E) Medullary collecting duct

Questions 72–74

A person with normal body fluid volumes weighs 60 kg and has an extracellular fluid volume of approximately 12.8 L, a blood volume of 4.3 L, and a hematocrit of 0.4; 57% of his body weight is water. Answer the following three questions based on this information.

72. What is the approximate intracellular fluid volume?

    A) 17.1 L
    B) 19.6 L
    C) 21.4 L
    D) 23.5 L
    E) 25.6 L

73. What is the approximate plasma volume?

    A) 2.0 L
    B) 2.3 L
    C) 2.6 L
    D) 3.0 L
    E) 3.3 L

74. What is the approximate interstitial fluid volume?

    A) 6.4 L
    B) 8.4 L
    C) 10.2 L
    D) 11.3 L
    E) 12.0 L

75. Which of the following nephron segments is the primary site of magnesium reabsorption under normal conditions?

    A) Proximal tubule
    B) Descending limb of the loop of Henle
    C) Ascending limb of the loop of Henle
    D) Distal convoluted tubule
    E) Collecting ducts

76. Which of the following changes would you expect to find in a newly diagnosed 10-year-old patient with type I diabetes and uncontrolled hyperglycemia (plasma glucose = 300 mg/dL).

	Thirst (water intake)	Urine volume	Glomerular filtration rate	Afferent arteriolar resistance
A)	↑	↓	↑	↓
B)	↑	↑	↓	↑
C)	↑	↑	↑	↓
D)	↓	↑	↑	↑
E)	↓	↓	↓	↓

Questions 77 and 78

To evaluate kidney function in a 45-year-old woman with type II diabetes, you ask her to collect her urine over 24 hours. She collects 3600 ml of urine in that period. The clinical laboratory returns the following results after analyzing the patient's urine and plasma samples: plasma creatinine = 4 mg/dL, urine creatinine = 32 mg/dL, plasma potassium = 5 mmol/L, and urine potassium = 10 mmol/L.

77. What is this patient's approximate GFR, assuming that she collected all her urine in the 24-hour period?

    A) 10 ml/min
    B) 20 ml/min
    C) 30 ml/min
    D) 40 ml/min
    E) 80 ml/min

78. What is the net renal tubular reabsorption rate of potassium in this patient?

    A) 1.050 mmol/min
    B) 0.100 mmol/min
    C) 0.037 mmol/min
    D) 0.075 mmol/min
    E) Potassium is not reabsorbed in this example

Questions 79–83

Match each of the patients described in questions 79 to 83 with the correct set of blood values in the following table (the same values may be used for more than one patient).

	pH	HCO_3^- (mEq/L)	P_{CO_2} (mm Hg)	Na^+ (mEq/L)	Cl^- (mEq/L)
A)	7.66	22	20	143	111
B)	7.28	30	65	142	102
C)	7.24	12	29	144	102
D)	7.29	14	30	143	117
E)	7.52	38	48	146	100
F)	7.07	14	50	144	102

79. A patient with severe diarrhea.

80. A patient with primary aldosteronism.

81. A patient with proximal renal tubular acidosis.

82. A patient with diabetic ketoacidosis and emphysema.

83. A patient treated chronically with a carbonic anhydrase inhibitor.

84. Which of the following changes would you expect to find in a patient who developed acute renal failure after ingesting poisonous mushrooms that caused renal tubular necrosis?

    A) Increased plasma bicarbonate concentration
    B) Metabolic acidosis
    C) Decreased plasma potassium concentration
    D) Decreased blood urea nitrogen concentration
    E) Decreased hydrostatic pressure in Bowman's capsule

85. An elderly patient complains of muscle weakness and lethargy. A urine specimen reveals a Na^+ concentration of 600 mmol/L and an osmolarity of 1200 mOsm/L. Additional laboratory tests provide the following information: plasma Na^+ concentration = 167 mmol/L, plasma renin activity = 4 ng angiotensin I/ml/hr (normal = 1), plasma antidiuretic hormone (ADH) = 60 pg/ml (normal = 3 pg/ml), and plasma aldosterone = 15 ng/dL (normal = 6 ng/dL). Which of the following is the most likely reason for this patient's hypernatremia?

    A) Dehydration caused by decreased fluid intake
    B) Syndrome of inappropriate ADH
    C) Nephrogenic diabetes insipidus
    D) Primary aldosteronism
    E) Renin-secreting tumor

86. A patient complains that he is always thirsty, and his breath has an acetone smell. You suspect that he has diabetes mellitus, and that diagnosis is confirmed by a urine sample that tests very positive for glucose and a blood sample that shows a fasting blood glucose concentration of 400 mg/dL. You would expect to find which of the following sets of changes in his plasma, compared with normal?

	Plasma HCO_3^-	Plasma pH	Plasma P_{CO_2}	Plasma anion gap
A)	↓	↓	↓	↓
B)	↓	↓	↓	↑
C)	↓	↓	↑	↓
D)	↑	↓	↑	↑
E)	↑	↓	↓	↑

87. Which of the following has similar values for both intracellular and interstitial body fluids?

    A) Potassium ion concentration
    B) Colloid osmotic pressure
    C) Sodium ion concentration
    D) Chloride ion concentration
    E) Total osmolarity

88. In a patient with very high levels of aldosterone and otherwise normal kidney function, approximately what percentage of the filtered load of sodium would be reabsorbed by the distal convoluted tubule and collecting duct?

    A) More than 66%
    B) 40% to 60%
    C) 20% to 40%
    D) 10% to 20%
    E) Less than 10%

89. Which of the following statements is true?

    A) Antidiuretic hormone (ADH) increases water reabsorption from the ascending loop of Henle
    B) Water reabsorption from the descending loop of Henle is normally less than that from the ascending loop of Henle
    C) Sodium reabsorption from the ascending loop of Henle is normally less than that from the descending loop of Henle
    D) Osmolarity of fluid in the early distal tubule would be less than 300 mOsm/L in a dehydrated person with normal kidneys and increased ADH levels
    E) ADH decreases the urea permeability in the medullary collecting tubules

90. Which of the following changes tends to increase urinary Ca^{++} excretion?

    A) Extracellular fluid volume expansion
    B) Increased plasma parathyroid hormone concentration
    C) Decreased blood pressure
    D) Increased plasma phosphate concentration
    E) Metabolic acidosis

91. A patient's one remaining kidney has moderate renal artery stenosis that reduces renal artery pressure distal to the stenosis to 85 mm Hg, compared with the normal level of 100 mm Hg. Which of the following is most likely decreased in this patient 2 weeks after the stenosis has occurred, assuming that his diet is unchanged?

    A) Efferent arteriolar resistance
    B) Afferent arteriolar resistance
    C) Renin secretion
    D) Sodium excretion rate
    E) Plasma aldosterone concentration

92. Which of the following changes would you expect to find in a patient consuming a high-sodium diet (200 mEq/day) compared with the same patient on a normal-sodium diet (100 mEq/day), assuming steady-state conditions?

    A) Increased plasma aldosterone concentration
    B) Increased urinary potassium excretion
    C) Decreased plasma renin activity
    D) Decreased plasma atrial natriuretic peptide
    E) An increase in plasma sodium concentration of at least 5 mmol/L

93. A 26-year-old construction worker is brought to the emergency room with a change in mental status after working a 10-hour shift on a hot summer day (average outside temperature was 97°F). The man had been sweating profusely during the day but did not drink fluids. He has a fever of 102°F, heart rate of 140 beats/min, and blood pressure of 100/55 mm Hg in the supine position. On examination, he has no perspiration, appears to have dry mucous membranes, and is poorly oriented to person, place, and time. Assuming that his kidneys were normal yesterday, which of the following sets of hormone levels describes his condition, compared with normal?

A) High antidiuretic hormone (ADH), high renin, low angiotensin II, low aldosterone
B) Low ADH, low renin, low angiotensin II, low aldosterone
C) High ADH, low renin, high angiotensin II, low aldosterone
D) High ADH, high renin, high angiotensin II, high aldosterone
E) Low ADH, high renin, low angiotensin II, high aldosterone

94. Acute metabolic acidosis tends to _____ in intracellular K⁺ concentration and _____ in K⁺ secretion by the cortical collecting tubules.

A) Increase, increase
B) Increase, decrease
C) Decrease, increase
D) Decrease, decrease
E) Cause no change in, increase
F) Cause no change in, cause no change in

95. Which part of the renal tubule would have the lowest tubular fluid osmolarity in a patient who has complete lack of antidiuretic hormone due to "central" diabetes insipidus?

A) Medullary collecting duct
B) Collecting tubule
C) Early distal tubule
D) Descending loop of Henle
E) Proximal tubule

96. If GFR suddenly decreases from 150 ml/min to 75 ml/min and tubular fluid reabsorption simultaneously decreases from 149 ml/min to 75 ml/min, which of the following changes will occur (assuming that the changes in GFR and tubular fluid reabsorption are maintained)?

A) Urine flow rate will decrease to 0
B) Urine flow rate will decrease by 50%
C) Urine flow rate will not change
D) Urine flow rate will increase by 50%

97. Given the following measurements, calculate the *filtration fraction*: glomerular capillary hydrostatic pressure = 50 mm Hg; Bowman's space hydrostatic pressure = 15 mm Hg; colloid osmotic pressure in the glomerular capillaries = 30 mm Hg; glomerular capillary filtration coefficient (K_f) = 12 ml/min/mm Hg; and renal plasma flow = 400 ml/min.

A) 0.15
B) 0.20
C) 0.25
D) 0.30
E) 0.35
F) 0.40

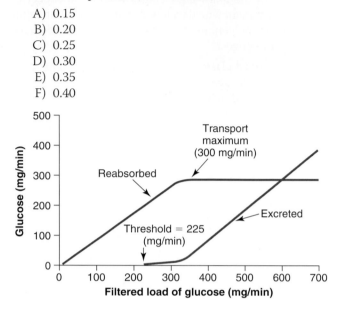

98. A 55-year-old overweight male patient complains of frequent urination and his blood pressure is 165/98 mm Hg. Based on 24-hour creatinine clearance, you estimate his GFR to be 150 ml/min. His plasma glucose is 400 mg/100 ml. Assuming that his renal transport maximum for glucose is normal, as shown in the figure, what would be the approximate rate of urinary glucose excretion for this patient?

A) 0 mg/min
B) 100 mg/min
C) 150 mg/min
D) 225 mg/min
E) 300 mg/min
F) Information provided is inadequate to estimate glucose excretion rate

99. You have been following a patient with type 2 diabetes and chronic renal disease and his GFR has decreased from 80 ml/min to 40 ml/min over the past 4 years. Which of the following changes would you expect to find compared to 4 years ago, before the decline in GFR, assuming steady-state conditions and no change in electrolyte intake or protein metabolism?

	Sodium excretion rate	Creatinine excretion rate	Creatinine clearance	Filtered load creatinine	Plasma creatinine conc.
A)	↓	↓	↔	↔	↑
B)	↓	↓	↓	↓	↑
C)	↔	↔	↓	↓	↑
D)	↔	↔	↓	↓	↔
E)	↔	↔	↓	↔	↑
F)	↔	↔	↔	↔	↑

100. In a person on a high (200 mmol/day) potassium diet, which part of the nephron would be expected to secrete the most potassium?

A) Proximal tubule
B) Descending loop of Henle
C) Ascending loop of Henle
D) Early distal tubule
E) Collecting tubules

101. Which of the following would tend to decrease plasma potassium concentration by causing a shift of potassium from the extracellular fluid into the cells?

A) Strenuous exercise
B) Aldosterone deficiency
C) Acidosis
D) Beta adrenergic blockade
E) Insulin excess

102. A 23-year-old male runs a 10-km race in July and loses 2 L of fluid by sweating. He also drinks 2 L of water during the race. Which of the following changes would you expect, compared to normal, after he absorbs the water and assuming osmotic equilibrium and no excretion of water or electrolytes?

	Intracellular volume	Intracellular osmolarity	Extracellular volume	Extracellular osmolarity
A)	↓	↑	↓	↑
B)	↓	↓	↓	↓
C)	↔	↓	↔	↓
D)	↔	↑	↓	↑
E)	↑	↓	↓	↓
F)	↑	↓	↑	↓

Questions 103–105

The following test results were obtained: urine flow rate = 2.0 ml/min; urine inulin concentration = 60 mg/ml; plasma inulin concentration = 2 mg/ml; urine potassium concentration = 20 μmol/ml; plasma potassium concentration = 4.0 μmol/ml; urine osmolarity = 150 mOsm/L; and plasma osmolarity = 300 mOsm/L.

103. What is the approximate GFR?

A) 20 ml/min
B) 25 ml/min
C) 30 ml/min
D) 60 ml/min
E) 75 ml/min
F) 150 ml/min

104. What is the net potassium reabsorption rate?

A) 0 μmol/min
B) 20 μmol/min
C) 60 μmol/min
D) 200 μmol/min
E) 240 μmol/min
F) 300 μmol/min
G) Potassium is not reabsorbed in this case

105. What is the free water clearance rate?

A) +1.0 ml/min
B) +1.5 ml/min
C) +2.0 ml/min
D) −1.0 ml/min
E) −1.5 ml/min
F) −2.0 ml/min

106. A patient has the following laboratory values: arterial pH = 7.04, plasma HCO_3^- = 13 mEq/L, plasma chloride concentration = 120 mEq/L, arterial PCO_2 = 30 mm Hg, and plasma sodium = 141 mEq/L. What is the most likely cause for his acidosis?

A) Emphysema
B) Methanol poisoning
C) Salicylic acid poisoning
D) Diarrhea
E) Diabetes mellitus

107. A young man is found comatose, having taking an unknown number of sleeping pills an unknown time before. An arterial blood sample yields the following values: pH = 7.02, HCO_3^- = 14 mEq/L, and PCO_2 = 68 mm Hg. This patient's acid–base status is most accurately described as

A) uncompensated metabolic acidosis
B) uncompensated respiratory acidosis
C) simultaneous respiratory and metabolic acidosis
D) respiratory acidosis with partial renal compensation
E) respiratory acidosis with complete renal compensation

108. In chronic respiratory acidosis with partial renal compensation, you would expect to find the following changes, compared to normal:___ urinary excretion of NH_4^+; _____ plasma HCO_3^- concentration; and _____ urine pH.

A) increased, increased, decreased
B) increased, decreased, decreased
C) no change in, increased, decreased
D) no change in, no change in, decreased
E) increased, no change in, increased

109. At which renal tubular sites would the concentration of creatinine be expected to be highest in a normally hydrated person?

A) The concentration would be the same in all of the above, since creatinine is neither secreted or reabsorbed
B) Glomerular filtrate
C) End of the proximal tubule
D) End of the loop of Henle
E) Distal tubule
F) Collecting duct

Questions 110 and 111

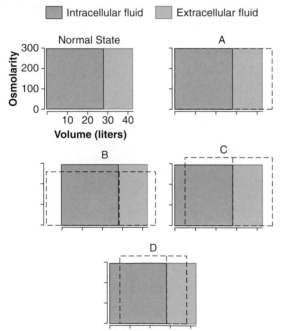

The diagrams represent various states of abnormal hydration. In each diagram, the normal (solid lines) is superimposed on the abnormal state (dashed lines) to illustrate the shifts in the volumes (width of rectangles) and total osmolarities (height of rectangles) of the extracellular fluid and intracellular fluid compartments.

110. Which of the diagrams would represent the changes (after osmotic equilibrium) in extracellular and intracellular fluid volumes and osmolarities after infusion of 2 L of 3.0% dextrose?

A)
B)
C)
D)

111. Which of the diagrams would represent the changes (after osmotic equilibrium) in extracellular and intracellular fluid volumes and osmolarities in a patient with severe "central" diabetes insipidus?

A)
B)
C)
D)

112. In a patient who has chronic diabetic ketoacidosis, you would expect to find which of the following?

A) Decreased renal HCO_3^- excretion, increased NH_4^+ excretion, increased plasma anion gap
B) Increased respiration rate, decreased arterial PCO_2, decreased plasma anion gap
C) Increased NH_4^+ excretion, increased plasma anion gap, increased urine pH
D) Increased renal HCO_3^- production, increased NH_4^+ excretion, decreased plasma anion gap
E) Decreased urine pH, decreased renal HCO_3^- excretion, increased arterial PCO_2

113. Increases in both renal blood flow and GFR are caused by which of the following?

A) Dilation of the afferent arterioles
B) Increased glomerular capillary filtration coefficient
C) Increased plasma colloid osmotic pressure
D) Dilation of the efferent arterioles
E) Increased blood viscosity due to increased hematocrit

114. If the cortical collecting tubule tubular fluid inulin concentration is 40 mg/100 ml and plasma concentration of inulin is 2.0 mg/100 ml, what is the approximate percentage of the filtered water that remains in the tubule at that point?

A) 0%
B) 2%
C) 5%
D) 10%
E) 20%
F) 100%

115. Which of the following changes would tend to increase Ca^{2+} reabsorption in the renal tubule?

   A) Extracellular fluid volume expansion
   B) Increased plasma parathyroid hormone concentration
   C) Increased blood pressure
   D) Decreased plasma phosphate concentration
   E) Metabolic alkalosis

116. Which of the following diuretics inhibits Na^+-$2Cl^-$-K^+ co-transport in the loop of Henle as its primary action?

   A) Thiazide diuretic
   B) Furosemide
   C) Carbonic anhydrase inhibitor
   D) Osmotic diuretic
   E) Amiloride
   F) Spironolactone

117. A 55-year-old male patient with hypertension has had his blood pressure reasonably well controlled by administration of a thiazide diuretic. During his last visit (6 months ago) his blood pressure was 130/75 mm Hg and his serum creatinine was 1 mg/100 ml. He has been exercising regularly for the past 2 years, but recently has complained of knee pain and began taking large amounts of a non-steroidal anti-inflammatory drug. When he arrives at your office, his blood pressure is 155/85 and his serum creatinine is now 2.5 mg/100 ml. Which of the following best explains his increased serum creatinine?

   A) Increased efferent arteriolar resistance that reduced GFR
   B) Increased afferent arteriolar resistance that reduced GFR
   C) Increased glomerular capillary filtration coefficient that reduced GFR
   D) Increased angiotensin II formation that decreased GFR
   E) Increased muscle mass due to the exercise

118. Which of the following would tend to decrease GFR by more than 10% in a normal kidney?

   A) Decrease in renal arterial pressure from 100 to 85 mm Hg
   B) 50% decrease in afferent arteriolar resistance
   C) 50% decrease in efferent arteriolar resistance
   D) 50% increase in the glomerular capillary filtration coefficient
   E) Decrease in plasma colloid osmotic pressure from 28 to 20 mm Hg

1. **B)** GFR is equal to inulin clearance, which is calculated as the urine inulin concentration (100 mg/ml) × urine flow rate (1 ml/min) ÷ plasma inulin concentration (2 mg/ml), which is equal to 50 ml/min.
   TMP12 340

2. **D)** The net urea reabsorption rate is equal to the filtered load of urea (GFR [50 ml/min] × plasma urea concentration [2.5 mg/ml]) − urinary excretion rate of urea (urine urea concentration [50 mg/ml] × urine flow rate [1 ml/min]). Therefore, net urea reabsorption = (50 ml/min × 2.5 mg/ml) − (50 mg/ml × 1 ml/min) = 75 mg/min.
   TMP12 340

3. **C)** A 3% sodium chloride (NaCl) solution is hypertonic and when infused intravenously would increase extracellular fluid volume and osmolarity, thereby causing water to flow out of the cell. This would decrease intracellular fluid volume and further increase extracellular fluid volume. The 0.9% NaCl solution and 5% dextrose solution are isotonic, and therefore would not reduce intracellular fluid volume. Pure water and the 0.45% NaCl solution are hypotonic, and when infused would increase both intracellular and extracellular fluid volumes.
   TMP12 291–294

4. **C)** Because the patient has a low plasma pH (normal = 7.4), he has acidosis. The fact that his plasma bicarbonate concentration is also low (normal = 24 mEq/L) indicates that he has metabolic acidosis. However, he also appears to have respiratory acidosis because his plasma P_{CO_2} is high (normal = 40 mm Hg). The rise in P_{CO_2} is due to his impaired breathing as a result of cardiopulmonary arrest. Therefore, the patient has a mixed acidosis with combined metabolic and respiratory acidosis.
   TMP12 392–395

5. **D)** An important compensation for respiratory acidosis is increased renal production of ammonia (NH_4^+) and increased NH_4^+ excretion. In acidosis, urinary excretion of HCO_3^- would be reduced, as would urine pH, and urinary titratable acid would be slightly increased as a compensatory response to the acidosis.
   TMP12 388–389

6. **B)** As water flows up the ascending limb of the loop of Henle, solutes are reabsorbed, but this segment is relatively impermeable to water; progressive dilution of the tubular fluid occurs so that the osmolarity decreases to approximately 100 mOsm/L by the time the fluid reaches the early distal tubule. Even during maximal antidiuresis, this portion of the renal tubule is relatively impermeable to water and is therefore called the diluting segment of the renal tubule.
   TMP12 352–353

7. **B)** A 1% solution of dextrose is hypotonic and when infused would increase both intracellular and extracellular fluid volumes while decreasing osmolarity of these compartments.
   TMP12 291–293

8. **C)** A 3% solution of sodium chloride is hypertonic and when infused into the extracellular fluid would raise osmolarity, thereby causing water to flow out of the cells into the extracellular fluid until osmotic equilibrium is achieved. In the steady state, extracellular fluid volume would increase, intracellular fluid volume would decrease, and osmolarity of both compartments would increase.
   TMP12 291–293

9. **B)** Excessive secretion of antidiuretic hormone would increase renal tubular reabsorption of water, thereby increasing extracellular fluid volume and reducing extracellular fluid osmolarity. The reduced osmolarity, in turn, would cause water to flow into the cells and raise intracellular fluid volume. In the steady state, both extracellular and intracellular fluid volumes would increase, and osmolarity of both compartments would decrease.
   TMP12 294–295, 355–356

10. **D)** A severe renal artery stenosis that reduces GFR to 25% of normal would also decrease renal blood flow but would cause only a transient decrease in urinary creatinine excretion. The transient decrease in creatinine excretion would increase serum creatinine (to about four times normal), which would restore the filtered creatinine load to normal and therefore return urinary creatinine excretion to normal levels under steady-state conditions. Urinary sodium secretion would also decrease transiently but would be restored to normal so that intake and excretion of sodium are balanced. Plasma sodium concentration would not change significantly because it is carefully regulated by the antidiuretic hormone–thirst mechanism.
    TMP12 341, 404–405

11. **C)** Aldosterone stimulates potassium secretion by the principal cells of the collecting tubules. Therefore, blockade of the action of aldosterone with spironolactone would inhibit potassium secretion. Other factors that stimulate potassium secretion by the cortical collecting tubule include increased potassium concentration, increased cortical collecting tubule flow rate (as would occur with high sodium intake or a diuretic that reduces proximal tubular sodium reabsorption), and acute alkalosis.

    TMP12 364–367

12. **A)** K^+ excretion rate = urine K^+ concentration (60 mEq/L) × urine flow rate (0.001 L/min) = 0.06 mEq/min.

    TMP12 340

13. **C)** In the absence of ADH secretion, there is a marked increase in urine volume because the late distal and collecting tubules are relatively impermeable to water. As a result of increased urine volume, there is dehydration and increased plasma osmolarity and high plasma sodium concentration. The resulting decrease in extracellular fluid volume stimulates renin secretion, resulting in an increase in plasma renin concentration.

    TMP12 354

14. **C)** In a patient with a very high rate of renin secretion, there would also be increased formation of angiotensin II, which in turn would stimulate aldosterone secretion. The increased levels of angiotensin II and aldosterone would cause a transient decrease in sodium excretion, which would cause expansion of the extracellular fluid volume and increased arterial pressure. The increased arterial pressure as well as other compensations would return sodium excretion to normal so that intake and output are balanced. Therefore, under steady-state conditions, sodium excretion would be normal and equal to sodium intake. The increased aldosterone concentration would cause hypokalemia (decreased plasma potassium concentration), whereas the high level of angiotensin II would cause renal vasoconstriction and decreased renal blood flow.

    TMP12 370–372

15. **D)** Impairment of proximal tubular NaCl reabsorption would increase NaCl delivery to the macula densa, which in turn would cause a tubuloglomerular feedback–mediated increase in afferent arteriolar resistance. The increased afferent arteriolar resistance would decrease the GFR. Initially there would be a transient increase in sodium excretion, but after 3 weeks, steady-state conditions would be achieved. Sodium excretion would equal sodium intake, and no significant change would occur in urinary sodium excretion.

    TMP12 319–321

16. **C)** When potassium intake is doubled (from 80 to 160 mmol/day), potassium excretion also approximately doubles within a few days, and the plasma potassium concentration increases only slightly. Increased potassium excretion is achieved largely by increased secretion of potassium in the cortical collecting tubule. Increased aldosterone concentration plays a significant role in increasing potassium secretion and in maintaining a relatively constant plasma potassium concentration during increases in potassium intake. Sodium excretion does not change markedly during chronic increases in potassium intake.

    TMP12 364–367

17. **A)** The patient described has protein in the urine (proteinuria) and reduced plasma protein concentration secondary to glomerulonephritis caused by an untreated streptococcal infection ("strep throat"). The reduced plasma protein concentration, in turn, decreased the plasma colloid osmotic pressure and resulted in leakage from the plasma to the interstitium. The extracellular fluid edema raised interstitial fluid pressure and interstitial fluid volume, causing increased lymph flow and decreased interstitial fluid protein concentration. Increasing lymph flow causes a "washout" of the interstitial fluid protein as a safety factor against edema. The decreased blood volume would tend to lower blood pressure and stimulate the secretion of renin by the kidneys, raising the plasma renin concentration.

    TMP12 297–298

18. **C)** A 50% reduction in afferent arteriolar resistance with no change in arterial pressure would increase renal blood flow and glomerular hydrostatic pressure, thereby increasing GFR. At the same time, the reduction in afferent arteriolar resistance would raise peritubular capillary hydrostatic pressure.

    TMP12 315– 316

19. **C)** The filtered load of glucose in this example is determined as follows: GFR (150 ml/min) × plasma glucose (300 mg/dL) = 450 mg/min. The transport maximum for glucose in this example is 300 mg/min. Therefore, the maximum rate of glucose reabsorption is 300 mg/min. The urinary glucose excretion is equal to the filtered load (450 mg/min) minus the tubular reabsorption of glucose (300 mg/min), or 150 mg/min.

    TMP12 326–327, 340

Characteristics of Primary Acid–Base Disturbances

	pH	H^+	P_{CO_2}	HCO_3^-
Normal	7.4	40 mEq/L	40 mm Hg	24 mEq/L
Respiratory acidosis	↓	↑	↑↑	↑
Respiratory alkalosis	↑	↓	↓↓	↓
Metabolic acidosis	↓	↑	↓	↓↓
Metabolic alkalosis	↑	↓	↑	↑↑

The primary event is indicated by the double arrows (↑↑ or ↓↓). Note that respiratory acid–base disorders are initiated by an increase or decrease in Pco_2, whereas metabolic disorders are initiated by an increase or decrease in HCO_3^-.

20. **B)** This patient has respiratory acidosis because the plasma pH is lower than the normal level of 7.4 and the plasma Pco_2 is higher than the normal level of 40 mm Hg. The elevation in plasma bicarbonate concentration above normal (~24 mEq/L) is due to partial renal compensation for the respiratory acidosis. Therefore, this patient has respiratory acidosis with partial renal compensation.
    TMP12 391

21. **C)** Peritubular capillary fluid reabsorption is determined by the balance of hydrostatic and colloid osmotic forces in the peritubular capillaries. Increased efferent arteriolar resistance reduces peritubular capillary hydrostatic pressure and therefore increases the net force favoring fluid reabsorption. Increased blood pressure tends to raise peritubular capillary hydrostatic pressure and reduce fluid reabsorption. Decreased filtration fraction increases the peritubular capillary colloid osmotic pressure and tends to reduce peritubular capillary reabsorption. Decreased angiotensin II causes vasodilatation of efferent arterioles, raising peritubular capillary hydrostatic pressure, decreasing reabsorption, and decreasing tubular transport of water and electrolytes. Increased renal blood flow also tends to raise peritubular capillary hydrostatic pressure and decrease fluid reabsorption.
    TMP12 335–337

22. **B)** Inhibition of aldosterone causes hyperkalemia by two mechanisms: (1) shifting potassium out of the cells into the extracellular fluid, and (2) decreasing cortical collecting tubular secretion of potassium. Increasing potassium intake from 60 to 180 mmol/day would cause only a very small increase in plasma potassium concentration in a person with normal kidneys and normal aldosterone feedback mechanisms (see TMP11 Figures 29-7 and 29-8). A reduction in sodium intake also has very little effect on plasma potassium concentration. Chronic treatment with a diuretic that inhibits loop of Henle Na^+-$2Cl^-$-K^+ co-transport would tend to cause potassium loss in the urine and hypokalemia. However, chronic treatment with a diuretic that inhibits sodium reabsorption in the collecting ducts, such as amiloride, would have little effect on plasma potassium concentration.
    TMP12 362, 364

23. **C)** The filterability of solutes in the plasma is inversely related to the size of the solute (molecular weight). Also, positively charged molecules are filtered more readily than are neutral molecules or negatively charged molecules of equal molecular weight. Therefore, the positively charged polycationic dextran with a molecular weight of 25,000 would be the most readily filtered substance of the choices provided. Red blood cells are not filtered at all by the glomerular capillaries under normal conditions.
    TMP12 313

24. **B)** Approximately 30% to 40% of the filtered urea is reabsorbed in the proximal tubule. However, the tubular fluid urea concentration increases because urea is not nearly as permeant as water in this nephron segment. Urea concentration increases further in the tip of the loop of Henle because water is reabsorbed in the descending limb of the loop of Henle. Under conditions of antidiuresis, urea is further concentrated as water is reabsorbed and as fluid flows along the collecting ducts. Therefore, the final urine concentration of urea is substantially greater than the concentration in the proximal tubule or in the plasma.
    TMP12 350–351

25. **D)** Excessive activity of the amiloride-sensitive sodium channel in the collecting tubules would cause a transient decrease in sodium excretion and expansion of extracellular fluid volume, which in turn would increase arterial pressure and decrease renin secretion, leading to decreased aldosterone secretion. Under steady-state conditions, sodium excretion would return to normal so that intake and renal excretion of sodium are balanced. One of the mechanisms that re-establishes this balance between intake and output of sodium is the rise in arterial pressure that induces a "pressure natriuresis."
    TMP12 370–372, 409

26. **B)** Free water clearance is calculated as urine flow rate (600 ml/2 hr, or 5 ml/min) − osmolar clearance (urine osmolarity × urine flow rate/plasma osmolarity). Therefore, free water clearance is equal to +2.5 ml/min.
    TMP12 354

27. **A)** Primary excessive secretion of aldosterone (Conn's syndrome) would be associated with marked hypokalemia and metabolic alkalosis (increased plasma pH). Because aldosterone stimulates sodium reabsorption and potassium secretion by the cortical collecting tubule, there could be a transient decrease in sodium excretion and an increase in potassium excretion, but under steady-state conditions, both urinary sodium and potassium excretion would return to normal to match the intake of these electrolytes. However, the sodium retention as well as the hypertension associated with aldosterone excess would tend to reduce renin secretion.
    TMP12 364, 375

28. B) A doubling of plasma creatinine implies that the creatinine clearance and GFR have been reduced by approximately 50%. Although the reduction in creatinine clearance would initially cause a transient decrease in filtered load of creatinine, creatinine excretion rate, and sodium excretion rate, the plasma concentration of creatinine would increase until the filtered load of creatinine and the creatinine excretion rate returned to normal. However, creatinine clearance would remain reduced, because creatinine clearance is the urinary excretion rate of creatinine divided by the plasma creatinine concentration. Urinary sodium excretion would also return to normal and would equal the sodium intake, under steady-state conditions, as a result of compensatory mechanisms that reduce renal tubular reabsorption of sodium.

TMP12 341, 404–405

29. C) The glomerular capillary filtration coefficient is the product of the hydraulic conductivity and surface area of the glomerular capillaries. Therefore, increasing the glomerular capillary filtration coefficient tends to increase GFR. Increased afferent arteriolar resistance, decreased efferent arteriolar resistance, increased Bowman's capsule hydrostatic pressure, and decreased glomerular hydrostatic pressure tend to decrease GFR.

TMP12 314–316

30. D) If a substance is completely cleared from the plasma, the clearance rate of that substance would equal the total renal plasma flow. In other words, the total amount of substance delivered to the kidneys in the blood (renal plasma flow × concentration of substance in the blood) would equal the amount of that substance excreted in the urine. Complete renal clearance of a substance would require both glomerular filtration and tubular secretion of that substance.

TMP12 340–343

31. C) The patient has a lower than normal pH and is therefore acidotic. Because the plasma bicarbonate concentration is also lower than normal, the patient has metabolic acidosis with respiratory compensation (P_{CO_2} is lower than normal). The plasma anion gap (Na^+-Cl^--HCO_3^- = 10 mEq/L) is in the normal range, suggesting that the metabolic acidosis is not caused by excess nonvolatile acids such as salicylic acid or ketoacids caused by diabetes mellitus. Therefore, the most likely cause of the metabolic acidosis is diarrhea, which would cause a loss of HCO_3^- in the feces and would be associated with a normal anion gap and a hyperchloremic (increased chloride concentration) metabolic acidosis.

TMP12 392–395

32. A) A 50% reduction of GFR would approximately double the plasma creatinine concentration, because creatinine is not reabsorbed or secreted and its excretion depends largely on glomerular filtration. Therefore,

when GFR decreases the plasma concentration of creatinine increases until the renal excretion of creatinine returns to normal. Plasma concentrations of glucose, potassium, sodium, and hydrogen ions are closely regulated by multiple mechanisms that keep them relatively constant even when GFR falls to very low levels. Plasma phosphate concentration is also maintained near normal until GFR falls to below 20% to 30% of normal.

TMP12 341, 404–405

33. D) Excessive ingestion of aspirin (salicylic acid) causes metabolic acidosis characterized by reductions in plasma HCO_3^- concentration and increased plasma anion gap. The acidosis stimulates respiration, causing a compensatory decrease in plasma P_{CO_2}. The acidosis also increases renal reabsorption of HCO_3^-, leading to decreased urine HCO_3^- excretion. Finally, the acidosis also stimulates a compensatory increase in renal tubular NH_4^+ production.

TMP12 392–395.

Step 1. Initial conditions

	Volume (L)	Concentration (mOsm/L)	Total (mOsm)
Extracellular fluid	12	260	3120
Intracellular fluid	24	260	6240
Total body water	36	260	9360

Step 2. Effect of adding 2 L of 3% sodium chloride after osmotic equilibrium

	Volume (L)	Concentration (mOsm/L)	Total (mOsm)
Extracellular fluid	17.2	300	3120 + 2052 = 5172
Intracellular fluid	20.8	300	6240
Total body water	36 + 2 = 38	300	9360 + 2052 = 11,412

34. C) Calculation of fluid shifts and osmolarities after infusion of hypertonic saline is discussed in Chapter 25 of TMP12. The tables shown above represent the initial conditions and the final conditions after infusion of 2 L of 3% NaCl and osmotic equilibrium. Three percent NaCl is equal to 30 g NaCl/L, or 0.513 mol/L (513 mmol/L). Because NaCl has two osmotically active particles per mole, the net effect is to add a total of 2052 millimoles in 2 L of solution. As an approximation, one can assume that cell membranes are impermeable to the NaCl and that the NaCl infused remains in the extracellular fluid compartment.

TMP12 291–294

35. **B)** Extracellular fluid volume is calculated by dividing the total milliosmoles in the extracellular compartment (5172 mOsm) by the concentration after osmotic equilibrium (300 mOsm/L) to give 17.2 L.

   TMP12 291–294

36. **C)** A large increase in aldosterone secretion combined with a high sodium intake would cause severe hypokalemia. Aldosterone stimulates potassium secretion and causes a shift of potassium from the extracellular fluid into the cells, and a high sodium intake increases the collecting tubular flow rate, which also enhances potassium secretion. In normal persons, potassium intake can be reduced to as low as one-fourth of normal with only a mild decrease in plasma potassium concentration (for further information, see TMP12, Figure 29-8). A low sodium intake would tend to oppose aldosterone's hypokalemic effect, because a low sodium intake would reduce the collecting tubular flow rate and thus tend to reduce potassium secretion. Patients with Addison's disease have a deficiency of aldosterone secretion and therefore tend to have hyperkalemia.

   TMP12 361, 364–367

37. **A)** The net filtration pressure at the glomerular capillaries is equal to the sum of the forces favoring filtration (glomerular capillary hydrostatic pressure) minus the forces that oppose filtration (hydrostatic pressure in Bowman's space and glomerular colloid osmotic pressure). Therefore, the net pressure driving glomerular filtration is $50 - 12 - 30 = 8$ mm Hg.

   TMP12 314

38. **D)** Uncontrolled diabetes mellitus results in increased blood acetoacetic acid levels, which in turn cause metabolic acidosis and decreased plasma HCO_3^- and pH. The acidosis causes several compensatory responses, including increased respiratory rate, which reduces plasma P_{CO_2}; increased renal NH^+ production, which leads to increased NH^+ excretion; and increased phosphate buffering of hydrogen ions secreted by the renal tubules, which increases titratable acid excretion.

   TMP12 391–393

39. **B)** Infusion of a hypotonic solution of NaCl would initially increase extracellular fluid volume and decrease extracellular fluid osmolarity. The reduction in extracellular fluid osmolarity would cause osmotic flow of fluid into the cells, thereby increasing intracellular fluid volume and decreasing intracellular fluid osmolarity after osmotic equilibrium.

   TMP12 292–294

40. **D)** The tubular fluid–plasma ratio of inulin concentration is 4 in the early distal tubule, as shown in the question's figure. Because inulin is not reabsorbed from the tubule, this means that water reabsorption must have concentrated the inulin to four times the level in the plasma that was filtered. Therefore, the amount of water remaining in the tubule is only one-fourth of what was filtered, indicating that 75% of the water has been reabsorbed prior to the distal convoluted tubule.

   TPM12 334

41. **B)** Potassium secretion by the cortical collecting ducts is stimulated by (1) aldosterone, (2) increased plasma potassium concentration, (3) increased flow rate in the cortical collecting tubules, and (4) alkalosis. Therefore, a diuretic that inhibits aldosterone, decreased plasma potassium concentration, acute acidosis, and low sodium intake would all tend to decrease potassium secretion by the cortical collecting tubules. A diuretic that decreases loop of Henle sodium reabsorption, however, would tend to increase the flow rate in the cortical collecting tubule and therefore stimulate potassium secretion.

   TMP12 364–367

42. **B)** Excessive secretion of aldosterone stimulates sodium reabsorption and potassium secretion in the principal cells of the collecting tubules, causing a transient reduction in urinary sodium excretion and expansion of extracellular fluid volume, as well as a transient increase in potassium excretion rate. Sodium retention raises blood pressure and decreases renin secretion. However, under steady-state conditions, sodium and potassium excretion would return to normal, so that intake and output of these electrolytes are balanced. Excess aldosterone excretion would cause a marked reduction in plasma potassium concentration because of the transient increase in potassium excretion, as well as aldosterone's effect of shifting potassium from the extracellular fluid into the cells.

   TMP12 337–338, 375

43. **B)** This patient with diabetes mellitus and chronic renal disease has a reduction in creatinine clearance to 40% of normal, implying a marked reduction in GFR. He also has acidosis, as evidenced by a plasma pH of 7.14. The decrease in creatinine clearance would cause only a transient reduction in sodium excretion and creatinine excretion rate. As the plasma creatinine concentration increased, the urinary creatinine excretion rate would return to normal, despite the sustained decrease in creatinine clearance (creatinine excretion rate/plasma concentration of creatinine). Diabetes is associated with increased production of acetoacetic acid, which would cause metabolic acidosis and decreased plasma HCO_3^- concentration, as well as a compensatory increase in renal NH_4^+ production and increased NH_4^+ excretion rate.

   TMP12 391–393, 404–405

44. **C)** A reduction in plasma protein concentration to 3.6 g/dL would increase the capillary filtration rate,

thereby raising interstitial fluid volume and interstitial fluid hydrostatic pressure. The increased interstitial fluid pressure would, in turn, increase the lymph flow rate and reduce the interstitial fluid protein concentration ("washout" of interstitial fluid protein).
TMP12 297–300

45. **B)** The most likely diagnosis for this patient is diabetes insipidus, which can account for the polyuria and the fact that her urine osmolarity is very low (80 mOsm/L) despite overnight water restriction. In many patients with diabetes insipidus, the plasma sodium concentration can be maintained relatively close to normal by increasing fluid intake (polydipsia). When water intake is restricted, however, the high urine flow rate leads to rapid depletion of extracellular fluid volume and severe hypernatremia, as occurred in this patient. The fact that she has no glucose in her urine rules out diabetes mellitus. Neither primary aldosteronism nor a renin-secreting tumor would lead to an inability to concentrate the urine after overnight water restriction. Syndrome of inappropriate antidiuretic hormone would cause excessive fluid retention and increased urine osmolarity.
TMP12 354, 358–359

46. **D)** Furosemide (Lasix) inhibits the Na^+-$2Cl^-$-K^+ co-transporter in the ascending limb of the loop of Henle. This not only causes marked natriuresis and diuresis but also reduces the urine concentrating ability. Furosemide does not cause edema; in fact, it is often used to treat severe edema and heart failure. Furosemide also increases the renal excretion of potassium and calcium and therefore tends to cause hypokalemia and hypocalcemia rather than increasing the plasma concentrations of potassium and calcium.
TMP12 331, 348, 366–368, 397–398

47. **A)** Excessive secretion of renin leads to the formation of large amounts of angiotensin II, which in turn causes marked constriction of efferent arterioles. This reduces renal blood flow, increases glomerular hydrostatic pressure, and decreases peritubular capillary hydrostatic pressure. Because constriction of efferent arterioles reduces renal blood flow more than GFR, the filtration fraction (ratio of GFR to renal plasma flow) increases.
TMP12 315–316, 318

48. **D)** Most of the daily variation in potassium excretion is caused by changes in potassium secretion in the late distal tubules and collecting tubules. Therefore, when the dietary intake of potassium increases, the total body balance of potassium is maintained primarily by an increase in potassium secretion in these tubular segments. Increased potassium intake has little effect on GFR or on reabsorption of potassium in the proximal tubule and loop of Henle. Although high potassium intake may cause a slight shift of potassium into

the intracellular compartment, a balance between intake and output must be achieved by increasing the excretion of potassium during high potassium intake.
TMP12 362–363

49. **B)** Hypernatremia can be caused by excessive sodium retention or water loss. The fact that the patient has large volumes of dilute urine suggests excessive urinary water excretion. Of the two possible disturbances listed that could cause excessive urinary water excretion (nephrogenic diabetes insipidus and central diabetes insipidus), nephrogenic diabetes insipidus is the most likely cause. Central diabetes insipidus (decreased ADH secretion) is not the correct answer because plasma ADH levels are markedly elevated. Simple dehydration due to decreased water intake is unlikely because the patient is excreting large volumes of dilute urine.
TMP12 295–296, 354

50. **C)** High urine flow occurs in type I diabetes because the filtered load of glucose exceeds the renal threshold, resulting in an increase in glucose concentration in the tubule, which decreases the osmotic driving force for water reabsorption. Increased urine flow reduces extracellular fluid volume and stimulates the release of antidiuretic hormone.
TMP12 326–327, 355–356

51. **C)** Diuretics that inhibit loop of Henle sodium reabsorption are used to treat conditions associated with excessive fluid volume (e.g., hypertension and heart failure). These diuretics initially cause an increase in sodium excretion that reduces extracellular fluid volume and blood pressure, but under steady-state conditions, the urinary sodium excretion returns to normal, due in part to the fall in blood pressure. One of the important side effects of loop diuretics is hypokalemia that is caused by the inhibition of Na^+-$2Cl^-$-K^+ co-transport in the loop of Henle and by the increased tubular flow rate in the cortical collecting tubules, which stimulates potassium secretion.
TMP12 366, 397–398

52. **C)** Approximately 80% to 90% of bicarbonate reabsorption occurs in the proximal tubule under normal conditions as well as in acidosis (see above). For each bicarbonate ion reabsorbed, there must also be a hydrogen ion secreted. Therefore, about 80% to 90% of the hydrogen ions secreted are normally used for bicarbonate reabsorption in the proximal tubules.
TMP12 387, 389–390

53. **A)** Thiazide diuretics inhibit NaCl co-transport in the luminal membrane of the early distal tubules. (For further information, see TMP12 Table 31-1.)
TMP12 398

54. C) Reducing the renal perfusion pressure to 80 mm Hg (within the range of autoregulation) would cause only a transient decrease in GFR, renal blood flow, and sodium excretion and a transient increase in renin secretion. The decreased sodium excretion and increased renin secretion would raise arterial pressure, thereby restoring renal perfusion pressure toward normal and returning renal function toward normal. As long as renal perfusion pressure is not reduced below the range of autoregulation, GFR and renal blood flow are returned to normal within minutes after renal artery constriction.

TMP12 319 (see also chapter 19, page 223)

55. C) Phosphate excretion by the kidneys is controlled by an overflow mechanism. When the transport maximum for reabsorbing phosphate is exceeded, the remaining phosphate in the renal tubules is excreted in the urine and can be used to buffer hydrogen ions and form titratable acid. Phosphate normally begins to spill into the urine when the concentration of extracellular fluid rises above a threshold of 0.8 mmol/L, which is usually exceeded.

TMP12 369

56. A) A reduction in the number of functional nephrons to 25% of normal would cause a compensatory increase in GFR and urine flow rate of the surviving nephrons and decreased urine concentrating ability. Under steady-state conditions, the urinary creatinine excretion rate and sodium excretion rate would be maintained at normal levels. (For further information, see TMP12 Table 31-6.)

TMP12 404–405

57. C) With excessive secretion of ADH, there is a marked increase in water permeability in the late distal tubules and collecting tubules, resulting in water retention, volume expansion, and decreased sodium and protein concentrations in the extracellular fluid. Plasma renin activity and aldosterone concentrations are also decreased because of the volume expansion. Although excessive ADH secretion initially causes a marked reduction in urine flow rate, as volume expansion occurs and as blood pressure increases, there is an "escape" from volume retention, so that urine flow rate returns to normal to match fluid intake.

TMP12 375–376

58. A) Excessive secretion of antidiuretic hormone increases water reabsorption by the renal collecting tubules, which reduces extracellular fluid sodium concentration (hyponatremia). Restriction of fluid intake, excessive aldosterone secretion, or administration of hypertonic 3% NaCl solution would all cause increased plasma sodium concentration (hypernatremia), whereas administration of 0.9% NaCl (an isotonic solution) would cause no major changes in plasma osmolarity.

TMP12 293–295

59. E) In the absence of ADH, the late distal tubule and collecting tubules are not permeable to water (see above). Therefore, the tubular fluid, which is already dilute when it leaves the loop of Henle (about 100 mOsm/L), becomes further diluted as it flows through the late distal tubule and collecting tubules as electrolytes are reabsorbed. Therefore, the final urine osmolarity in the complete absence of ADH is less than 100 mOsm/L.

TMP12 352, Figure 28-8

60. A) About 65% of the filtered potassium is reabsorbed in the proximal tubule, and another 20% to 30% is reabsorbed in the loop of Henle. Although most of the daily variation in potassium excretion is caused by changes in potassium secretion in the distal and collecting tubules, only a small percentage of the filtered potassium load can be reabsorbed in these nephron segments. (For further information, see TMP12 Figure 29-2.)

TMP12 362–363

61. A) The proximal tubule normally absorbs approximately 65% of the filtered water, with much smaller percentages being reabsorbed in the descending loop of Henle and in the distal and collecting tubules. The ascending limb of the loop of Henle is relatively impermeable to water and therefore reabsorbs very little water.

TMP12 329, 352–353

62. C) The thick ascending limb of the loop of Henle is relatively impermeable to water even under conditions of maximal antidiuresis. The proximal tubule and descending limb of the loop of Henle are highly permeable to water under normal conditions as well as during antidiuresis. Water permeability of the late distal and collecting tubules increases markedly during antidiuresis owing to the effects of increased levels of antidiuretic hormone.

TMP12 352–353

63. D) Interstitial fluid volume is equal to extracellular fluid volume minus plasma volume. Extracellular fluid volume can be estimated from the distribution of inulin or ^{22}Na, whereas plasma volume can be estimated from ^{125}I-albumin distribution. Therefore, interstitial fluid volume is calculated from the difference between the inulin distribution space and the ^{125}I-albumin distribution space.

TMP12 289–290, Table 25-3

64. D) Dehydration due to water deprivation decreases extracellular fluid volume, which in turn increases renin secretion and decreases plasma atrial natriuretic peptide. Dehydration also increases the plasma sodium concentration, which stimulates the secretion of ADH. The increased ADH increases water permeability in the collecting ducts. The ascending limb of

the loop of Henle is relatively impermeable to water, and this low permeability is not altered by water deprivation or increased levels of ADH.
TMP12 349–350, 355–356

65. **E)** A 50% reduction in renal efferent arteriolar resistance would reduce glomerular capillary hydrostatic pressure (upstream from the efferent arterioles) and therefore reduce GFR, while increasing hydrostatic pressure in peritubular capillaries (downstream from the efferent arterioles) and increasing renal blood flow.
TMP12 315–316, 336

Factors that can alter potassium distribution between the intra- and extra-cellular fluid

Factors that shift K^+ into cells (decrease extracellular $[K^+]$)	Factors that shift K^+ out of cells (increase extracellular $[K^+]$)
Insulin	Insulin deficiency (diabetes mellitus)
Aldosterone	Aldosterone deficiency (Addison's disease)
β-adrenergic stimulation	β-adrenergic blockade
Alkalosis	Acidosis
	Cell lysis
	Strenuous exercise
	Increased extracellular fluid osmolarity

66. **E)** Metabolic alkalosis is associated with hypokalemia due to a shift of potassium from the extracellular fluid into the cells. β-adrenergic blockade, insulin deficiency, strenuous exercise, and aldosterone deficiency all cause hyperkalemia due to a shift of potassium out of the cells into the extracellular fluid.
TMP12 361–362, Table 29-1

67. **B)** Fluid entering the early distal tubule is almost always hypotonic because sodium and other ions are actively transported out of the thick ascending loop of Henle, whereas this portion of the nephron is virtually impermeable to water. For this reason, the thick ascending limb of the loop of Henle and the early part of the distal tubule are often called the diluting segment.
TMP12 330–331

68. **D)** In this example, the filtered load of glucose is equal to GFR (100 ml/min) × plasma glucose (150 mg/dL), or 150 mg/min. If there is no detectable glucose in the urine, the reabsorption rate is equal to the filtered load of glucose, or 150 mg/min.
TMP12 340

69. **D)** The patient has classic symptoms of diabetes mellitus: increased thirst, breath smelling of acetone (due to increased acetoacetic acids in the blood), high fasting blood glucose concentration, and glucose in the urine. The acetoacetic acids in the blood cause metabolic acidosis that leads to a compensatory decrease in renal HCO_3^- excretion, decreased urine pH, and increased renal production of ammonium and HCO_3^-. The high level of blood glucose increases the filtered load of glucose, which exceeds the transport maximum for glucose, causing an osmotic diuresis (increased urine volume) due to the unreabsorbed glucose in the renal tubules acting as an osmotic diuretic.
TMP12 326–327, 391–392

70. **D)** Approximately 40% to 50% of the filtered urea is reabsorbed in the proximal tubule. The distal convoluted tubule and the cortical collecting tubules are relatively impermeable to urea, even under conditions of antidiuresis; therefore, little urea reabsorption takes place in these segments. Likewise, very little urea reabsorption takes place in the thick ascending limb of the loop of Henle. Under conditions of antidiuresis, the concentration of urea in the renal medullary interstitial fluid is markedly increased because of reabsorption of urea from the collecting ducts, which contributes to the hyperosmotic renal medulla.
TMP12 350–351

71. **A)** Under normal conditions as well as during antidiuresis, most of the filtered water is reabsorbed in the proximal tubule (approximately 60% to 65%). Although dehydration markedly increases water permeability in the cortical and medullary collecting ducts, these segments reabsorb a relatively small (albeit important) fraction of the filtered water.
TMP12 352–353

72. **C)** Intracellular fluid volume is calculated as the difference between total body fluid (0.57 × 60 kilograms = 34.2 kilograms, or approximately 34.2 L) and extracellular fluid volume (12.8 L), which equals 21.4 L.
TMP12 289–290

73. **C)** Plasma volume is calculated as blood volume (4.3 L) × (1.0 − hematocrit), which is 4.3 × 0.6 = 2.58 L (rounded up to 2.6).
TMP12 289–290

74. **C)** Interstitial fluid volume is calculated as the difference between extracellular fluid volume (12.8 L) and plasma volume (2.6 L), which is equal to 10.2 L.
TMP12 289–290

75. **C)** The primary site of reabsorption of magnesium is in the loop of Henle, where about 65% of the filtered load of magnesium is reabsorbed. The proximal tubule normally reabsorbs only about 25% of filtered magnesium, and the distal and collecting tubules reabsorb less than 5%.
TMP12 369–370

76. **C)** A plasma glucose concentration of 300 mg/dL would increase the filtered load of glucose above the renal tubular transport maximum and therefore increase urinary glucose excretion. The unreabsorbed glucose in the renal tubules would also cause an osmotic diuresis, increased urine volume, and decreased extracellular fluid volume, which would stimulate thirst. Increased glucose also causes vasodilatation of afferent arterioles, which increases GFR.
    TMP12 321, 327, 358

77. **B)** GFR is approximately equal to the clearance of creatinine. Creatinine clearance = urine creatinine concentration (32 mg/dL) × urine flow rate (3600 ml/24 hr, or 2.5 ml/min) ÷ plasma creatinine concentration (4 mg/dL) = 20 ml/min.
    TMP12 340–341

78. **D)** The net renal tubular reabsorption rate is the difference between the filtered load of potassium (GFR × plasma potassium concentration) and the urinary excretion of potassium (urine potassium concentration × urine flow rate). Therefore, the net tubular reabsorption of potassium is 0.075 mmol/min.
    TMP12 340–343

79. **D)** Severe diarrhea would result in loss of HCO_3^- in the stool, thereby causing metabolic acidosis that is characterized by low plasma HCO_3^- and low pH. Respiratory compensation would reduce PCO_2. The plasma anion gap would be normal, and the plasma chloride concentration would be elevated (hyperchloremic metabolic acidosis) in metabolic acidosis caused by HCO_3^- loss in the stool.
    TMP12 392, 394–395

80. **E)** Primary excessive secretion of aldosterone causes metabolic alkalosis due to increased secretion of hydrogen ions and HCO_3^- reabsorption by the intercalated cells of the collecting tubules. Therefore, the metabolic alkalosis would be associated with increases in plasma pH and HCO_3^-, with a compensatory reduction in respiration rate and increased PCO_2. The plasma anion gap would be normal, with a slight reduction in plasma chloride concentration.
    TMP12 393–395

81. **D)** Proximal tubular acidosis results from a defect of renal secretion of hydrogen ions, reabsorption of bicarbonate, or both. This leads to increased renal excretion of HCO_3^- and metabolic acidosis characterized by low plasma HCO_3^- concentration, low plasma pH, a compensatory increase in respiration rate and low PCO_2, and a normal anion gap with an increased plasma chloride concentration.
    TMP12 392, 395

82. **F)** A patient with diabetic ketoacidosis and emphysema would be expected to have metabolic acidosis (due to excess ketoacids in the blood caused by diabetes) as well as increased plasma PCO_2 due to impaired pulmonary function. Therefore, the patient would be expected to have decreased plasma pH, decreased HCO_3^-, increased PCO_2, and an increased anion gap (Na^+-Cl^--$HCO_3^- > 10-12$ mEq/L) due to the addition of ketoacids to the blood.
    TMP12 393–394

83. **D)** Secretion of hydrogen ions and reabsorption of HCO_3^- depend critically on the presence of carbonic anhydrase in the renal tubules. After inhibition of carbonic anhydrase, renal tubular secretion of hydrogen ions and reabsorption of HCO_3^- would decrease, leading to increased renal excretion of HCO_3^-, reduced plasma HCO_3^- concentration, and metabolic acidosis. The metabolic acidosis, in turn, would stimulate the respiration rate, leading to decreased PCO_2. The plasma anion gap would be within the normal range.
    TMP12 386–387, 394–395

84. **B)** Acute renal failure caused by tubular necrosis would cause the rapid development of metabolic acidosis due to the kidneys' failure to rid the body of the acid waste products of metabolism. The metabolic acidosis would lead to decreased plasma HCO_3^- concentration. Acute renal failure would also lead to a rapid increase in blood urea nitrogen concentration and a significant increase in plasma potassium concentration due to the kidneys' failure to excrete electrolytes or nitrogenous waste products. Necrosis of the renal epithelial cells causes them to slough away from the basement membrane and plug up the renal tubules, thereby increasing hydrostatic pressure in Bowman's capsule and decreasing GFR.
    TMP12 401, 407

85. **A)** In this example, the plasma sodium concentration is markedly increased, but the urine sodium concentration is relatively normal, and urine osmolarity is almost maximally increased to 1200 mOsm/L. In addition, there are increases in plasma renin, ADH, and aldosterone, which is consistent with dehydration caused by decreased fluid intake. The syndrome of inappropriate ADH would result in a decrease in plasma sodium concentration, as well as suppression of renin and aldosterone secretion. Nephrogenic diabetes insipidus, caused by the kidneys' failure to respond to ADH, would also be associated with dehydration, but urine osmolarity would be reduced rather than increased. Primary aldosteronism would tend to cause sodium and water retention with only a modest change in plasma sodium concentration and a marked reduction in the secretion of renin. Likewise, a renin-secreting tumor would be associated with increases in plasma aldosterone concentration and plasma renin activity, but only a modest change in plasma sodium concentration.
    TMP12 354, 359–360

86. **B)** This diabetic patient has metabolic acidosis characterized by a low HCO_3^-, decreased plasma pH, and increased plasma anion gap. The acidosis stimulates respiration, resulting in a compensatory decrease in plasma P_{CO_2}.
  TMP12 391, 395

87. **E)** Intracellular and extracellular body fluids have the same total osmolarity under steady-state conditions because the cell membrane is highly permeable to water. Therefore, water flows rapidly across the cell membrane until osmotic equilibrium is achieved. The colloid osmotic pressure is determined by the protein concentration, which is considerably higher inside the cell. The cell membrane is also relatively impermeable to potassium, sodium, and chloride, and active transport mechanisms maintain low intracellular concentrations of sodium and chloride and a high intracellular concentration of potassium.
  TMP12 290–292

88. **E)** Although aldosterone is one of the body's most potent sodium-retaining hormones, it stimulates sodium reabsorption only in the late distal tubule and collecting tubules, which together reabsorb much less than 10% of the filtered load of sodium. Therefore, the maximum percentage of the filtered load of sodium that could be reabsorbed in the distal convoluted tubule and collecting duct, even in the presence of high levels of aldosterone, would be less than 10%.
  TMP12 331–333, 337–338

89. **D)** In a dehydrated person, osmolarity in the early distal tubule is usually less than 300 mOsm/L because the ascending limb of the loop of Henle and the early distal tubule are relatively impermeable to water, even in the presence of ADH. Therefore, the tubular fluid becomes progressively more dilute in these segments, compared with plasma. ADH does not influence water reabsorption in the ascending limb of the loop of Henle. The ascending limb, however, reabsorbs sodium to a much greater extent than does the descending limb. Another important action of ADH is to increase the urea permeability in the medullary collecting ducts, which contributes to the hyperosmotic renal medullary interstitium in antidiuresis.
  TMP12 352–353

90. **A)** In the proximal tubule, calcium reabsorption usually parallels sodium and water reabsorption. With extracellular volume expansion or increased blood pressure, proximal sodium and water reabsorption is reduced, and there is also a reduction in calcium reabsorption, causing increased urinary excretion of calcium. Increased parathyroid hormone, increased plasma phosphate concentration, and metabolic acidosis all tend to decrease the renal excretion of calcium.
  TMP12 367–369

91. **B)** A moderate degree of renal artery stenosis that reduces renal artery pressure distal to the stenosis to 85 mm Hg would result in an autoregulatory response that decreases afferent arteriolar resistance. The decreased renal perfusion pressure would stimulate renin secretion, which in turn would increase angiotensin II formation and cause constriction of efferent arterioles. Increased angiotensin II formation would also tend to increase aldosterone secretion.
  TMP12 320

92. **C)** Increasing sodium intake would decrease renin secretion and plasma renin activity, as well as reduce plasma aldosterone concentration and increase plasma atrial natriuretic peptide owing to a modest expansion of extracellular fluid volume. Although a high sodium intake would initially increase distal sodium chloride delivery, which would tend to increase potassium excretion, the decrease in aldosterone concentration would offset this effect, resulting in no change in potassium excretion under steady-state conditions. Even very large increases in sodium intake cause only minimal changes in plasma sodium concentration as long as the antidiuretic hormone–thirst mechanisms are fully operative.
  TMP12 366–367

93. **D)** This patient is severely dehydrated as a result of sweating and lack of adequate fluid intake. The dehydration markedly stimulates the release of ADH and renin secretion, which in turn stimulates the formation of angiotensin II and aldosterone secretion.
  TMP12 337–338, 355–356

94. **D)** Acute metabolic acidosis reduces intracellular potassium concentration which, in turn, decreases potassium secretion by the principal cells of the collecting tubules. The primary mechanism by which increased hydrogen ion concentration inhibits potassium secretion is by reducing the activity of the sodium-potassium ATPase pump. This then reduces intracellular potassium concentration which, in turn, decreases the rate of passive diffusion of potassium across the luminal membrane into the tubule.
  TMP12 367

95. **A)** As the dilute fluid in the early distal tubule passes into late distal tubules and the cortical and medullary collecting tubules, there is additional reabsorption of sodium chloride. In the complete absence of antidiuretic hormone (ADH), this portion of the tubule is also relatively impermeable to water and the additional reabsorption of solutes causes the tubular fluid to become even more dilute than in the diluting segment (early distal tubule), decreasing its osmolarity to as low as 50 mOsm/L. Therefore, in a person with complete absence of ADH, the part of the renal tubule that would have the lowest tubular fluid osmolarity is the medullary collecting duct.
  TMP12 352–353, Figure 28-8

96. **A)** Urine flow rate is calculated as the difference between GFR and tubular fluid reabsorption rate. If GFR decreases from 150 to 75 ml/min and tubular fluid reabsorption rate simultaneously decreases from 149 to 75 ml/min, the urine flow rate would be the GFR minus the tubular reabsorption rate, or 75–75 ml/min, which would equal 0 ml/min.
    TMP12 323, 340–341

97. **A)** Filtration fraction is calculated as the GFR divided by the renal plasma flow. GFR is equal to the net filtration pressure (glomerular hydrostatic pressure minus Bowman's hydrostatic pressure minus colloid osmotic pressure in glomerular capillaries) multiplied by the capillary filtration coefficient. Thus, the filtration fraction is equal to the GFR (60 ml/min) divided by the renal plasma flow (400 ml/min), or 0.15.
    TMP12 314, 342

98. **E)** The kidneys excrete little or no glucose as long as the filtered load of glucose (the product of the GFR and the plasma glucose concentration) does not exceed the tubular transport maximum for glucose. Once the filtered load of glucose rises above the transport maximum, the excess glucose filtered is not reabsorbed and passes into the urine. Therefore, the urinary excretion rate of glucose can be calculated as the filtered load of glucose minus the transport maximum. In this example, the filtered load of glucose is the GFR (150 ml/min) multiplied by the plasma glucose concentration (400 mg/100 ml, or 4 mg/ml) which is equal to 600 mg/min. Since the transport maximum is only 300 mg/min, the rate of glucose excretion would be 600 minus 300 mg/min, or 300 mg/min.
    TMP12 326–327, 340–342

99. **E)** A 50% reduction in GFR (from 80 to 40 ml/min) would result in an approximate 50% reduction in creatinine clearance rate, since creatinine clearance is approximately equal to the GFR. This would, in turn, lead to doubling of plasma creatinine concentration. This rise in plasma creatinine concentration results from an initial decrease in creatinine excretion rate, but as the plasma creatinine concentration increases, the filtered load of creatinine (the product of GFR × plasma creatinine concentration) returns to normal and creatinine excretion rate returns to normal under steady-state conditions. Thus, under the steady state conditions, a 50% reduction in GFR is associated with a doubling of plasma creatinine concentration, a 50% decrease in creatinine clearance, a normal filtered load of creatinine, as well as no change in load of filtered creatinine and no change in creatinine excretion rate as long as the person's protein metabolism is not altered. Likewise, sodium excretion rate returns to normal even when the GFR is reduced because of multiple feedback systems that eventually reestablish sodium balance. Under steady-state conditions sodium excretion must equal sodium intake in order to maintain life.
    TMP12 341, 370

100. **E)** Most of the potassium secretion occurs in the collecting tubules. A high potassium diet stimulates potassium secretion by the collecting tubules through multiple mechanisms, including small increases in extracellular potassium concentration as well as increased levels of aldosterone.
    TMP12 364–365

101. **E)** Increased levels of insulin cause a shift of potassium from the extracellular fluid into the cells. All of the other conditions have the reverse effect of shifting potassium out of the cells into the extracellular fluid.
    TMP12 361–362

102. **E)** After running the race and losing fluid as well as electrolytes, this person replaces his fluid volume by drinking 2 L of water. However, he did not replace the electrolytes. Therefore, he would be expected to experience a decrease in plasma sodium concentration resulting in a decrease in both intracellular and extracellular fluid osmolarity. The decrease in extracellular fluid osmolarity would lead to an increase in intracellular volume as fluid diffused into the cells from the extracellular compartment. Therefore, after drinking the water and absorbing it, the total body volume would be normal but intracellular volume would be increased and extracellular volume would be reduced.
    TMP12 292

103. **D)** GFR is equal to the clearance of inulin. Inulin clearance = urine inulin concentration (60 mg/ml) × urine flow rate (2 ml/min)/plasma inulin concentration (2 mg/ml) = 60 ml/min.
    TMP12 340–342

104. **D)** The net renal tubular potassium reabsorption rate is the difference between the filtered load of potassium (GFR × plasma potassium concentration) and the urinary excretion rate of potassium (urine potassium concentration × urine flow rate). Therefore, the net tubular reabsorption rate of potassium is 200 μmol/min.
    TMP12 340–342

105. **A)** Free water clearance is calculated as urine flow rate (2.0 ml/min) − osmolar clearance (urine osmolarity × urine flow rate/plasma osmolarity). Therefore, free water clearance is equal to +1.0 ml/min.
    TMP12 354

106. **D)** The patient has metabolic acidosis as evidenced by the reduced plasma HCO_3^- concentration (normal = 24 mEq/L) and decreased arterial PCO_2 (normal is approximately 40 mm Hg). Because the plasma anion

gap (plasma sodium − HCO_3^- − chloride) is normal (approximately 10 mEq/L), the acidosis is not caused by excess nonvolatile acids caused by salicylic acid poisoning, diabetes, or methanol poisoning. Therefore, the most likely cause of the metabolic acidosis is diarrhea, which leads to loss of bicarbonate in the feces. With emphysema, the acidosis would be associated with the increase in PCO_2.

TMP12 390–391, 395

107. **C)** In this example the acidosis is associated with a reduced plasma bicarbonate concentration, signifying metabolic acidosis. In addition, the patient also has an elevated PCO_2 signifying respiratory acidosis. Therefore, the patient has simultaneous respiratory and metabolic acidosis.

TMP12 391–394

108. **A)** Chronic respiratory acidosis is caused by insufficient pulmonary ventilation, resulting in an increase in PCO_2. Acidosis, in turn, stimulates the secretion of hydrogen ions into the tubular fluid and increased renal tubular production of NH_4^+, which further contributes to the excretion of hydrogen ions and the renal production of HCO_3^-, thereby increasing plasma bicarbonate concentration. The increased tubular secretion of hydrogen ions also reduces urine pH.

TMP12 391

109. **F)** Because creatinine is not reabsorbed significantly in the renal tubules, the concentration of creatinine progressively increases as water is reabsorbed along the renal tubular segments. Therefore, in a normally hydrated person the concentration of creatinine would be greatest in the collecting ducts.

TMP12 334, Figure 27-14

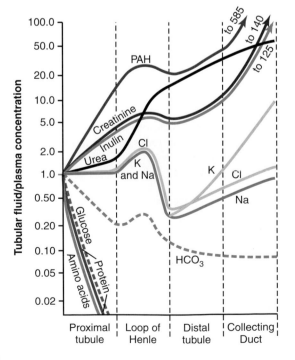

110. **B)** Three percent dextrose is a hypotonic solution. Therefore, infusing the 3% dextrose would decrease extracellular fluid osmolarity which, in turn, would lead to diffusion of water into the cells. Under steady-state conditions, there would be a reduction in intracellular and extracellular osmolarity as well as an increase in the fluid volume of both compartments.

TMP12 292–294

111. **D)** In a patient with central diabetes insipidus there would be deficient secretion of antidiuretic hormone, resulting in excretion of large volumes of water. This, in turn, would cause dehydration and hypernatremia (increased plasma osmolarity). The hypernatremia would result in decreased intracellular volume. Therefore, the primary loss of water would lead to increases in both extracellular and intracellular fluid osmolarity as well as decreases in intracellular and extracellular fluid volumes.

TMP12 293–296

112. **A)** Diabetic ketoacidosis results in a metabolic acidosis that is characterized by a decrease in plasma bicarbonate concentration, increased anion gap (due to the addition of unmeasured anions to the extracellular fluid along with the keto acids), and a renal compensatory response that includes increased secretion of $NH4^+$. There is also an increased respiratory rate with a reduction in arterial PCO_2, as well as decreased urine pH and decreased renal HCO_3^- excretion.

TMP12 392–395

113. **A)** Dilation of the afferent arterioles leads to an increase in the glomerular hydrostatic pressure and therefore an increase in GFR as well as an increase in renal blood flow. Increased glomerular capillary filtration coefficient would also raise the GFR but would not be expected to alter renal blood flow. Increased plasma colloid osmotic pressure or dilation of the efferent arterioles would both tend to reduce the GFR. Increased blood viscosity would tend to reduce renal blood flow and GFR.

TMP12 314–317

114. **C)** Since inulin is not reabsorbed or secreted by the renal tubules, increasing concentration of inulin in the renal tubules reflects water reabsorption. Thus, an increase of inulin concentration from a level 2 mg/100 ml in the plasma to 40 mg/100 ml in the cortical collecting tubule implies that there has been a 20-fold increase in concentration of inulin. In other words, only 1/20th (5%) of the water that was filtered into the renal tubule remains in the collecting tubule.

TMP12 334

115. B) Increased levels of parathyroid hormone stimulate calcium reabsorption in the thick ascending loops of Henle and distal tubules. Extracellular fluid volume expansion, increased blood pressure, decreased plasma phosphate concentration, and metabolic alkalosis are all associated with decreased calcium reabsorption by the renal tubules.

  TMP12 368–369

116. B) Furosemide is a powerful inhibitor of the Na^+-$2Cl^-$-K^+ co-transporter in the loop of Henle. Thiazide diuretics primarily inhibit sodium chloride reabsorption into the distal tubule, whereas carbonic andydrase inhibitors decrease bicarbonate reabsorption in the tubules. Amiloride inhibits sodium channel activity whereas spironolactone inhibits the action of mineralocorticoids in the renal tubules. Osmotic diuretics inhibit water and solute reabsorption by increasing osmolarity of the tubular fluid.

  TMP12 398

117. B) Nonsteroidal anti-inflammatory drugs inhibit the synthesis of prostaglandins, which, in turn, causes constriction of afferent arterioles that can reduce the GFR. The decrease in GFR, in turn, leads to an increase in serum creatinine. Increased efferent arteriole resistance, and increased glomerular capillary filtration coefficient would both tend to increase rather than reduce GFR. Increasing muscle mass due to exercise would cause very little change in serum creatinine.

  TMP12 314–316, 321

118. C) A 50% reduction in efferent arteriolar resistance would cause a large decrease in GFR, greater than 10%. A decrease in renal artery pressure from 100 to 85 mm Hg would cause only a slight decrease in GFR in a normal, autoregulating kidney. A decrease in afferent arteriole resistance, a decrease in plasma colloid osmotic pressure, or an increase in the glomerular capillary filtration coefficient would all tend to increase GFR.

  TMP12 314–316, 319, Figures 26-15 and 26-17

Blood Cells, Immunity, and Blood Coagulation

The following table of normal test values can be referenced throughout Unit VI.

Test	Normal Values
Bleeding time (template)	2–7 minutes
Erythrocyte count	Male: 4.3–5.9 million/μl^3
	Female: 3.5–5.5 million/μl^3
Hematocrit	Male: 41–53%
	Female: 36–46%
Hemoglobin, blood	Male: 13.5–17.5 g/dL
	Female: 12.0–16.0 g/dL
Mean corpuscular hemoglobin	25.4–34.6 pg/cell
Mean corpuscular hemoglobin concentration	31–36% Hb/cell
Mean corpuscular volume	80–100 fl
Reticulocyte count	0.5–1.5% of red cells
Platelet count	150,000–400,000/μl^3
Leukocyte count and differential	
Leukocyte count	4500–11,000/μl^3
Neutrophils	54–62%
Eosinophils	1–3%
Basophils	0–0.75%
Lymphocytes	25–33%
Monocytes	3–7%
Partial thromboplastin time (activated)	25–40 seconds
Prothrombin time	11–15 seconds
Bleeding time	2–7 minutes

1. During the second trimester of pregnancy, where is the predominant site of red blood cell production?

   A) Yolk sac
   B) Bone marrow
   C) Lymph nodes
   D) Liver

2. Following a blood donation, red cell production begins to increase in

   A) 30 minutes
   B) 24 hours
   C) 2 days
   D) 5 days
   E) 2 weeks

Questions 3–6

Which points in the following graph most closely define the following conditions? Normal erythropoietin (EPO) levels are approximately 10.

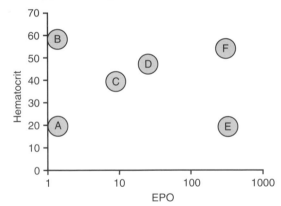

3. Olympic marathoner D
4. Aplastic anemia E
5. End-stage renal disease A
6. Polycythemia vera B

7. A 62-year-old female arrives for her annual physical. She complains of itching in her hands along with headaches and vertigo. A routine complete blood count (CBC) shows red blood cells (RBCs) of 8.2 million/μl, white blood cells (WBCs) 37,000/μl, and platelets 640,000/μl. Her erythropoietin levels are lower than normal. The primary diagnosis would be

   A) thrombocytopenia
   B) relative polycythemia
   C) secondary polycythemia
   D) polycythemia vera
   E) myeloid leukemia

8. A 40-year-old woman visits the clinic complaining of fatigue. She had recently been treated for an infection. Her laboratory values are RBC $1.8 \times 10^6/\mu l$, Hb 5.2 g/dL, hematocrit (Hct) 15, WBC $7.6 \times 10^3/\mu l$, platelet count $320,000/\mu l$, mean corpuscular volume (MCV) 92 fL, and reticulocyte count 24%. What is the most likely explanation for this presentation?

   A) Aplastic anemia
   B) Hemolytic anemia
   C) Hereditary spherocytosis
   D) B_{12} deficiency

9. Which of the following would describe the condition in a patient with aplastic anemia?

	Hct	Blood Hemoglobin	MCV	EPO
A)	↔	↔	↔	↔
B)	↔	↓	↓	↑
C)	↓	↓	↔	↑
D)	↓	↔	↔	↔
E)	↔	↔	↑	↑
F)	↓	↓	↑	↔
G)	↓	↔	↔	↑

10. A 34-year-old man with schizophrenia has had chronic fatigue for 6 months. He has a good appetite, but has refused to eat vegetables for 1 year because he hears voices saying that vegetables are poisoned. His physical and neurological examinations are normal. His hemoglobin level is 9.1 g/dL, leukocyte count is $10,000/\mu l^3$, and MCV is 122. Which of the following is the most likely diagnosis?

   A) Acute blood loss
   B) Sickle cell
   C) Aplastic anemia
   D) Hemolytic anemia
   E) Folic acid deficiency

11. A 24-year-old African-American man comes to the emergency room 3 hr after the onset of severe back and chest pain. These problems started while he was skiing. He lives in Los Angeles and had a previous episode of these symptoms 5 years ago while visiting Wyoming. He is in obvious pain. Laboratory studies show the following:

Hemoglobin	11 gm/dl
Leukocyte count	$22,000/\mu l^3$
Reticulocyte count	25%

   What is the diagnosis of this patient?

   A) Acute blood loss
   B) Sickle cell anemia
   C) Anemia of chronic disease
   D) End-stage renal disease

12. A 62-year-old man complains of headaches, visual difficulties, and chest pains. His examination shows a red complexion and a large spleen. His complete blood count follows: hematocrit, 58%, WBC $13,300/\mu l$, and platelets $600,000/\mu l$. His arterial oxygen saturation is 97% on room air. Which of the following would you recommend as a treatment?

   A) Chemotherapy
   B) Phlebotomy
   C) Iron supplement
   D) Inhaled oxygen therapy

13. A 45-year-old woman developed fatigue in July and had blood counts that were reported to be normal. She was hospitalized because of a very severe headache in December, and was found to have a blood pressure of 175/90. Her laboratory values were as follows: hemoglobin (8.3 g/dL), RBC count ($2.2 \times 10^6/\mu l$), Hct (23%), MCV (89 fL), WBCs ($5100/\mu l$), platelets ($262 \times 10^3/\mu l$), and reticulocyte count 0.8%. What is the diagnosis for this patient?

   A) Folic acid deficiency
   B) Iron deficiency
   C) Hemolytic anemia
   D) End-stage renal disease

14. A 38-year-old healthy female comes to you for a routine visit. She has spent the last 2 months hiking through the Himalayas and climbed to the base camp of Mount Everest. Which of the following would you expect to see on her CBC (complete blood count)?

	Hct	RBC count	WBC count	MCV
A)	↑	↑	↑	↑
B)	↑	↑	↔	↑
C)	↑	↑	↔	↔
D)	↑	↔	↔	↔
E)	↔	↑	↑	↔
F)	↑	↔	↑	↑
G)	↔	↑	↔	↑

15. A patient presents to your office complaining of extreme fatigue and shortness of breath on exertion that has gradually worsened over the past 2 weeks. On physical examination, you observe a well-nourished woman who appears comfortable but somewhat short of breath. Her vital signs include a pulse of 120, respiratory rate of 20, and blood pressure of 120/70. When she stands up her pulse increases to 150 and her blood pressure falls to 80/50. Her hematologic values are Hgb 7 g/dL, Hct 20%, RBC count $2 \times 10^6/\mu l$, platelet count of $400,000/\mu l$. On a peripheral smear, her RBCs are microcytic and hypochromic. What would be your diagnosis of this patient?

   A) Aplastic anemia
   B) Renal failure
   C) Iron deficiency anemia
   D) Sickle cell anemia
   E) Megaloblastic anemia

16. After a person is placed in an atmosphere with low oxygen, how long does it take before there are increased numbers of reticulocytes?

    A) 6 hours
    B) 12 hours
    C) 3 days
    D) 5 days
    E) 2 weeks

17. Over the past 12 weeks, a 75-year-old man with a moderate aortic stenosis has developed shortness of breath and chest pains during exertion. He appears pale. Test of his stool for blood is positive. Laboratory studies show the following: hemoglobin 7.2 g/dL, and mean corpuscular volume 75. A blood smear shows microcytic, hypochromic erythrocytes. Which of the following is the most likely diagnosis?

    A) Vitamin B_{12} deficiency
    B) Autoimmune hemolytic anemia
    C) Folate deficiency anemia
    D) Iron deficiency anemia

18. A 24-year-old man came into the ER with a broken leg. A blood test was ordered and his WBC count was $22 \times 10^3/\mu l$. Five hours later, a second blood test resulted in values of $7 \times 10^3/\mu l$. What is the cause of the increased WBC count with the first test?

    A) Increased production of WBC by the bone marrow
    B) Shift of WBCs from the marginated pool to the circulating pool
    C) Decreased destruction of WBCs
    D) Increased production of selectins

19. Adhesion of white blood cells to the endothelium is

    A) due to a decrease in selectins
    B) dependent on activation of integrins
    C) due to the inhibition of histamine release
    D) greater on the arterial than venous side of the circulation

20. During an inflammatory response, which is the correct order for cellular events?

    A) Filtration of monocytes from blood, increased production of neutrophils, activation of tissue macrophages, infiltration of neutrophils from the blood
    B) Activation of tissue macrophages, infiltration of neutrophils from the blood, infiltration of monocytes from blood, increased production of neutrophils
    C) Increased production of neutrophils, activation of tissue macrophages, infiltration of neutrophils from the blood, infiltration of monocytes from blood
    D) Infiltration of neutrophils from the blood, activation of tissue macrophages, infiltration of monocytes from blood, increased production of neutrophils

21. In a normal healthy person, which of the following blood components has the shortest life span?

    A) Macrophages
    B) Memory T cells
    C) Erythrocytes
    D) Memory B lymphocytes

22. A 45-year-old man presents to the emergency room with a 2-week history of diarrhea that has gotten progressively worse over the last several days. He has minimal urine output and is admitted to the hospital for dehydration. His stool specimen is positive for parasitic eggs. Which type of WBCs would have an elevated number?

    A) Eosinophils
    B) Neutrophils
    C) T lymphocytes
    D) B lymphocytes
    E) Monocytes

23. An 8-year-old male is frequently coming to the clinic for persistent skin infections that do not heal within a normal time frame. He had a normal recovery from the measles. Checking his antibodies following immunizations yielded normal antibody responses. A defect in which of the following cells would most like be the cause of the continual infections?

    A) B lymphocytes
    B) Plasma cells
    C) Neutrophils
    D) Macrophages
    E) CD4 T lymphocytes

24. Where does the transmigration of WBCs occur in response to infectious agents?

    A) Arterioles
    B) Lymphatic ducts
    C) Venules
    D) Inflamed arteries

25. A 65-year-old alcoholic developed chest pain and cough with an expectoration of sputum. A blood sample revealed that his white blood cell count was $42,000/\mu l$. What is the origin of these WBCs?

    A) Pulmonary alveoli
    B) Bronchioles
    C) Bronchi
    D) Trachea
    E) Bone marrow

26. A 26-year-old man received a paper cut. What substance is the major cause of pain of this acute inflammatory response?

    A) Platelet-activating factor (PAF)
    B) Bradykinin
    C) Interleukin-1
    D) Tumor necrosis factor (TNF)

27. A patient visits his dentist, who notices a sore on the patient's lip. The sore was unusual in that there was no pain or drainage from the sore. The patient was subsequently admitted to the hospital with a violent shaking chill. His lab values were Hct 30%, platelets 400,000/μl, WBC 4200/μl, 68% lymphocytes, and 20% neutrophils. What is the diagnosis of this patient?

    A) A mild, nontreatable, infection
    B) Agranulocytosis
    C) Aplastic anemia
    D) Acute leukemia

28. What occurs following activation of basophils?

    A) Decreased diapedesis of neutrophils
    B) Decreased ameboid motion
    C) Contraction of blood vessels
    D) Increased capillary permeability

29. Fluid exudation into the tissue in the acute inflammatory reaction is due to

    A) decreased blood pressure
    B) decreased protein in the interstitium
    C) obstruction of the lymph vessels
    D) increased clotting factors
    E) increased vascular permeability

30. Which of the following applies to AIDS patients?

    A) Able to generate a normal antibody response
    B) Increased helper T cells
    C) Increased secretion of interleukins
    D) Decrease in helper T cells

31. Presentation of antigen on MHC-I by a cell will result in

    A) generation of antibodies
    B) activation of cytotoxic T cells
    C) increase in phagocytosis
    D) release of histamine by mast cells

32. What is the term for adhesion of an invading microbe with IgG and complement to facilitate recognition?

    A) Chemokinesis
    B) Opsonization
    C) Phagolysosome fusion
    D) Signal transduction

33. Interleukin-2 (IL-2) is an important molecule in the immune response. What is the function of IL-2?

    A) Binds to and presents antigen
    B) Stimulates proliferation of cytotoxic T cells
    C) Kills virus-infected cells
    D) Is required for replication of helper T cells

34. CD4 is a marker of

    A) B cells
    B) Cytotoxic T cells
    C) Helper T cells
    D) An activated macrophage
    E) A neutrophil precursor

35. What will occur following presentation of antigen by a macrophage?

    A) Direct generation of antibodies
    B) Activation of cytotoxic T cells
    C) Increase in phagocytosis
    D) Activation of helper T cells

36. Activation of the complement system results in which of the following actions?

    A) Binding of the invading microbe with IgG
    B) Inactivation of eosinophils
    C) Decreased tissue levels of complement
    D) Generation of chemotaxic substances

37. A 9-year-old female has nasal discharge and itching of the eyes in the spring every year. An allergist performs a skin test using a mixture of grass pollens. Within a few minutes she develops a focal redness and a swelling at the test site. This response is most likely due to

    A) antigen–antibody complexes being formed in blood vessels in the skin
    B) activation of neutrophils due to injected antigens
    C) activation of CD4 helper cells and the resultant generation of specific antibodies
    D) activation of cytotoxic T lymphocytes to destroy antigens

38. Which of the following applies to cytotoxic T cells?

    A) Cytotoxic T cells require the presence of a competent B-lymphocyte system
    B) Cytotoxic T cells require the presence of a competent suppressor T-lymphocyte system
    C) Cytotoxic T cells are activated by the presentation of antigen by an infected cell
    D) Cytotoxic T cells destroy bacteria by initiating macrophage phagocytosis

39. Helper T cells

    A) are activated by the presentation of antigen by an infected cell
    B) require the presence of a competent B-cell system
    C) destroy bacteria by phagocytosis
    D) are activated by the presentation of antigen by macrophage or dendritic cells

40. Which of the following transfusions will result in an immediate transfusion reaction?

    A) O Rh− whole blood to an O Rh+ patient
    B) A Rh− whole blood to a B Rh− patient
    C) AB Rh− whole blood to an AB Rh+ patient
    D) B Rh− whole blood to an B Rh− patient

41. Which of the following is a TRUE statement?

   A) In a transfusion reaction, there is agglutination of the recipient blood

   B) Shutdown of the kidneys following a transfusion reaction occurs slowly

   C) Blood transfusion of Rh+ blood into any Rh− recipient will result in an immediate transfusion reaction

   D) A person with type AB blood is considered to be a universal recipient

42. Which blood type is depicted in the following figure?

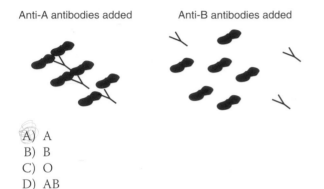

Anti-A antibodies added   Anti-B antibodies added

   A) A
   B) B
   C) O
   D) AB

43. A couple requests blood typing of their 2-year-old child (father AB, Rh-negative; mother B, Rh-negative). Results of hemagglutination assays of the child's blood are shown in the next figure. Which of the following conclusions concerning the child's parentage is valid?

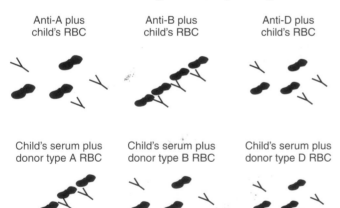

Anti-A plus   Anti-B plus   Anti-D plus
child's RBC   child's RBC   child's RBC

Child's serum plus   Child's serum plus   Child's serum plus
donor type A RBC   donor type B RBC   donor type D RBC

   A) The child could be the natural offspring of this couple
   B) The mother could be the natural mother, but the father could not be the natural father
   C) The father could be the natural father, but the mother could not be the natural mother
   D) Neither the father nor the mother could be the natural parents

44. A 21-year-old female, blood type B, is undergoing surgery. Her platelet count is 75,000/μl. She will need platelet infusions before and during surgery. Which of the following blood types would be used to collect platelets that are compatible with the patient?

   A) Type A only
   B) Type B only
   C) Type O only
   D) Types B and O
   E) Types A and B
   F) Types A and B only
   G) Types A, B, and AB only

45. Which of the following is TRUE concerning erythroblastosis fetalis (hemolytic disease of the newborn, HDN)?

   A) This occurs when a Rh+ mother has an Rh− child
   B) This is prevented by giving the mother a blood transfusion
   C) A complete blood transfusion after the first birth will prevent HDN
   D) The father of the child has to be Rh+

46. Which of the following will result in a transfusion reaction? Assume that the patient has never had a transfusion.

   A) Type O Rh− packed cells to an AB Rh+ patient
   B) Type A Rh+ packed cells to an A Rh− patient
   C) Type AB Rh+ packed cells to an AB Rh+ patient
   D) Type A Rh+ packed cells to an O Rh+ patient

47. A mother of blood type A+ who has always been perfectly healthy just delivered her second child. The father is of blood group O−. Knowing that the child is of blood group O− (O, Rh−), what would you expect to find in this child?

   A) The child will suffer from erythroblastosis fetalis due to rhesus incompatibility
   B) The child will suffer from erythroblastosis fetalis due to ABO blood group incompatibility
   C) The child will suffer from both A and B
   D) The child has no chance of developing HDN

48. Which of the following blood units carries the least risks for inducing an immediate transfusion reaction into a B+ (B, rhesus positive) recipient?

   A) Whole blood A+
   B) Whole blood O+
   C) Whole blood AB+
   D) Packed red cells O+
   E) Packed red cells AB−

49. A pregnant woman comes in for a visit. She is AB Rh− and her husband is A Rh+. This is her first child. What should be done at this time?

   A) Nothing
   B) Administer anti-D immunoglobulin to the mother at this time
   C) Administer anti-D immunoglobulin to the mother after delivery
   D) Administer anti-D immunoglobulin to the child after delivery
   E) Administer anti-D immunoglobulin to the child if the child is Rh+

50. What is the proper pathway for the extrinsic clotting pathway?

 A) Contact of blood with collagen, formation of pro-thrombin activator, conversion of prothrombin into thrombin, conversion of fibrinogen into fibrin threads
 B) Tissue trauma, formation of prothrombin activator, conversion of prothrombin into thrombin, conversion of fibrinogen into fibrin threads
 C) Activation of platelets, formation of prothrombin activator, conversion of prothrombin into thrombin, conversion of fibrinogen into fibrin threads
 D) Trauma to the blood, formation of prothrombin activator, conversion of prothrombin into thrombin, conversion of fibrinogen into fibrin threads

51. What condition leads to a deficiency in factor IX that can be corrected by an intravenous injection of vitamin K?

 A) Classic hemophilia
 B) Hepatitis B
 C) Bile duct obstruction
 D) Genetic deficiency in antithrombin III

52. A patient suffers from a congenital deficiency in factor XIII (fibrin-stabilizing factor). What would analysis of his blood reveal?

 A) Prolonged prothrombin time
 B) Prolonged whole blood clotting time
 C) Prolonged partial thromboplastin time
 D) Easily breakable clot

53. A 2-year-old boy bruises easily and has previously had bleeding gums. The maternal grandfather has a bleeding disorder. His physical examination shows several small bruises on the legs. Of which coagulation factor would you suspect this patient to be deficient?

 A) Prothrombin activator
 B) Factor II
 C) Factor VIII
 D) Factor X

54. An 11-year-old premenstrual female presents with a painful knee after mild trauma. Upon further evaluation you observe soft tissue bruises. The child is an orphan and there is no family history. The foster mother reports no other problems. The aPTT is prolonged and the PT is normal. A complete hematologic workup would yield

 A) decreased plasma Ca^{2+}
 B) elevated plasmin
 C) lack of factor VIII
 D) decreased platelet number

55. The coagulation pathway that begins with tissue thromboplastin is

 A) extrinsic pathway
 B) intrinsic pathway
 C) common pathway
 D) fibrin stabilization

56. A 63-year-old woman returned to work following a vacation in New Zealand. Several days after returning home, she awoke with swelling and pain in her right leg and her leg was blue. She went immediately to the emergency room where an examination showed an extensive deep vein thrombosis involving the femoral and iliac veins on the right side. Following resolution of the clot, this patient will require which treatment in the future?

 A) Continual heparin infusion
 B) Warfarin
 C) Aspirin
 D) Vitamin K

57. Which of the following would most likely be used for prophylaxis of transient ischemic heart attack?

 A) Heparin
 B) Warfarin
 C) Aspirin
 D) Streptokinase

58. Which of the following would be appropriate therapy for massive pulmonary embolism?

 A) Heparin
 B) Warfarin
 C) Aspirin
 D) Tissue plasminogen activator

59. Which of the following would best explain a prolonged bleeding time test?

 A) Hemophiliac A
 B) Hemophilia B
 C) Thrombocytopenia
 D) Coumarin use

60. Why do some malnourished patients bleed excessively when injured?

 A) Vitamin K deficiency
 B) Platelet sequestration by fatty liver
 C) Serum bilirubin raises neutralizing thrombin
 D) Low serum-protein levels cause factor XIII problems

61. A teenaged boy with numerous nosebleeds was referred to a physician for evaluation prior to a minor surgery. His prothrombin time (PT) was 11 sec (11–15 sec normal), partial thromboplastin time (PTT) was 58 sec (25–40 sec normal), and bleeding time was 6.5 min (2–7 min normal). Which of the following is most likely abnormal in this young man?

 A) Decreased platelet number
 B) Defective platelets
 C) Intrinsic pathway
 D) Extrinsic pathway
 E) Production of clotting factors by the liver

1. **D)** Red blood cell production begins in the yolk sac for the first trimester. Production in the yolk sac decreases at the beginning of the second trimester and the liver becomes the predominate source of red cell production. During the third trimester red cell production increases from the bone marrow and continues throughout life.
   TMP12 414

2. **B)** Red cell production increases rapidly within 24 hours; however, new red cells do appear in the blood for 5 days.
   TMP12 416

3. **D)** A well-trained athlete will have a slightly elevated EPO level and the hematocrit will be elevated up to a value of 50%. A hematocrit higher than 50% suggests EPO treatment.
   TMP12 416

4. **E)** Aplastic anemia is a condition in which the bone marrow has a decreased production but does not respond to erythropoietin. Therefore, a person with aplastic anemia would have a low hematocrit and an elevated erythropoietin level.
   TMP12 420

5. **A)** With end-stage renal disease there is a decrease in erythropoietin level due to decreased release from the diseased kidneys. As a consequence of the decreased erythropoietin level, the hematocrit will be decreased.
   TMP12 416

6. **B)** With polycythemia vera the bone marrow produces red blood cells without a stimulus from erythropoietin. The hematocrit is very high, even up to 60%. With the elevated hematocrit there is a feedback suppression of erythropoietin and the erythropoietin levels are very low.
   TMP12 421

7. **D)** The increase in RBC, WBC, and platelets suggests that the patient is suffering from polycythemia vera. Renal disease would result in a low EPO level, but the RBC count would be low. Myeloid leukemia would result in an increase in WBCs, with no increase in RBCs. Secondary polycythemia would have an elevated EPO level. Relative is due to dehydration.
   TMP12 421

8. **B)** This patient has decreased production of red blood cells as confirmed by the anemia (low number, Hb, and Hct), yet the red blood cells being produced have a normal size, MCV = 90. Therefore, the patient does not have spherocytosis (small red cells) or vitamin B_{12} deficiency (large red cells). The normal WBC count and the increased reticulocyte count suggest that the bone marrow is functioning. The increased reticulocyte count means that a large number of red cells are being produced. These laboratory values support an anemia due to some type of blood loss; in this case an anemia due to hemolysis.
   TMP12 420

9. **C)** With aplastic anemia the person has minimal or no red cell production. The Hct and hemoglobin would be low, the MCV would be normal (normal red cells just low production), and an elevated EPO level.
   TMP12 420

10. **E)** This patient is anemic: Hg < 14 g/dL. White count is normal, suggesting a normal bone marrow. His red cells are considerably larger than normal (normal MCV = 90). His lack of vegetable consumption suggests either a vitamin B_{12} or folic acid deficiency. However, the body has sufficient stores of vitamin B_{12} to last 4 to 5 years, so he does not appear to have vitamin B_{12} deficiency. The body only stores folic acid for 3 to 6 months, so 1 year of not eating vegetables would result in a folic acid deficiency.
    TMP12 417, 420

11. **B)** This African-American man has anemia as seen by his decreased hemoglobin concentration and his elevated reticulocyte count. He has some infectious/inflammatory response as seen with the elevated white count. The high altitude was the stimulus for a hypoxic episode that caused sickling of his red cells. This patient has sickle cell anemia.
    TMP12 418, 420

12. **B)** This patient has polycythemia vera: increased RBCs, WBCs, and platelets. His increased Hct also increases the viscosity of the blood resulting in increased afterload for the heart. This is probably the reason for his chest pain. Thus, a phlebotomy (bleeding) is needed to decrease his elevated blood count.
    TMP12 421

13. **D)** This patient is anemic, but the RBCs being produced are normal (note normal MCV). The overall production of the RBCs is decreased (reticulocyte

count is low). WBCs and platelets are normal, suggesting a normal bone marrow. Folic acid and iron deficiency anemia would result in a lower RBC MCV. Hemolytic anemia would result in an increase reticulocyte count. The elevated blood pressure provides evidence of renal disease. This patient has end-stage renal disease and decreased erythropoietin production.
   TMP12 416

14. **C)** She has developed secondary polycythemia due to exposure to low oxygen. She will have increased HCT, and thus increased RBC count, but normal WBC count. The cells are normal so the MCV will be normal.
   TMP12 421

15. **C)** The blood count values show that the patient is anemic. Her bone marrow is functioning and she has a normal platelet count, but is generating a decreased number of abnormal RBCs. The microcytic (small), hypochromic (decreased intracellular hemoglobin) is a classic description of iron deficiency anemia. With renal failure the patient would be anemic with normal RBCs. Sickle cell anemia has misshapen RBCs. Megaloblastic anemia is characterized by macrocytic (large) RBCs.
   TMP12 418

16. **C)** Erythropoietin levels increase following a decreased arterial oxygen level with the maximum erythropoietin production occurring within 24 hours. It takes 5 days for the production of new erythrocytes. However, since it takes 1–2 days for a reticulocyte to become an erythrocyte, the correct answer is 3 days until there are an increased number of reticulocytes.
   TMP12 414-416

17. **D)** This patient is anemic and has low hemoglobin with small red cells. Vitamin B_{12} and folic acid deficiency will result in macrocytic red blood cells. His WBC and platelet counts are normal, suggesting a normal bone marrow. The positive stool shows a gastrointestinal blood loss. A person can be anemic from a blood loss and have normal-sized RBCs as long as there is enough iron in the body. The microcytic and hypochromic RBCs are classic signs of iron deficient anemia.
   TMP12 417-417

18. **B)** The majority of WBCs are stored in the bone marrow, waiting for an increased level of cytokines to stimulate the release from the bone marrow. However, trauma to bone can result in a release of WBCs into the circulation. This increase in WBC count is not due to any inflammatory response, but instead to mechanical trauma.
   TMP12 424

19. **B)** Activation of selections or integrins results in adhesion of white cells to endothelium.
   TMP12 425, 429

20. **B)** The first cellular event during an inflammatory state is activation of the tissue macrophages. Then there is invasion of neutrophils and monocytes in that order, and finally there is an increase in production of WBCs by the bone marrow.
   TMP12 428

21. **C)** Macrophages last for many years. T- and B-memory cells will last the life of the patient. Erythrocytes last about 120 days and then are destroyed during passage through the spleen.
   TMP12 424

22. **A)** Eosinophils constitute about 2% of the total WBC count, but are produced in large numbers in people with parasitic infections.
   TMP12 430

23. **C)** For the acquired immune response, T and B lymphocytes, and plasma cells, along with macrophages are needed. Basophils are not required to fight mild infections. Neutrophils are needed for routine infections.
   TMP12 428-429

24. **C)** Transmigration of WBCs occurs through parts of the vasculature that have very thin walls and minimal vascular smooth muscle layers. This includes capillaries and venules.
   TMP12 425, 429

25. **E)** All white blood cells originate from the bone marrow from myelocytes or lymphocytes.
   TMP12 424

26. **B)** There are several factors that can cause pain and initiate pain. These include histamine, bradykinin, and prostaglandins. PAF activates platelets during the clotting process. Interleukin and TNF are factors involved in the inflammatory response and control of macrophages.
   TMP12 428

27. **B)** The patient has a slightly decreased red cell count and normal platelet count. This would suggest that the bone marrow is working properly. His white count is within the normal range, but the percentage of cells is not normal. He should have 60% neutrophils. The 66% lymphocytes (30% normal value) would suggest that the patient has an acute leukemia.
   TMP12 431

28. **D)** Basophils release heparin, histamine, and a series of activating factors. The histamine acts to increase capillary permeability while the heparin prevents clotting. Substances released from basophils also attract neutrophils and increase capillary permeability.
   TMP12 431

29. **E)** Fluid leaks into the tissue due to an increase in capillary permeability.
TMP12 428

30. **D)** Helper T cells are destroyed by the AIDS virus, leaving the patient unprotected against infectious diseases.
TMP12 440

31. **B)** Presentation of an antigen on an infected cell will result in activation of the cytotoxic T cells to kill the infected cell. Presentation of an antigen by macrophages will activate helper T cells, leading to antibody formation.
TMP12 441

32. **B)** One of the products of the complement cascade activates phagocytosis of the bacteria to which the antigen-antibody complex is attached. This is called opsonization.
TMP12 439

33. **B)** Interleukin-2 (IL-2) is secreted by helper T cells when the T cells are activated by specific antigens. IL-2 plays a specific role in the growth and proliferation of both cytotoxic and suppressor T cells.
TMP12 440–441

34. **C)** CD4 helper T cells recognize the MHC class II + peptide on the presenting cell. CD8 T cells recognize the MHC class I + peptide on the infected cell.
TMP12 440

35. **D)** Presentation of an antigen on the surface of macrophages or dendritic cells results in the activation of helper T cells. Activation of helper T cells then initiates the release of lymphokines that stimulate cytotoxic T-cell activation along with activation of B cells and the generation of antibodies.
TMP12 440–441

36. **D)** Activation of the complement system results in a series of actions. These include opsonization and phagocytosis by neutrophils, lysis of bacteria, agglutination of organisms, activation of basophils and mast cells, and chemotaxis. Fragment C5a of the complement system causes chemotaxis of neutrophils and macrophages.
TMP12 439

37. **A)** Since the person has demonstrated allergic reactions the initial reaction would be due to an antigen-antibody reaction, and the activation of the complement system. Influx of neutrophils, activation of T-helper cells, and sensitized lymphocytes would take some time.
TMP12 443

38. **C)** Cytotoxic cells act on infected cells when the cells have the appropriate antigen located on the surface. The cytotoxic T cells are stimulated by lymphokines

generated by activation of helper T cells. Cytotoxic T cells destroy an infected cell by releasing proteins that punch large holes in the membrane of the infected cells. There is no interaction between cytotoxic T cells and B cells.
TMP12 441

39. **D)** Helper T cells are activated by the presentation of antigens on the surface of antigen presenting cells. Helper T cells activate B cells to form antibodies, but B cells are not required for activation of helper T cells. Helper T cells help macrophages with phagocytosis but do not have the capability to phagocytize bacteria.
TMP12 440–441

40. **B)** Transfusion of Rh− blood into a Rh+ person with the same ABO type will not result in any reaction. Type A blood has A antigen on the surface and type B antibodies. Type B blood has B antigens and A antibodies. Therefore, transfusing A blood into a person with type B blood will cause the A antibodies in the type B person to react with the donor blood.
TMP12 445–448

41. **D)** The recipient blood has the larger amount of plasma and thus antibodies. These antibodies will act on the donor red blood cells. The donor's plasma will be diluted and have minimal effect on the recipient's red blood cells. With any antigen–antibody transfusion reaction there is a rapid breakdown of red blood cells, releasing hemoglobin into the plasma, which can cause rapid acute renal shutdown. Transfusion of Rh+ blood will only result in a transfusion reaction if the Rh− person has previously been transfused or exposed to Rh+ antibodies. A type AB person has no AB antibodies in their plasma, so they can receive any blood type.
TMP12 448

42. **A)** There is an antigen and antibody reaction between the anti-A antibodies and the red cells. There is no reaction between the anti-B antibodies and the red cells. Therefore the red cells have the A antigen and the cells must be type A.
TMP12 446-447

43. **A)** There is no antigen and antibody reaction between the anti-B antibodies and the red cells. There is a reaction between the anti-B antibodies and the red cells. Therefore the red cells have the B antigen and must be type B. There is no antigen and antibody reaction between the anti-D antibodies and the red cells. Therefore the red cells must be Rh-negative. The child is blood type B−. Since father is AB− and the mother is B−, the child could be B−.
TMP12 446–447

44. **B)** Since the plasma contains antibodies the wrong plasma could contain antibodies against the B antigen.

Therefore, he could receive B plasma (containing anti-A antibodies) or AB (containing neither anti-A or anti-B antibodies.)

TMP12 448

45. **D)** HDN occurs when an Rh− mother gives birth to a second Rh+ child. Therefore, the father has to be Rh+. The mother becomes sensitized to the Rh antigens following the birth of the first Rh+ child. HDN is prevented by treating the mother with antibodies against Rh antigen after the birth of each Rh+ child. This will destroy all fetal RBCs in the mother and prevent the mother from being sensitized to the Rh antigen. A complete blood transfusion of the mother would be required to prevent the formation of Rh antibodies, but this is impractical. A transfusion of the first child after the birth will not accomplish anything as the mother has been exposed to the Rh+ antigen during the birth process.

TMP12 447–448

46. **D)** Type O RBCs are considered to be universal donor blood. Reactions occur between the recipient's antibody and donor antigen as shown in the following table.

Donor	Donor Antigen	Recipient	Recipient Antibody	Reaction
O−	None	AB+	None	None
A+	A, Rh	A−	B	None
AB+	A, B, Rh	AB+	None	None
A+	A, Rh	O+	A, B	A (antigen) and A (antibody)

TMP12 445–447

47. **D)** HDN occurs when the mother is Rh−, the father is Rh+, resulting in an Rh− child. Since the child is O− and the father is Rh−, there is no chance of HDN.

TMP12 447-448

48. **D)** In any patient, transfusion of O-type packed cells will minimize a transfusion reaction since the antibodies will be removed with the plasma removal. If the Rh factor is matched, then this will also minimize transfusion reaction. Therefore, in a B+ patient, a B+ transfusion or an O+ transfusion will elicit no transfusion reaction.

TMP12 445–448

49. **A)** An Rh− mother will generate antibodies to the Rh+ red blood cells after the birth of the first child that is Rh+. In the scenario presented, the mother has not been exposed to Rh+ RBCs so she has not developed antibodies. However, after the birth of this child, and if the child is found to be Rh+, then anti-D immunoglobulin should be administered to the mother to destroy any fetal RBCs to which she has been exposed and to prevent her from forming antibodies to the Rh+ (D) antigen.

TMP12 447-448

50. **B)** The extrinsic pathway involves damage to the tissue, then the subsequent formation of prothrombin activator. Tissue trauma results in the release of tissue factor or tissue thromboplastin, which functions as a proteolytic enzyme. Tissue factor binding with factor VII results in an activation of factor X. There is a subsequent activation of prothrombin activator, conversion of prothrombin to thrombin, then the conversion of fibrinogen into fibrin threads. Activation of the extrinsic pathway is very fast because of the small number of enzymatic reactions.

TMP12 453–455

51. **C)** Hemophilia is due to a genetic loss of clotting factor VIII. Most clotting factors are formed in the liver. If a vitamin K injection will correct the problem, this implies that the liver is working fine, and that the patient does not have hepatitis. Vitamin K is a fat-soluble vitamin and is absorbed from the intestine along with fats. Bile secreted by the gallbladder is required for the absorption of fats. If the patient is deficient in vitamin K, then clotting deficiency can be corrected by an injection of vitamin K. Antithrombin II has no relationship to factor IX.

TMP12 457–458

52. **D)** Fibrin monomers polymerize to form a clot. To make a strong clot requires the presence of fibrin-stabilizing factor that is released from platelets within the clot. The other clotting tests determine the activation of extrinsic and intrinsic pathways or number of platelets.

TMP12 452, 454, 460–461

53. **C)** A young man with bleeding disorders and a history of bleeding disorders in the males of his family would lead one to suspect hemophilia A, a deficiency of factor VIII.

TMP12 458

54. **D)** Factor VIII is classical hemophilia which occurs in males. Plasma Ca^{2+} does not change. Plasminogen breaks up clots. The bruises suggest that there is abnormal platelet number or function.

TMP12 457-458, 460–461

55. **A)** The extrinsic pathway begins with the release of tissue thromboplastin in response to vascular injury or contact between traumatized extravascular tissue and blood. Tissue thromboplastin is composed of phospholipids from the membranes of tissue.

TMP12 455

56. **B)** This clot is due to stasis of blood flow in her venous circulation. Heparin is used for the prevention of a clot, but has to be infused. This anticoagulation occurs by heparin binding to antithrombin III and the subsequent inactivation of thrombin. A continuous heparin drip is impractical. Warfarin is used to inhibit

the formation of vitamin K clotting factors and would prevent the formation of any clot. Aspirin is used to prevent activation of platelets. The current clot is not due to activation of platelets. Vitamin K will be used to restore clotting factors that may be decreased after warfarin treatment. This patient has sufficient clotting factors as evidenced by her venous clot.
TMP12 459–460

57. **C)** Heparin is used for the prevention of a clot, but has to be infused. This occurs by binding to antithrombin III and the subsequent inactivation of thrombin. Warfarin is used to inhibit the formation of vitamin K clotting factors. Aspirin is used to prevent activation of platelets. Activation of platelets following exposure to an atherosclerotic plaque and the formation of a platelet plug will impede blood flow and result in an ischemic heart attack. Streptokinase is used to break down an already formed clot, which is appropriate therapy for a pulmonary embolus.
TMP12 459–460

58. **D)** Heparin is used for the prevention of a clot. This occurs by binding to antithrombin III and the subsequent inactivation of thrombin. Warfarin is used to inhibit the formation of vitamin K clotting factors. Aspirin is used to prevent activation of platelets. Streptokinase is used to break down an already formed clot, which is appropriate therapy for a pulmonary embolus.
TMP12 459

59. **C)** There are three major tests used to determine coagulation defects. Prothrombin time is used to test the extrinsic pathway and is based on the time required for the formation of a clot following the addition of tissue thromboplastin. Bleeding time following a small cut is used to test for several clotting factors, but is especially prolonged by a lack of platelets.
TMP12 460

60. **A)** The clotting factors are formed in the liver and require vitamin K. Vitamin K is a fat-soluble vitamin and absorption is dependent on adequate fat digestion and absorption. Therefore, any state of malnutrition would have a decreased fat absorption, and results in decreased vitamin K absorption and decreased synthesis of clotting factors.
TMP12 457–458

61. **C)** The prothrombin time, test of extrinsic pathway, is the time required for clot formation following addition of tissue thromboplastin. This is normal so no problem with extrinsic. Partial thromboplastin time is a test of the intrinsic pathway. This is longer than normal so there is a problem with the intrinsic pathway. Bleeding time tests platelets, and since this is normal there is no problem with the platelets.
TMP12 460–461

1. A healthy, 45-year-old man is reading the newspaper. Which of the following muscles are used for quiet breathing?

   A) Diaphragm and external intercostals
   B) Diaphragm and internal intercostals
   C) Diaphragm only
   D) Internal intercostals and abdominal recti
   E) Scaleni
   F) Sternocleidomastoid muscles

2. A healthy, 25-year-old medical student participates in a 10-km charity run for the American Heart Association. Which of the following muscles does the student use (contract) during expiration?

   A) Diaphragm and external intercostals
   B) Diaphragm and internal intercostals
   C) Diaphragm only
   D) Internal intercostals and abdominal recti
   E) Scaleni
   F) Sternocleidomastoid muscles

3. The pleural pressure of a normal 56-year-old woman is approximately −5 cm H_2O during resting conditions immediately before inspiration (i.e., at functional residual capacity). What is the pleural pressure (in cm H_2O) during inspiration?

   A) +1
   B) +4
   C) 0
   D) −3
   E) −7

4. The alveolar pressure of a normal 77-year-old woman is approximately 1 cm H_2O during expiration. What is the alveolar pressure during inspiration (in cm H_2O)?

   A) +0.5
   B) +1
   C) +2
   D) 0
   E) −1
   F) −5

5. A man inspires 1000 ml from a spirometer. The intrapleural pressure was −4 cm H_2O before inspiration and −12 cm H_2O the end of inspiration. What is the compliance of the lungs?

   A) 50 ml/cm H_2O
   B) 100 ml/cm H_2O
   C) 125 ml/cm H_2O
   D) 150 ml/cm H_2O
   E) 250 ml/cm H_2O

6. The diagram above shows three different compliance curves (S, T, and U) for isolated lungs subjected to various transpulmonary pressures. Which of the following best describe the relative compliances for the three curves?

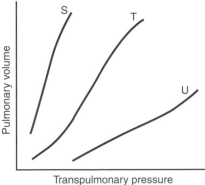

   A) S < T < U
   B) S < T > U
   C) S = T = U
   D) S > T < U
   E) S > T > U

7. A liquid-ventilated lung compared to a gas-ventilated lung

   A) has a reduced airway resistance
   B) has increased residual volume
   C) has a more pronounced hysteresis
   D) is more compliant
   E) requires greater pressure to inflate

8. A 22-year-old woman has a pulmonary compliance of 0.2 L/cm H_2O and a pleural pressure of −4 cm H_2O. What is the pleural pressure (in cm H_2O) when the woman inhales 1.0 L of air?

   A) −6
   B) −7
   C) −8
   D) −9
   E) −10

9. A preterm infant has a surfactant deficiency. Without surfactant, many of the alveoli collapse at the end of each expiration, which in turn leads to pulmonary failure. Which of the following sets of changes are present in the preterm infant, compared to a normal infant?

	Alveolar surface tension	Pulmonary compliance
A)	Decreased	Decreased
B)	Decreased	Increased
C)	Decreased	No change
D)	Increased	Decreased
E)	Increased	Increased
F)	Increased	No change
G)	No change	No change

10. A patient has a dead space of 150 ml, functional residual capacity of 3 L, tidal volume of 650 ml, expiratory reserve volume of 1.5 L, total lung capacity of 8 L, and respiratory rate of 15 breaths/min. What is the residual volume?

    A) 500 ml
    B) 1000 ml
    C) 1500 ml
    D) 2500 ml
    E) 6500 ml

Questions 11 and 12

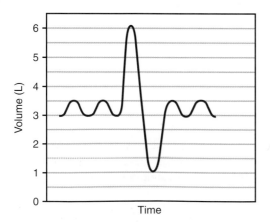

11. A 27-year-old man is breathing quietly. He then inhales as much air as possible and exhales as much air as he can, producing the spirogram shown in the previous figure. What is his expiratory reserve volume (in liters)?

    A) 2.0
    B) 2.5
    C) 3.0
    D) 3.5
    E) 4.0
    F) 5.0

12. A 22-year-old woman inhales as much air as possible and exhales as much air as she can producing the spirogram shown in the figure. A residual volume of 1.0 L was determined using the helium dilution technique. What is her functional residual capacity (in liters)?

    A) 2.0
    B) 2.5
    C) 3.0
    D) 3.5
    E) 4.0
    F) 5.0

13. The various lung volumes and capacities include the total lung volume (TLC), vital capacity (VC), inspiratory capacity (IC), tidal volume (VT), expiratory capacity (EC), expiratory reserve volume (ERV), inspiratory reserve volume (IRV), functional residual capacity (FRC), and residual volume (RV). Which of the following lung volumes and capacities can be measured using direct spirometry without additional methods?

	TLC	VC	IC	VT	EC	ERV	IRV	FRC	RV
A)	No	No	Yes	No	Yes	No	Yes	No	No
B)	No	Yes	Yes	Yes	Yes	Yes	Yes	No	No
C)	No	Yes	Yes	Yes	Yes	Yes	Yes	Yes	No
D)	Yes	Yes	Yes	Yes	Yes	Yes	Yes	No	Yes
E)	Yes	Yes	Yes	Yes	Yes	Yes	Yes	Yes	Yes

14. A patient has a dead space of 150 ml, functional residual capacity of 3 L, tidal volume of 650 ml, expiratory reserve volume of 1.5 L, a total lung capacity of 8 L, respiratory rate of 15 breaths/min. What is the alveolar ventilation?

    A) 5 L/min
    B) 7.5 L/min
    C) 6.0 L/min
    D) 9.0 L/min

15. At the end of inhalation, with an open glottis, the pleural pressure is

    A) greater than atmospheric pressure
    B) equal to atmospheric pressure
    C) less than alveolar pressure
    D) equal to alveolar pressure
    E) greater than alveolar pressure

16. An experiment is conducted in two individuals (subjects T and V) with identical tidal volumes (1000 ml), dead space volumes (200 ml), and ventilation frequencies (20 breaths per minute). Subject T doubles his tidal volume and reduces his ventilation frequency by 50%. Subject V doubles his ventilation frequency and reduces his tidal volume by 50%. Which of the following best described the total ventilation (also called minute ventilation) and alveolar ventilation of subjects T and V?

	Total ventilation	Alveolar ventilation
A)	T < V	T = V
B)	T < V	T > V
C)	T = V	T < V
D)	T = V	T = V
E)	T = V	T > V
F)	T > V	T < V
G)	T > V	T = V

17. A healthy 10-year-old boy breathes quietly under resting conditions. His tidal volume is 400 ml and ventilation frequency is 12/min. Which of the following best describes the ventilation of the upper, middle, and lower lung zones in this boy?

	Upper zone	Middle zone	Lower zone
A)	Highest	Lowest	Intermediate
B)	Highest	Intermediate	Lowest
C)	Intermediate	Lowest	Highest
D)	Lowest	Intermediate	Highest
E)	Same	Same	Same

18. A 34-year-old male sustains a bullet wound to the chest that causes a pneumothorax. Which of the following best describes the changes in lung volume and thoracic volume in this man, compared to normal?

	Lung volume	Thoracic volume
A)	Decreased	Decreased
B)	Decreased	Increased
C)	Decreased	No change
D)	Increased	Decreased
E)	Increased	Increased
F)	No change	Decreased

19. The resistance of the pulmonary tree is so low that a 1 cm of water pressure gradient is sufficient to cause normal air flow during resting conditions. Which of the following often has a substantial resistance during pulmonary disease states that can limit alveolar ventilation?

A) Alveoli
B) Bronchioles
C) Large bronchi
D) Small bronchi
E) Trachea

20. The following diagram shows pulmonary airway resistance expressed as a function of pulmonary volume. Which relationship best describes the normal lung?

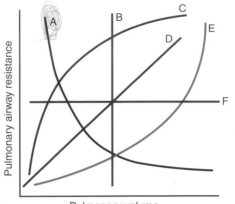

21. The respiratory passageways have smooth muscle in their walls. Which of the following best describes the effect of acetylcholine and epinephrine on the respiratory passageways?

	Acetylcholine	Epinephrine
A)	Constrict	Constrict
B)	Constrict	Dilate
C)	Constrict	No effect
D)	Dilate	Constrict
E)	Dilate	Dilate
F)	Dilate	No effect
G)	No effect	Constrict
H)	No effect	Dilate

22. A 67-year-old man is admitted as an emergency to University Hospital because of severe chest pain. A Swan-Ganz catheter is floated into the pulmonary artery, the balloon is inflated, and the pulmonary wedge pressure is measured. The pulmonary wedge pressure is used clinically to monitor which of the following pressures?

A) Left atrial pressure
B) Left ventricular pressure
C) Pulmonary artery diastolic pressure
D) Pulmonary artery systolic pressure
E) Pulmonary capillary pressure

23. Which of the following sets of differences best describes the hemodynamics of the pulmonary circulation when compared to the system circulation?

	Flow	Resistance	Arterial pressure
A)	Higher	Higher	Higher
B)	Higher	Lower	Lower
C)	Lower	Higher	Lower
D)	Lower	Lower	Lower
E)	Same	Higher	Lower
F)	Same	Lower	Lower

24. Which diagram best illustrates the pulmonary vasculature when the cardiac output has increased to a maximum extent?

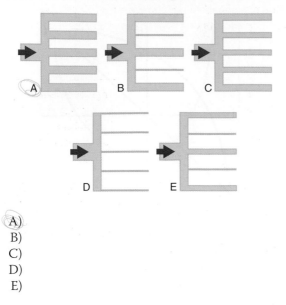

   (A)
   B)
   C)
   D)
   E)

25. A 30-year-old woman performs a valsalva maneuver about 30 min after eating lunch. Which of the following best describes the changes in pulmonary and systemic blood volumes that occur in this woman?

	Pulmonary volume	Systemic volume
A)	Decreases	Decreases
B)	Decreases	Increases
C)	Decreases	No change
D)	Increases	Decreases
E)	Increases	Increases
F)	Increases	No change
G)	No change	Decreases
H)	No change	Increases
I)	No change	No change

26. A 32-year-old man drives to the top of Pikes Peak where the oxygen tension is 85 mm Hg. Which of the following best describes the effects of a hypoxic environment on the pulmonary and systemic vascular resistances?

	Pulmonary vascular resistance	Systemic vascular resistance
A)	Decreases	Decreases
B)	Decreases	Increases
C)	Decreases	No change
D)	Increases	Decreases
E)	Increases	Increases
F)	Increases	No change
G)	No change	Decreases
H)	No change	Increases
I)	No change	No change

27. Going from a quiet, standing position to climbing a set of stairs, which of the following conditions will be present?

	Apical flow	Basal flow
A)	↑	↑
B)	↑	↓
C)	↓	↑
D)	↓	↓
E)	↑	↔
F)	↓	↔

28. A 65-year-old man with emphysema due to 34 years of cigarette smoking is admitted to hospital due to dyspnea. With further tests the mean pulmonary arterial pressure is determined to be 45 mm Hg at rest. He is hypoxic (Po_2 = 49 mm Hg), hypercapnic (85 mm Hg), and slightly acidotic. The cardiovascular and oxygen changes are due to which of the following?

   A) Increased arterial Pco_2
   B) Increased parasympathetic activity
   C) Decreased alveolar Po_2
   D) Decreased pH
   E) Decreased pulmonary resistance

29. Which of the following will decrease pulmonary blood flow resistance?

   A) IV injection of norepinephrine
   B) Inhalation to total lung capacity
   C) Breathing 5% O_2
   D) Having the lung at FRC

30. A 19-year-old man suffers a full-thickness burn over 60% of his body surface area. A systemic *Pseudomonas aeruginosa* infection occurs and severe pulmonary edema follows 7 days later. Data collected from the patient follow: plasma colloid osmotic pressure, 19 mm Hg; pulmonary capillary hydrostatic pressure, 7 mm Hg; and interstitial fluid hydrostatic pressure, 1 mm Hg. Which of the following sets of changes has occurred in the lungs of this patient as a result of the burn and subsequent infection?

	Lymph flow	Plasma colloid osmotic pressure	Pulmonary capillary permeability
A)	Decrease	Decrease	Decrease
B)	Increase	Decrease	Decrease
C)	Increase	Decrease	Increase
D)	Increase	Increase	Decrease
E)	Increase	Increase	Increase

31. A person's normal tidal volume is 400 ml with a dead space of 100 ml. The respiratory rate is 12 breaths/min. The person is placed on ventilator for surgery and the tidal volume is 700 with a rate of 12. What is the approximate alveolar P_{CO_2} for this person?

A) 10
B) 20
C) 30
D) 40
E) 45

32. The forces governing the diffusion of a gas through a biological membrane include the pressure difference across the membrane (ΔP), the cross-sectional area of the membrane (A), the solubility of the gas (S), the distance of diffusion (d), and the molecular weight of the gas (MW). Which of the following changes increases the diffusion of a gas through a biological membrane?

	ΔP	A	S	d	MW
A)	Increase	Increase	Increase	Increase	Increase
B)	Increase	Increase	Increase	Increase	Decrease
C)	Increase	Decrease	Increase	Decrease	Decrease
D)	Increase	Increase	Increase	Decrease	Increase
E)	Increase	Increase	Increase	Decrease	Decrease

33. A person with normal lungs at sea level (760 mm Hg) is breathing 50% oxygen. What is the approximate alveolar P_{O_2}?

A) 100
B) 159
C) 268
D) 330
E) 380

34. A child has been eating round candies approximately 1 and 1.5 cm in diameter and inhaled one down his airway blocking his left bronchiole. Which of the following will describe the changes that occur?

	Left lung alveolar P_{CO_2}	Left lung alveolar P_{O_2}	Systemic arterial P_{O_2}
A)	↑	↑	↔
B)	↑	↔	↑
C)	↓	↓	↓
D)	↑	↑	↑
E)	↑	↓	↓

35. During exercise, the oxygenation of blood is increased not only by increased alveolar ventilation but also by a greater diffusing capacity of the respiratory membrane for transporting oxygen into the blood. Which of the following sets of changes occur during exercise?

	Surface area of respiratory membrane	Ventilation-perfusion ratio
A)	Decrease	Improvement
B)	Increase	Improvement
C)	Increase	No change
D)	No change	Improvement
E)	No change	No change

36. The diffusing capacity of a gas is the volume of gas that will diffuse through a membrane each minute for a pressure difference of 1 mm Hg. Which of the following gases is often used to estimate the oxygen diffusing capacity of the lungs?

A) Carbon dioxide
B) Carbon monoxide
C) Cyanide gas
D) Nitrogen
E) Oxygen

37. A 23-year-old medical student has mixed venous oxygen and carbon dioxide tensions of 40 mm Hg and 45 mm Hg, respectively. A group of alveoli are not ventilated in this student because mucus blocks a local airway. What are the alveolar oxygen and carbon dioxide tensions distal to the mucus block (in mm Hg)?

	Carbon dioxide	Oxygen
A)	40	100
B)	40	40
C)	45	40
D)	50	50
E)	90	40

38. A 45-year-old man at sea level has an inspired oxygen tension of 149 mm Hg, nitrogen tension of 563 mm Hg, and water vapor pressure of 47 mm Hg. A small tumor pushes against a pulmonary blood vessel that completely blocks the blood flow to a small group of alveoli. What are the oxygen and carbon dioxide tensions of the alveoli that are not perfused (in mm Hg)?

	Carbon dioxide	Oxygen
A)	0	0
B)	0	149
C)	40	104
D)	47	149
E)	45	149

39. The O_2-CO_2 diagram here shows a ventilation-perfusion ratio line for the normal lung. Which of the following best describes the effect of decreasing ventilation-perfusion ratio on the alveolar P_{O_2} and P_{CO_2}?

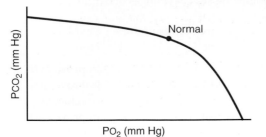

PCO₂ (mm Hg) — Normal — PO₂ (mm Hg)

	Carbon dioxide tension	Oxygen tension
A)	Decrease	Decrease
B)	Decrease	Increase
C)	Decrease	No change
D)	Increase	Decrease
E)	Increase	Increase

40. In which of the following conditions is alveolar P_{O_2} increased and alveolar P_{CO_2} decreased?

A) Increased alveolar ventilation and unchanged metabolism

B) Decreased alveolar ventilation and unchanged metabolism

C) Increased metabolism and unchanged alveolar ventilation

D) Proportional increase in metabolism and alveolar ventilation

Questions 41 and 42

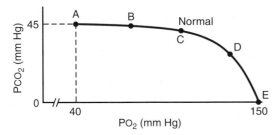

PCO₂ (mm Hg) — 45 — A — B — Normal — C — D — E — 0 — 40 — 150 — PO₂ (mm Hg)

41. A 67-year-old man has a solid tumor that pushes against an airway partially obstructing air flow to the distal alveoli. Which point on the ventilation-perfusion line of the O_2-CO_2 diagram corresponds to the alveolar gas of these distal alveoli?

A)
B)
C)
D)
E)

42. A 55-year-old male has a pulmonary embolism that partially blocks the blood flow to his right lung. Which point on the ventilation-perfusion line of the O_2-CO_2 diagram corresponds to the alveolar gas of his right lung?

A)
B)
C)
D)
E)

43. The following diagram shows a lung with a large shunt in which mixed venous bypasses the oxygen exchange areas of the lung. Breathing room air produces the oxygen partial pressures shown on the diagram. What is the oxygen tension of the arterial blood (in mm Hg) when the person breathes 100% oxygen and the inspired oxygen tension is over 600 mm Hg?

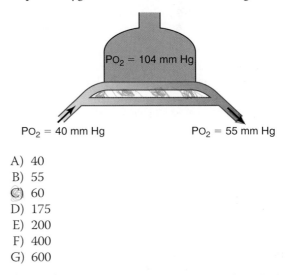

P_{O_2} = 104 mm Hg

P_{O_2} = 40 mm Hg P_{O_2} = 55 mm Hg

A) 40
B) 55
C) 60
D) 175
E) 200
F) 400
G) 600

44. The next diagram shows two lung units (S and T) with their blood supplies. Lung unit S has an ideal relationship between blood flow and ventilation. Lung unit T has a comprised blood flow. What is the relationship between alveolar dead space (D_{ALV}), physiologic dead space (D_{PHY}) and anatomic dead space (D_{ANAT}) for these lung units?

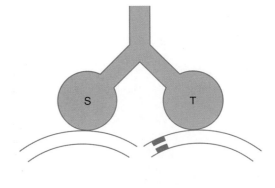

S   T

	Lung unit S	Lung unit T
A)	$D_{PHY} < D_{ANAT}$	$D_{PHY} = D_{ANAT}$
B)	$D_{PHY} = D_{ALV}$	$D_{PHY} > D_{ALV}$
C)	$D_{PHY} = D_{ANAT}$	$D_{PHY} < D_{ANAT}$
D)	$D_{PHY} = D_{ANAT}$	$D_{PHY} > D_{ANAT}$
E)	$D_{PHY} > D_{ANAT}$	$D_{PHY} < D_{ANAT}$

45. A 32-year-old medical student has a fourfold increase in cardiac output during strenuous exercise. Which of the curves on the following diagram most likely represents the changes in oxygen tension that occur as blood flows from the arterial end to the venous end of the pulmonary capillaries in this student?

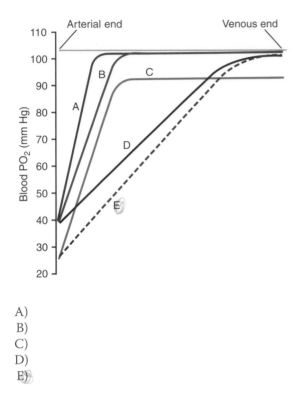

A)
B)
C)
D)
E)

46. The diagrams show changes in the partial pressures of oxygen and carbon dioxide as blood flows from the arterial end to the venous of the pulmonary capillaries. Which diagram best depicts the normal relationship between Po_2 (red line) and Pco_2 (green line) during resting conditions?

47. A 17-year-old female was bicycling without a helmet when she fell and hit her head. In the emergency room, she was not conscious and was receiving ventilator assistance. Her blood gases follow:

$PaO_2 = 52$ mm Hg,
$PaCO_2 = 75$ mm Hg, pH = 7.15, and
$HCO_3^- = 31$ mM

The majority of the CO_2 was being transported as

A) CO_2 bound to plasma proteins
B) CO_2 bound to hemoglobin
C) Bicarbonate ions
D) Dissolved

48. The following diagram shows a normal oxygen-hemoglobin dissociation curve. Which of the following are approximate values of hemoglobin saturation (% Hb-O_2), oxygen partial pressure (Po_2), and oxygen content (O_2 content) for oxygenated blood leaving the lungs and reduced blood returning to the lungs from the tissues?

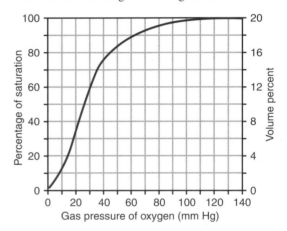

	Oxygenated blood			Reduced blood		
	% Hb-O_2	Po_2	O_2 content	% Hb-O_2	Po_2	O_2 content
A)	100	104	15	80	42	16
B)	100	104	20	30	20	6
C)	100	104	20	75	40	15
D)	90	100	16	60	30	12
E)	98	140	20	75	40	15

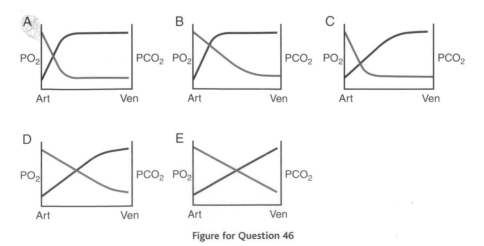

Figure for Question 46

49. Arterial P_{O_2} is 100 mm Hg and arterial P_{CO_2} is 40 mm Hg. Total blood flow to all muscle is 700 ml/min. There is a sympathetic activation resulting in a decrease in blood flow to 350 ml/min. Which of the following will occur?

	Venous P_{O_2}	Venous P_{CO_2}
A)	↑	↓
B)	↓	↑
C)	↓	↔
D)	↔	↑
E)	↑	↑
F)	↓	↓
G)	↔	↔

50. Which of the points on the following figures represent arterial blood in a severely anemic person?

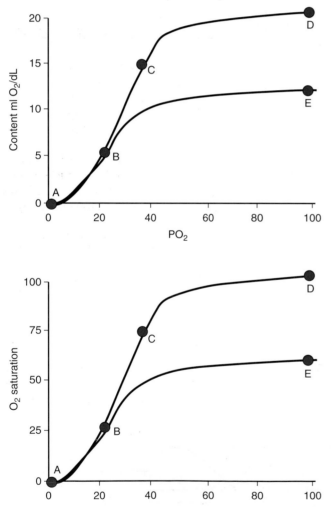

	Figure 1	Figure 2
A)	D	D
B)	E	E
C)	D	E
D)	E	D

51. A 34-year-old woman is anemic with a blood hemoglobin concentration of 7.1 g/dL. Which of the following sets of changes has occurred in this woman, compared to normal?

	Arterial P_{O_2}	Mixed venous P_{O_2}	2,3 diphophosphoglycerate
A)	Decreased	Decreased	Increased
B)	Decreased	Decreased	Normal
C)	Decreased	Normal	Decreased
D)	Increased	Decreased	Normal
E)	Increased	Increased	Increased
F)	Increased	Normal	Decreased
G)	Normal	Decreased	Decreased
H)	Normal	Decreased	Increased
I)	Normal	Normal	Normal

52. Which of the following oxygen-hemoglobin dissociation curves corresponds to normal blood (red line) and blood containing carbon monoxide (green line)?

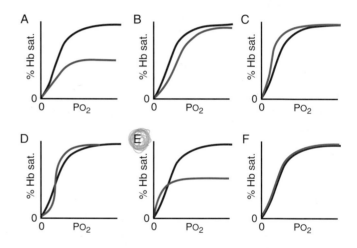

53. Which of the following oxygen-hemoglobin dissociation curves corresponds to blood during resting conditions (red line) and blood during exercise (green line)?

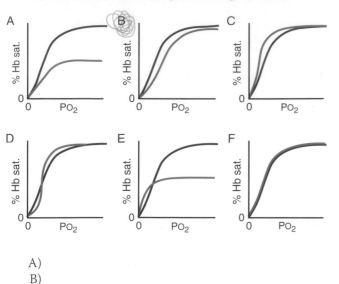

A)
B)
C)
D)
E)
F)

54. Which of the following oxygen-hemoglobin dissociation curves corresponds to blood from an adult (red line) and blood from a fetus (green line)?

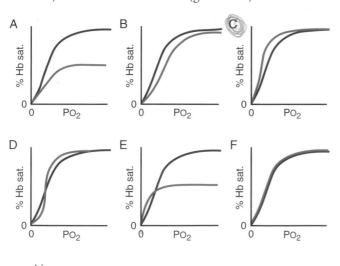

A)
B)
C)
D)
E)
F)

55. A person with anemia has a hemoglobin (Hb) concentration of 12 g/dL. He starts exercising and uses 12 ml O_2/dL. What is the mixed venous P_{O_2}?

   A) 0 mm Hg
   B) 10 mm Hg
   C) 20 mm Hg
   D) 40 mm Hg
   E) 100 mm Hg

56. Carbon dioxide is transported in the blood in the dissolved state, in the form of bicarbonate ion, and in combination with hemoglobin (carbaminohemoglobin). Which of the following best describes the quantitative relationship of these three mechanisms for transporting carbon dioxide in the venous blood under normal conditions (in percentages)?

	Dissolved state	Bicarbonate ion	Carbaminohemoglobin
A)	7	70	23
B)	70	23	7
C)	23	70	7
D)	7	23	70
E)	70	7	23
F)	23	7	70

57. A 26-year-old medical student on a normal diet has a respiratory exchange ratio of 0.8. How much oxygen and carbon dioxide are transported between the lungs and tissues of this student (in ml gas/100 ml blood)?

	Oxygen	Carbon dioxide
A)	4	4
B)	5	3
C)	5	4
D)	5	5
E)	6	3
F)	6	4

58. Carbon dioxide is transported from the tissues to the lungs predominantly in the form of bicarbonate ion. Compared to arterial red blood cells, which of the following best describes venous red blood cells?

	Intracellular chloride concentration	Cell volume
A)	Decreased	Decreased
B)	Decreased	Increased
C)	Decreased	No change
D)	Increased	Decreased
E)	Increased	No change
F)	Increased	Increased
G)	No change	Decreased
H)	No change	Increased
I)	No change	No change

59. The basic rhythm of respiration is generated by neurons located in the medulla. Which of the following limits the duration of inspiration and increases respiratory rate?

A) Apneustic center
B) Dorsal respiratory group
C) Nucleus of the tractus solitarius
D) Pneumotaxic center
E) Ventral respiratory group

60. When respiratory drive for increased pulmonary ventilation becomes greater than normal, a special set of respiratory neurons that are inactive during normal quiet breathing then becomes active, contributing to the respiratory drive. These neurons are located in which of the following structures?

A) Apneustic center
B) Dorsal respiratory group
C) Nucleus of the tractus solitarius
D) Pneumotaxic center
E) Ventral respiratory group

61. The Hering-Breuer inflation reflex is mainly a protective mechanism that controls ventilation under certain conditions. Which of the following best describes the effect of this reflex on inspiration and expiration as well as the location of the stretch receptors that initiate the reflex?

	Location of stretch receptors	Inspiration	Expiration
A)	Alveolar wall	No effect	Switches off
B)	Alveolar wall	Switches off	No effect
C)	Alveolar wall	Switches on	Switches on
D)	Bronchi/bronchioles	No effect	Switches off
E)	Bronchi/bronchioles	Switches off	No effect
F)	Bronchi/bronchioles	Switches on	Switches on
G.	Chest wall	No effect	Switches off
H.	Chest wall	Switches off	No effect
I.	Chest wall	Switches on	Switches on

62. At a fraternity party a 17-year-old male places a paper bag over his mouth and breathes in and out of the bag. As he continues to breathe into this bag, his rate of breathing continues to increase. Which of the following is responsible for the increased ventilation?

A) Increased alveolar P_{O_2}
B) Increased alveolar P_{CO_2}
C) Decreased arterial P_{CO_2}
D) Increased pH

63. Which of the following occurs with carbon monoxide inhalation?

	Alveolar P_{O_2}	Alveolar P_{CO_2}	Peripheral chemoreceptor activity
A)	↑	↔	↔
B)	↔	↔	↔
C)	↓	↔	↑
D)	↓	↓	↓
E)	↓	↓	↑
F)	↔	↓	↑

64. Which diagram best describes the relationship between alveolar ventilation (VA) and arterial carbon dioxide tension (P_{CO_2}) when the P_{CO_2} is changed acutely over a range of 35 to 75 mm Hg?

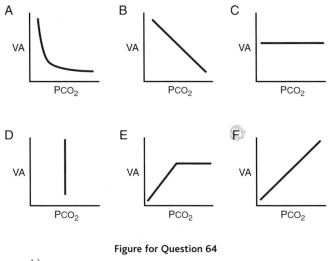

Figure for Question 64

A)
B)
C)
D)
E)
F)

65. Which diagram best describes the relationship between alveolar ventilation (VA) and arterial oxygen tension (P_{O_2}) when the P_{O_2} is changed acutely over a range of 0 to 160 mm Hg and the arterial P_{CO_2} and hydrogen ion concentration remain normal?

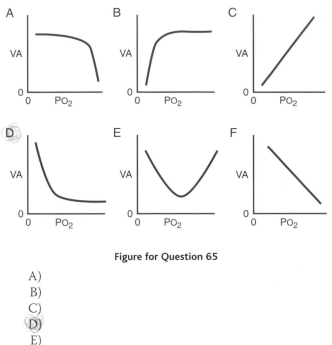

Figure for Question 65

A)
B)
C)
D)
E)
F)

66. An anesthetized male is breathing with no assistance. He is then artificially ventilated for 10 min at his normal tidal volume but at twice his normal frequency. He is ventilated with a gas mixture of 60% O_2 and 40% N_2. The artificial ventilation is stopped and he fails to breathe for several minutes. This apneic episode is due to which of the following?

A) High arterial P_{O_2} suppressing the activity of the peripheral chemoreceptors
B) Decrease in arterial pH suppressing the activity of the peripheral chemoreceptors
C) Low arterial P_{CO_2} suppressing the activity of the medullary chemoreceptors
D) High arterial P_{CO_2} suppressing the activity of the medullary chemoreceptors
B) Low arterial P_{CO_2} suppressing the activity of the peripheral chemoreceptors

67. In strenuous exercise, oxygen consumption and carbon dioxide formation can increase as much as 20-fold. Alveolar ventilation increases almost exactly in step with the increase in oxygen consumption. Which of the following best describes what happens to the mean arterial oxygen tension (P_{O_2}), carbon dioxide tension (P_{CO_2}) and pH in a healthy athlete during strenuous exercise?

	Arterial P_{O_2}	Arterial P_{CO_2}	Arterial pH
A)	Decreases	Decreases	Decreases
B)	Decreases	Increases	Decreases
C)	Increases	Decreases	Increases
D)	Increases	Increases	Increases
E)	No change	No change	No change

68. Alveolar ventilation increases several-fold during strenuous exercise. Which of the following factors is most likely to stimulate ventilation during strenuous exercise?

A) Collateral impulses from higher brain centers
B) Decreased mean arterial pH
C) Decreased mean arterial P_{O_2}
D) Decreased mean venous P_{O_2}
E) Increased mean arterial P_{CO_2}

69. The following diagram shows the depth of respiration of a 45-year-old man who suffered a head injury in an automobile accident. This "crescendo-decrescendo" pattern of breathing is called which of the following?

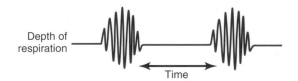

A) Apnea
B) Biot breathing
C) Cheyne-Stokes breathing
D) Hyperpnea
E) Tachypnea

70. Cheyne-Stokes breathing is an abnormal breathing pattern characterized by a gradual increase in the depth of breathing, followed by a progressive decrease in the depth of breathing that occurs again and again about every minute, as shown in the following diagram. Which of the following time points (V-Z) are associated with the highest Pco_2 of lung blood and highest Pco_2 of the neurons in the respiratory center?

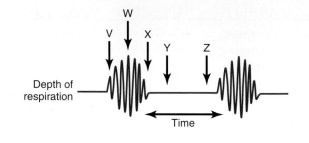

	Lung blood	Respiratory center
A)	V	V
B)	V	W
C)	W	W
D)	X	Z
E)	Y	Z

71. A 45-year-old man inhaled as much air as possible and then expired with a maximum effort until no more air could be expired. This produced the maximum expiratory flow-volume curve shown in the following diagram. What is the forced vital capacity of this man (in liters)?

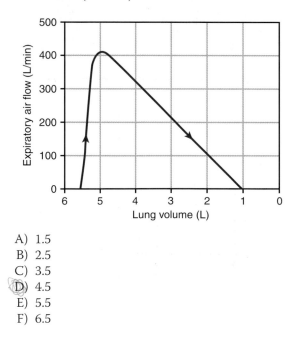

A) 1.5
B) 2.5
C) 3.5
D) 4.5
E) 5.5
F) 6.5

72. The maximum expiratory flow-volume curve shown in the following diagram is used as a diagnostic tool for identifying obstructive and restrictive lung diseases. At which of the following points on the curve does airway collapse limit maximum expiratory air flow?

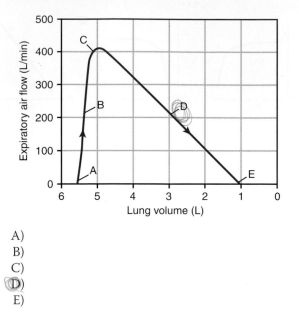

A)
B)
C)
D)
E)

73. The maximum expiratory flow-volume curves shown in the next diagram were obtained from a healthy individual (red curve) and a 57-year-old man who complains of shortness of breath (green curve). Which of the following disorders is most likely present in the man?

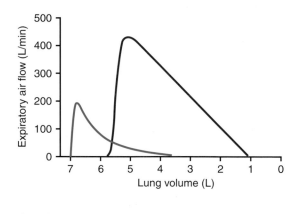

A) Asbestosis
B) Emphysema
C) Kyphosis
D) Scoliosis
E) Silicosis
F) Tuberculosis

74. A 62-year-old man complains to his physician that he has difficulty breathing. The following diagram shows a maximum expiratory flow-volume (MEFV) curve from the patient (green line) and from a typical healthy individual (red curve). Which of the following best explains the MEFV curve of the patient?

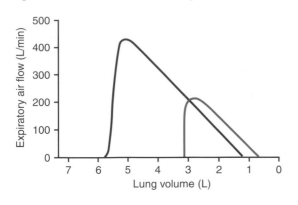

  A) Asbestosis
  B) Asthma
  C) Bronchospasm
  D) Emphysema
  E) Old age

75. The maximum expiratory flow-volume curve shown in the next diagram (red line) was obtained from a 75-year-old man who smoked 40 cigarettes per day for the past 60 years. The green flow-volume curve was obtained from the man during resting conditions. Which of the following sets of changes are most likely to apply to this man?

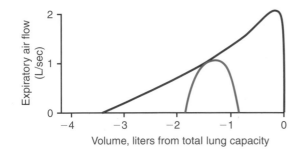

	Exercise tolerance	Total lung capacity	Residual volume
A)	Decreased	Decreased	Decreased
B)	Decreased	Increased	Increased
C)	Decreased	Normal	Normal
D)	Increased	Increased	Increased
E)	Normal	Decreased	Decreased

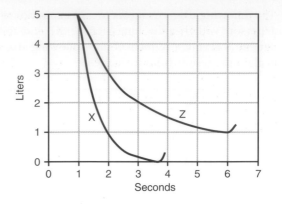

76. The diagram above shows a forced expiration for a healthy person (curve X) and a person with a pulmonary disease (curve Z). What is the FEV_1/FVC ratio (as a percent) in these individuals?

	Person X	Person Z
A)	80	50
B)	80	40
C)	100	80
D)	100	60
E)	90	50
F)	90	60

77. The next diagram shows forced expirations from a person with healthy lungs (curve X) and from a patient (curve Z). Which of the following is most likely present in the patient?

  A) Asthma
  B) Bronchospasm
  C) Emphysema
  D) Old age
  E) Silicosis

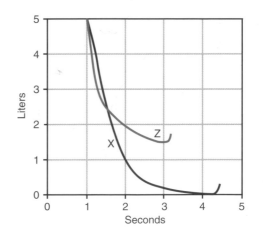

78. The following diagram shows forced expirations from a person with healthy lungs (curve X) and from a patient (curve Z). Which of the following can best explain the results from the patient?

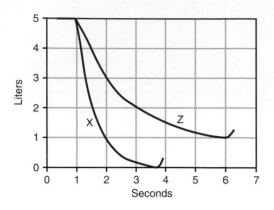

A) Asbestosis
B) Emphysema
C) Fibrotic pleurisy
D) Pleural effusion
E) Pneumothorax
F) Silicosis
G) Tuberculosis

79. The volume–pressure curves shown in the next diagram were obtained from a young, healthy subject and a patient. Which of the following best describes the condition of the patient?

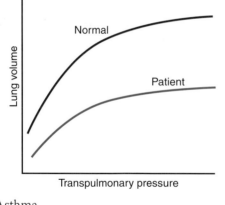

A) Asthma
B) Bronchospasm
C) Emphysema
D) Old age
E) Silicosis

80. The volume–pressure curves shown here were obtained from a normal subject and a patient suffering from a pulmonary disease. Which of the following abnormalities is most likely present in the patient?

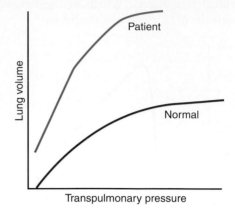

A) Asbestosis
B) Emphysema
C) Mitral obstruction
D) Rheumatic heart disease
E) Silicosis
F) Tuberculosis

81. A 34-year-old medical student generates the flow–volume curves shown in the next diagram. Curve W is a normal maximum expiratory flow–volume curve generated when the student was healthy. Which of the following can best explain curve X?

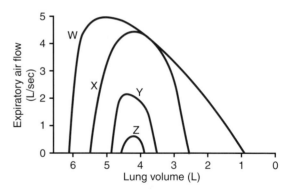

A) Asthma attack
B) Aspiration of meat into the trachea
C) Heavy exercise
D) Light exercise
E) Normal breathing at rest
F) Pneumonia
G) Tuberculosis

82. A 78-year-old man who smoked 60 cigarettes per day for 55 years complains of shortness of breath. The patient is diagnosed with chronic pulmonary emphysema. Which of the following sets of changes is present in this man, compared to a healthy, nonsmoker?

	Pulmonary compliance	Lung elastic recoil	Total lung capacity
A)	Decreased	Decreased	Decreased
B)	Decreased	Decreased	Increased
C)	Decreased	Increased	Increased
D)	Increased	Decreased	Decreased
E)	Increased	Decreased	Increased
F)	Increased	Increased	Increased

83. A 75-year-old man worked for 5 years in a factory in his early 40s where asbestos was used as an insulator. The man is diagnosed with asbestosis. Which of the following sets of changes is present in this man, compared to a person with healthy lungs?

	Pulmonary compliance	Lung elastic recoil	Total lung capacity
A)	Decreased	Decreased	Decreased
B)	Decreased	Increased	Increased
C)	Decreased	Increased	Decreased
D)	Increased	Decreased	Decreased
E)	Increased	Decreased	Increased
F)	Increased	Increased	Increased

84. Comparing a premature infant with respiratory distress syndrome to a normal full-term infant, how do lung compliance and surfactant levels compare?

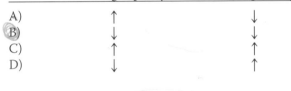

	Compliance in preterm compared to full term infant	Surfactant in preterm compared to full term infant
A)	↑	↓
B)	↑	↑
C)	↓	↓
D)	↓	↑
E)	↔	↑
F)	↔	↓

85. Which of the following decreases with emphysema?
   A) Alveolar P_{CO_2}
   B) Cardiac output
   C) Diffusion area
   D) Pulmonary artery pressure

86. Oxygen therapy is most beneficial in which of the following situations? Lung function is normal.
   A) Anemia
   B) CO_2 retention (COPD)
   C) Cyanide poisoning
   D) High altitude

87. Compared to a normal healthy person, how do total lung capacity and maximal expiratory flow patient change with restrictive lung disease?

	Total lung capacity	Maximal expiratory flow
A)	↑	↓
B)	↓	↓
C)	↑	↑
D)	↓	↑

1. **C)** The lungs can be expanded and contracted by increasing and decreasing the volume of the chest cavity. The volume of the chest cavity can be changed in two ways: (a) downward and upward movement of the diaphragm increases and decreases the length of the chest cavity, and (b) elevating and depressing the rib cage increases and decreases the anteroposterior diameter of the chest cavity. Normal breathing during resting conditions is accomplished entirely by the diaphragm. The diaphragm contracts causing inspiration and relaxes causing expiration. The other muscles listed in the question elevate or depress the rib cage and are used during heavy breathing associated with exercise as well as respiratory abnormalities characterized by excessive respiratory effort.

   TMP12 465–466

2. **D)** Contraction of the internal intercostals and abdominal recti pull the rib cage downward during expiration. The abdominal recti and other abdominal muscles compress the abdominal contents upward toward the diaphragm, which also helps to eliminate air from the lungs. The diaphragm relaxes during expiration. The external intercostals, sternocleidomastoid muscles, and scaleni increase the diameter of the chest cavity during exercise and thus assist with inspiration, but only the diaphragm is necessary for inspiration during quiet breathing.

   TMP12 465–466

3. **E)** The pleural pressure (sometimes called the intrapleural pressure) is the pressure of the fluid in the narrow space between the visceral pleura of the lungs and parietal pleura of the chest wall. The pleural pressure is normally about −5 cm H_2O immediately before inspiration (i.e., at functional residual capacity, FRC) when all of the respiratory muscles are relaxed. During inspiration, the volume of the chest cavity increases and the pleural pressure becomes more negative. The pleural pressure averages about −7.5 cm H_2O immediately before expiration when the lungs are fully expanded. The pleural pressure then returns to its resting value of −5 cm H_2O as the diaphragm relaxes and lung volume returns to FRC. Therefore, the intrapleural pressure is always subatmospheric under normal conditions varying between −5 and −7.5 cm H_2O during quiet breathing.

   TMP12 466

4. **E)** Alveolar pressure is the pressure of the air inside the lung alveoli. When the glottis is open and no air is flowing into or out of the lungs, the pressures in all parts of the respiratory tree are equal to zero. Expansion of the chest cavity during inspiration causes the alveolar pressure to become subatmospheric, averaging about −1 cm H_2O during quiet breathing: this creates a +1 cm H_2O pressure gradient for air to move into the lungs. Contraction of the chest cavity during expiration causes the alveolar pressure to achieve a positive value of about +1 cm H_2O, which again creates a +1 cm H_2O pressure gradient for air to move out of the lungs. The alveolar pressures become more negative during inspiration and more positive during expiration during heavy breathing associated with exercise as well as during various disease states.

   TMP12 466

5. **C)** Compliance is change in volume/change in pressure. This calculates to 1000 ml/8 cm H_2O equaling 125.

   TMP12 467

6. **E)** Compliance (C) is the change in lung volume (ΔV) that occurs for a given change in the transpulmonary pressure (ΔP), that is, $C = \Delta V/\Delta P$. (The transpulmonary pressure is the difference between the alveolar pressure and pleural pressure.) Because compliance is equal to the slope of the volume–pressure relationship, it should be clear that curve S represents the highest compliance, and that curve U represents the lowest compliance.

   TMP12 467

7. **D)** Compliance is the change in volume per change in pressure. Compliance is due to "elastic forces of the lung tissue and . . . elastic forces caused by surface tension of the fluid that lines the inside walls of the alveoli." If a person is being ventilated with a liquid then there is a lack of elastic forces due to surface tension. Therefore the compliance is decreased.

   TMP12 467–468

8. **D)** Because the compliance is 0.2 L/cm H_2O, it should be clear that a 1.0-L increase in volume will cause a 5 cm H_2O decrease in pleural pressure (1.0 L/0.2 L/cm H_2O = 5.0 cm H_2O); and, because the initial pleural pressure was −4 cm H_2O before inhalation, the pressure is reduced by 5 cm H_2O (to −9 cm H_2O) when 1.0 L air is inhaled.

   TMP12 466–467

9. **D)** Surfactant is formed relatively late in fetal life. Premature babies born without adequate amounts of surfactant can develop pulmonary failure and die. Surfactant is a surface active agent that greatly reduces the surface tension of the water lining the alveoli. Water is normally attracted to itself, which is why raindrops are round. By reducing the surface tension of the water lining the alveoli (and thus reducing the tendency of water molecules to coalesce), the surfactant reduces the work of breathing, i.e., less transpulmonary pressure is required to inhale a given volume of air. Because compliance is equal to the change in lung volume for a given change in transpulmonary pressure, it should be clear that pulmonary compliance is decreased in the absence of surfactant.
  TMP12 467–468

10. **C)** Residual volume = FRC − ERV = 3 L − 1.5 L = 1.5 L
  TMP12 469–471

11. **A)** The expiratory reserve volume (ERV) is the maximum extra volume of air that can be expired by forceful expiration after the end of a normal tidal expiration. ERV is equal to the difference between the functional residual capacity (FRC, 3 L) and the residual volume (RV, 1 L). Although neither FRC nor RV can be determined from a spirogram alone, the relative differences between these two volumes can still be determined from a spirogram and thus can be used to calculate ERV.
  TMP12 469–471

12. **C)** The functional residual capacity (FRC) equals the expiratory reserve volume (2 L) plus the residual volume (1.0 L). This is the amount of air that remains in the lungs at the end of a normal expiration. FRC is considered to be the resting volume of the lungs because none of the respiratory muscles are contracted at FRC. This problem illustrates an important point: a spirogram can measure changes in lung volume, but not absolute lung volumes. Thus, a spirogram alone cannot be used to determine residual volume, functional residual capacity, or total lung capacity.
  TMP12 469–471

13. **B)** A spirometer can be used to measure changes in lung volume, but cannot determine absolute volume. It consists of a drum filled with air inverted over a chamber of water. When the person breathes in and out, the drum moves up and down recording the changes in lung volume. The spirometer cannot be used to measure residual volume (RV) because the residual volume of air in the lungs cannot be exhaled into the spirometer. The functional residual capacity (FRC) is the amount of air left in the lungs after a normal expiration. FRC cannot be measured using a spirometer because it contains the RV. The total lung capacity (TLC) is the total amount of air that the lungs can hold after a maximum inspiration. Because the TLC includes the RV it cannot be measured using a spirometer. TLC, FRC, and RV can be determined using the helium dilution method or a body plethysmograph.
  TMP12 469–471

14. **B)** Alveolar ventilation = Frequency * $(V_T − V_D)$ = 15/min * (650 − 150) = 7.5 L/min
  TMP12 472

15. **C)** Pleural pressure during inhalation is always less than alveolar or atmospheric.
  TMP12 465–466

16. **E)** Total ventilation is equal to the tidal volume (V_T) times the ventilation frequency (Freq). Alveolar ventilation = $(V_T − V_D)$ × Frequency, where V_D is the dead space volume. Both individuals have the same total ventilation: subject T, 1000 × 10 = 10 L/min; subject V, 500 × 20 = 10 L/min. However, subject T has an alveolar ventilation of 18 L (that is, (2000 − 200) × 10)); whereas subject V has an alveolar ventilation of only 12 L (that is, (500 − 200) × 40)). This problem further illustrates that the most effective means of increasing alveolar ventilation is to increase the tidal volume, not the respiratory frequency.
  TMP12 471–472

17. **D)** The lower zones of the lung ventilate better than the upper zones and the middle zones have intermediate ventilation. These differences in regional ventilation can be explained by regional differences in pleural pressure. The pleural pressure is typically about −10 cm H_2O in the upper regions and about −2.5 cm H_2O in the lower regions. A less negative pleural pressure in the lower regions of the chest cavity causes less expansion of the lower zones of the lung during resting conditions. Therefore, the bottom of the lung is relatively compressed during rest but expands better during inspiration compared to the apex.
  TMP12 493–494

18. **B)** Both the lung and thoracic cage are elastic. Under normal conditions, the elastic tendency of the lungs to collapse is exactly balanced by the elastic tendency of the thoracic cage to expand. When air is introduced into the pleural space, the pleural pressure becomes equal to atmospheric pressure—the chest wall springs outward and the lungs collapse.
  TMP12 466–467

19. **B)** The larger bronchi near to the trachea have the greatest resistance to airflow in the healthy lung. However, in disease conditions, the smaller bronchioles often have a far greater role in determining resistance because (a) they are easily occluded because of their small size, and (b) they have an abundance of smooth muscle in their walls and therefore constrict easily.
  TMP12 473

20. **A)** An increase in pulmonary volume causes a decrease in airway resistance, which means that airway diameter increases. The airways are tethered to the surrounding tissues, which causes them to be pulled open when the lungs expand. This so-called "radial traction" phenomenon can explain why it is easier for a person with obstructive pulmonary disease to breathe at higher than normal lung volumes.
     TMP12 473, 516

21. **B)** Smooth muscle tone in the respiratory passageways is under the control of the autonomic nervous system as well as circulating epinephrine. Motor innervation is by the vagus nerve. Stimulation of adrenergic receptors by norepinephrine and epinephrine causes bronchodilation. Parasympathetic activity (as well as acetylcholine) causes bronchoconstriction. Note that these effects of the autonomic nervous system on the respiratory passageways are opposite to those on peripheral blood vessels.
     TMP12 473

22. **A)** It is usually not feasible to measure the left atrial pressure directly in the normal human being because it is difficult to pass a catheter through the heart chambers into the left atrium. The balloon-tipped, flow directed catheter (Swan-Ganz catheter) was developed nearly 30 years ago to estimate left atrial pressure for the management of acute myocardial infarction. When the balloon is inflated on a Swan-Ganz catheter, the pressure measured through the catheter, called the wedge pressure, approximates the left atrial pressure for the following reason: blood flow distal to the catheter tip has been stopped all the way to the left atrium, which allows left atrial pressure to be estimated. The wedge pressure is actually a few mm Hg higher than the left atrial pressure, depending on where the catheter is wedged, but this still allows changes in left atrial pressure to be monitored in patients with left ventricular failure.
     TMP12 478

23. **F)** The pulmonary and systemic circulations both receive about the same amount of blood flow because the lungs receive the entire cardiac output. [However, the output of the left ventricle is actually 1% to 2% higher than the right ventricle because the bronchial arterial blood originates from the left ventricle and the bronchial venous blood empties into the pulmonary veins.] The pulmonary blood vessels have a relatively low resistance allowing the entire cardiac output to pass through them without increasing the pressure to a great extent. The pulmonary artery pressure averages about 15 mm Hg, which is much lower than the systemic arterial pressure of about 100 mm Hg.
     TMP12 477–479

24. **A)** The pulmonary blood flow can increase severalfold without causing an excessive increase in pulmonary artery pressure for the following two reasons: previously closed vessels open up (recruitment), and the vessels enlarge (distension). Recruitment and distension of the pulmonary blood vessels both serve to lower the pulmonary vascular resistance (and thus to maintain low pulmonary blood pressures) when the cardiac output has increased.
     TMP12 480

25. **B)** When a person performs the valsalva maneuver (forcing air against a closed glottis), high pressure builds up in the lungs that can force as much as 250 ml of blood from the pulmonary circulation into the systemic circulation. The lungs have an important blood reservoir function, automatically shifting blood to the systemic circulation as a compensatory response to hemorrhage and other conditions in which the systemic blood volume is too low.
     TMP12 478

26. **D)** It is important for the blood to be distributed to those segments of the lungs where the alveoli are best oxygenated. When the oxygen tension of the alveoli decreases below normal, the adjacent blood vessels constrict causing their resistance to increase as much as fivefold at extremely low oxygen levels. This is opposite to the effect observed in systemic vessels, which dilate in response to low oxygen (i.e., resistance decreases).
     TMP12 479

27. **A)** During standing there will be an increase in blood flow to the base of the lung and a decrease in blood flow to the apex of the lung. With exercise there is a parallel increase in blood flow throughout the lung.
     TMP12 479-480

28. **C)** Decreased alveolar P_{O_2} will cause an increase in pulmonary vascular resistance, leading to pulmonary hypertension.
     TMP12 479

29. **B)** Inhalation to TLC or exhalation to residual volume will increase pulmonary blood flow resistance. Alveolar hypoxia will increase blood flow resistance. Having the lung at FRC pulmonary resistance is at the lowest level.
     TMP12 478–480

30. **C)** A *Pseudomonas* infection can increase the capillary permeability in the lungs and elsewhere in the body, which leads to excess loss of plasma proteins into the interstitial spaces. This leakage of plasma proteins from the vasculature caused the plasma colloid osmotic pressure to decrease from a normal value of about 28 mm Hg to 19 mm Hg. The capillary hydrostatic pressure remained at a normal value of 7 mm Hg, but

it can sometimes increase to higher levels, exacerbating the formation of edema. The interstitial fluid hydrostatic pressure has increased from a normal value of about −5 mm Hg to 1 mm Hg, which tends to decrease fluid loss from the capillaries. Excess fluid in the interstitial spaces (edema) causes lymph flow to increase.

TMP12 481–483

31. **B)** Answer. Normal alveolar P_{CO_2} is 40 mm Hg. Normal alveolar ventilation for this person is 3.6 L/min. On the ventilator the alveolar ventilation is 7.2 L/min. A doubling of alveolar ventilation results in a decrease in alveolar P_{CO_2} by one-half. Thus alveolar P_{CO_2} would be 20.

TMP12 488

32. **E)** Fick's law of diffusion states that the rate of diffusion (D) of a gas through a biological membrane is proportional to ΔP, A, and S, and inversely proportional to d and the square root of the MW of the gas (i.e., $D \alpha (\Delta P \times A \times S) / (d \times MW^{-2})$). The greater the pressure gradient there is a faster diffusion. The larger the cross-sectional area of the membrane, the higher will be the total number of molecules that can diffuse through the membrane. The higher the solubility of the gas, the higher will be the number of gas molecules available to diffuse for a given difference in pressure. When the distance of the diffusion pathway is shorter, it will take less time for the molecules to diffuse the entire distance. When the molecular weight of the gas molecule is decreased, the velocity of kinetic movement of the molecule will be higher, which also increases the rate of diffusion.

TMP12 486–487

33. **C)** To calculate inspired P_{O_2} one has to remember that the air is humidified when it enters the body. Therefore the humidified air has an effective total pressure of atmospheric pressure (760) − water vapor pressure (47). This yields a pressure of (760 − 47) = 713 mm Hg. The oxygen is 50% of the total gas so the partial pressure of oxygen is 716 * 0.5 = 316 mm Hg. To correct for the CO_2 in the alveolar, one has to then subtract the partial pressure of CO_2 divided by the respiratory quotient (normally 0.8). Therefore, the alveolar $P_{O_2} = PiO_2 - (P_{CO_2}/R) = 318 - (40/0.8) = 318 - 50 = 268$ mm Hg.

TMP12 487–489

34. **E)** When there is a blockage of an airway there is no movement of fresh air. Therefore the air in the alveoli reaches an equilibration with pulmonary arterial blood. Therefore, P_{O_2} will decrease from 100 to 40, P_{CO_2} will increase from 40 to 45, and systemic P_{O_2} will decrease because there is a decrease in oxygen uptake from the alveoli and thus decreased O_2 diffusion from the alveoli.

TMP12 492–493

35. **B)** The diffusing capacity of a gas is the volume of a gas that will diffuse through a membrane each minute for a pressure difference of 1 mm Hg. The diffusing capacity of oxygen is increased during exercise by (a) opening up of previously closed capillaries (recruitment) and dilating previously open capillaries (distension), both of which increase the surface area of the blood into which oxygen can diffuse, and (b) improving the ventilation-perfusion ratio which means improvement of the match between the ventilation of the alveoli and the perfusion of the alveolar capillaries with blood.

TMP12 491–492

36. **B)** It is not practical to measure the oxygen diffusing capacity directly because it is not possible to measure accurately the oxygen tension of the pulmonary capillary blood. However, the diffusing capacity for carbon monoxide (CO) can be measured accurately because the CO tension in pulmonary capillary blood is zero under normal conditions. The CO diffusing capacity is then used to calculate the oxygen diffusing capacity by taking into account the differences in diffusion coefficient between oxygen and CO. Knowing the rate of transfer of CO across the respiratory membrane is often helpful for evaluating the presence of possible parenchymal lung disease when spirometry and/or lung volume determinations suggest a reduced vital capacity, residual volume and/or total lung capacity.

TMP12 492

37. **C)** Because the blood that perfuses the pulmonary capillaries is venous blood returning to the lungs (i.e., mixed venous blood) from the systemic circulation, it is the gases in this blood with which the alveolar gases equilibrate. Therefore, when an airway is blocked, the alveolar air equilibrates with the mixed venous blood and the partial pressures of the gases in both the blood and alveolar air become identical.

TMP12 492–494

38. **B)** Alveolar air normally equilibrates with the mixed venous blood that perfuses them so that the gas composition of alveolar air and pulmonary capillary blood are identical. When a group of alveoli are not perfused, the composition of the alveolar air becomes equal to the inspired gas composition, which has an oxygen tension of 149 mm Hg and carbon dioxide tension of about 0 mm Hg.

TMP12 492–494

39. **D)** A decrease in the ventilation-perfusion ratio (VA/Q) is depicted by moving to the left along the normal ventilation-perfusion line shown in the diagram. Whenever the VA/Q is below normal, there is inadequate ventilation to provide the oxygen needed to fully oxygenate the blood flowing through the alveolar capillaries (i.e., alveolar P_{O_2} is low). Therefore, a

certain fraction of the venous blood passing through the pulmonary capillaries does not become oxygenated. Poorly ventilated areas of the lung also accumulate carbon dioxide diffusing into the alveoli from the mixed venous blood. The result of decreasing VA/Q (moving to the left along the VA/Q line) on alveolar P_{O_2} and P_{CO_2} is shown in the diagram, that is, P_{O_2} decreases and P_{CO_2} increases.

TMP12 492–494

40. **A)** Alveolar P_{O_2} is dependent on inspired gas and alveolar P_{CO_2}. Alveolar P_{CO_2} is a balance between alveolar ventilation and CO_2 production. To decrease alveolar P_{CO_2} there has to be increased alveolar ventilation in relation to metabolism. Low P_{O_2} will not directly affect P_{CO_2}, but can stimulate respiration (if P_{O_2} is sufficiently low) and this would then reduce P_{CO_2}). An increased metabolism with unchanged alveolar ventilation will increase P_{CO_2}. A doubling in metabolism with a doubling in alveolar ventilation will have no effect on P_{CO_2}.

TMP12 488–489

41. **A)** When the ventilation is reduced to zero (VA/Q = 0) alveolar air equilibrates with the mixed venous blood entering the lung, which causes the gas composition of the alveolar air to become identical to that of the blood. This occurs at point A, where the alveolar P_{O_2} is 40 mm Hg and the alveolar P_{CO_2} is 45 mm Hg, as shown on the diagram. A reduction in VA/Q (caused by the partially obstructed airway in this problem) causes the alveolar P_{O_2} and P_{CO_2} to approach the values achieved when VA/Q = 0.

TMP12 492–494

42. **E)** A pulmonary embolism decreases blood flow to the affected lung causing ventilation to exceed blood flow. When the embolism completely blocks all blood flow to an area of the lung, the gas composition of the inspired air entering the alveoli equilibrates with blood trapped in the alveolar capillaries so that within a short time, the gas composition of the alveolar air is identical to that of inspired air. This situation in which VA/Q is equal to infinity corresponds to point E on the diagram (inspired gas). An increase in VA/Q caused by the partially obstructed blood flow in this problem causes the alveolar P_{O_2} and P_{CO_2} to approach the values achieved when VA/Q = ∞.

TMP12 492–494

43. **C)** Breathing 100% oxygen has a limited effect on the arterial P_{O_2} when the cause of arterial hypoxemia is a vascular shunt. However, breathing 100% oxygen raises the arterial P_{O_2} to over 600 mm Hg in a normal subject. With a vascular shunt, the arterial P_{O_2} is determined by (a) highly oxygenated end-capillary blood (P_{O_2} > 600 mm Hg) that has passed through ventilated portions of the lung, and (b) shunted blood that has bypassed the ventilated portions of the lungs and thus has an oxygen partial pressure equal to that of mixed venous blood (P_{O_2} = 40 mm Hg). A mixture of the two bloods causes a large fall in P_{O_2} because the oxygen dissociation curve is so flat in its upper range.

TMP12 493–494

44. **D)** The anatomic dead space (D_{ANAT}) is the air that a person breathes in that fills the respiratory passageways but never reaches the alveoli. Alveolar dead space (D_{ALV}) is the air in the alveoli that are ventilated but not perfused. Physiologic dead space (D_{PHY}) is the sum of D_{ANAT} and D_{ALV} (i.e., $D_{PHY} = D_{ANAT} + D_{ALV}$). The D_{ALV} is zero in lung unit S (the ideal lung unit) and the D_{ANAT} and D_{PHY} are thus equal to each other. The diagram shows a group of alveoli with a poor blood supply (lung unit T), which means that the D_{ALV} is substantial. Thus, D_{PHY} is greater than either D_{ANAT} or D_{ALV} in lung unit T.

TMP12 489, 493–494

45. **E)** The P_{O_2} of mixed venous blood entering the pulmonary capillaries is normally about 40 mm Hg and the P_{O_2} at the venous end of the capillaries is normally equal to that of the alveolar gas (104 mm Hg). The P_{O_2} of the pulmonary blood normally rises to equal that of the alveolar air by the time the blood has moved a third of the distance through the capillaries, becoming almost 104 mm Hg. Thus, curve B represents the normal resting state. During exercise, the cardiac output can increase severalfold, but the pulmonary capillary blood still becomes almost saturated with oxygen during its transit through the lungs. However, because of the faster flow of blood through the lungs during exercise, the oxygen has less time to diffuse into the pulmonary capillary blood, and therefore the P_{O_2} of the capillary blood does not reach its maximum value until it reaches the venous end of the pulmonary capillaries. Although curves D and E both show that oxygen saturation of blood occurs near the venous end, note that only curve E shows a low P_{O_2} of 25 mm Hg at the arterial end of the pulmonary capillaries, which is typical of mixed venous blood during strenuous exercise.

TMP12 495–496

46. **A)** The P_{O_2} of mixed venous blood entering the pulmonary capillaries increases during its transit through the pulmonary capillaries (from 40 mm Hg to 104 mm Hg) and the P_{CO_2} decreases simultaneously from 45 mm Hg to 40 mm Hg. Thus, P_{O_2} is represented by the red lines and P_{CO_2} is represented by the green lines in the various diagrams. During resting conditions, oxygen has a 64 mm Hg pressure gradient (104 − 64 = 64 mm Hg) and carbon dioxide has a 5 mm Hg pressure gradient (45 − 40 = 5 mm Hg) between the blood at the arterial end of the capillaries and the alveolar air.

Despite this large difference in pressure gradients between oxygen and carbon dioxide, both gases equilibrate with the alveolar air by the time the blood has moved a third of the distance through the capillaries in the normal resting state (choice A). This is possible because carbon dioxide can diffuse about 20 times as rapidly as oxygen.
TMP12 496–497

47. C) CO_2 is transported in three forms, dissolved (7% of total), bound directly to hemoglobin (23%), or it is converted to carbonic acid and transported as HCO_3- with the H^+ bound to hemoglobin (70%). Therefore the majority of CO_2 is transported as bicarbonate ions.
TMP12 501–502

48. C) Pulmonary venous blood is nearly 100% saturated with oxygen, has a Po_2 of about 104 mm Hg, and each 100 ml of blood carries about 20 m/s of oxygen (i.e., oxygen content is about 20 vol%). Approximately 25% of the oxygen carried in the arterial blood is used by the tissues under resting conditions. Thus, reduced blood returning to the lungs is about 75% saturated with oxygen, has a Po_2 of about 40 mm Hg, and has an oxygen content of about 15 vol%. Note that it necessary to know only one value for oxygenated and reduced blood and that the other two values requested in the question can be read from the oxygen-hemoglobin dissociation curve.
TMP12 496, 498–499

49. B) Tissue Po_2 is a balance between delivery and usages. With a decrease in blood flow, with no change in metabolism there will be a decrease in venous Po_2 (less delivery but no change in metabolism) and an increase in venous Pco_2 (less washout).
TMP12 496–497

50. D) When a person is anemic, there is a decrease in content. The oxygen saturation of hemoglobin in the arterial blood and the arterial oxygen partial pressure are not affected by the hemoglobin concentration of the blood.
TMP12 498–499

51. H) The oxygen carrying capacity of the blood is reduced in an anemic person, but the arterial Po_2 and oxygen saturation of hemoglobin are both normal. The decrease in arterial oxygen content is compensated for by an increase in the extraction of oxygen from hemoglobin, which reduces the Po_2 of the venous blood. The unloading of oxygen at the tissue level is enhanced by increased levels of 2,3 diphophosphoglycerate (2,3 DPG) in an anemic patient because 2,3 DPG causes a right-shift of the oxygen-hemoglobin dissociation curve.
TMP12 498–500

52. E) Carbon monoxide (CO) combines with hemoglobin at the same point on the hemoglobin molecule as oxygen and therefore can displace oxygen from the hemoglobin, reducing the oxygen saturation of hemoglobin. Because CO binds with hemoglobin (to form carboxyhemoglobin) with about 250 times as much tenacity as oxygen, even small amounts of CO in the blood can severely limit the oxygen carrying capacity of the blood. The presence of carboxyhemoglobin also shifts the oxygen dissociation curve to the left (which means that oxygen binds more tightly to hemoglobin), which further limits the transfer of oxygen to the tissues.
TMP12 499, 501

53. B) In exercise, several factors shift the oxygen-hemoglobin curve to the right, which serves to deliver extra amounts of oxygen to the exercising muscle fibers. These factors include increased quantities of carbon dioxide released from the muscle fibers, increased hydrogen ion concentration in the muscle capillary blood, and increased temperature resulting from heat generated by the exercising muscle. The right shift of the oxygen-hemoglobin curve allows more oxygen to be released to the muscle at a given oxygen partial pressure in the blood.
TMP12 499–500

54. C) Structural differences between fetal hemoglobin and adult hemoglobin make fetal hemoglobin unable to react with 2,3 diphophosphoglycerate (2,3-DPG) and thus to have a higher affinity for oxygen at a given partial pressure of oxygen. The fetal dissociation curve is thus shifted to the left relative to the adult curve. Typically, fetal arterial oxygen pressures are low, and hence the leftward shift enhances the placental uptake of oxygen.
TMP12 499–500

55. C) Each gram of hemoglobin can normally carry 1.34 milliliters of oxygen. Hb= 12 g//dL. Arterial oxygen content = 12 * 1.34 = 16 ml O2/dL. Using 12 ml O_2/dL yields a mixed venous saturation of 25%. With a saturation of 25% the venous Po_2 should be close to 20 mm Hg.
TMP12 499–500

56. A) Most of the carbon dioxide (70%) is transported in the blood in the form of bicarbonate ion. Dissolved carbon dioxide reacts with water to form carbonic acid (mostly in red blood cells), which dissociates into bicarbonate and hydrogen ions. Carbon dioxide also reacts with amine radicals of the hemoglobin molecule to form the compound carbaminohemoglobin, which accounts for about 23% of the carbon dioxide transported in the blood. The remaining carbon dioxide (7%) is transported in the dissolved state.
TMP12 502–503

57. C) The respiratory exchange ratio (R) is equal to the rate of carbon dioxide output divided by the rate of oxygen uptake. A value of 0.8 therefore means

that the amount of carbon dioxide produced by the tissues is 80% of the amount of oxygen used by the tissues, which also means that the amount of carbon dioxide transported from the tissues to the lungs in each 100 ml of blood is 80% of the amount of oxygen transported from the lungs to the tissues in each 100 ml of blood. Choice C is the only answer in which the ratio of carbon dioxide to oxygen is 0.8 (4/5 = 0.8). Although R changes under different metabolic conditions, ranging from 1.00 in those who consume carbohydrates exclusively to 0.7 in those who consume fats exclusively, the average value for R is close to 0.8.
    TMP12 503

58. **F)** Dissolved carbon dioxide combines with water in red blood cells to form carbonic acid, which dissociates to form bicarbonate and hydrogen ions. Many of the bicarbonate ions diffuse out of the red blood cells while chloride ions diffuse into the red blood cells to maintain electrical neutrality. The phenomenon, called the chloride shift, is made possible by a special bicarbonate-chloride carrier protein in the red cell membrane that shuttles the ions in opposite directions. Water moves into the red blood cells to maintain osmotic equilibrium, which results in a slight swelling of the red blood cells in the venous blood.
    TMP12 502–503

59. **D)** The pneumotaxic center transmits signals to the dorsal respiratory group that "switch off" inspiratory signals, thus controlling the duration of the filling phase of the lung cycle. This has a secondary effect of increasing the rate of breathing, because limitation of inspiration also shortens expiration and the entire period of respiration.
    TMP12 505–506

60. **E)** The basic rhythm of respiration is generated in the dorsal respiratory group of neurons, located almost entirely within the nucleus of the tractus solitarius. When the respiratory drive for increased pulmonary ventilation becomes greater than normal, respiratory signals spill over into the ventral respiratory neurons, causing the ventral respiratory area to contribute to the respiratory drive. However, neurons of the ventral respiratory group remain almost totally inactive during normal quiet breathing.
    TMP12 505–506

61. **E)** The muscular walls of the bronchi and bronchioles contain stretch receptors that transmit signals through the vagi into the dorsal respiratory group of neurons when the lungs are overstretched. These signals "switch off" inspiration thus preventing excess lung inflation in much the same way as signals from the pneumotaxic center. The reflex does not have a direct effect on expiration.
    TMP12 506

62. **B)** In a normal person the alveolar gases are the same as the arterial blood. With rebreathing, the exhaled CO_2 is never removed and continues to accumulate in the bag. This increase in alveolar and thus arterial P_{CO_2} will be the stimulus for the increased breathing. He will have a decrease alveolar P_{O_2}, not increased, with the decreased P_{O_2} stimulating breathing. A decreased P_{CO_2} will not stimulate ventilation. An increased pH, alkalosis, will not stimulate ventilation.
    TMP12 507–509

63. **B)** With carbon monoxide there is only a small change in CO required to bind to hemoglobin. Therefore there is a minimal change in P_{O_2}. Thus, there will be no stimulus to increase respiration, and thus no change in P_{CO_2}.
    TMP12 501–502, 508–509

64. **F)** Alveolar ventilation can increase by more than eightfold when the arterial carbon dioxide tension is increased over a physiological range from about 35 to 75 mm Hg. This demonstrates the tremendous effect that carbon dioxide changes have in controlling respiration. By contrast, the change in respiration caused by changing the blood pH over a normal range from 7.3 to 7.5 is more than 10 times less effective.
    TMP12 508

65. **D)** The arterial oxygen tension has essentially no effect on alveolar ventilation when it is higher than about 100 mm Hg, but ventilation approximately doubles when the arterial oxygen tension falls to 60 mm Hg and can increase as much as fivefold at very low oxygen tensions. This quantitative relationship between arterial oxygen tension and alveolar ventilation was established in an experimental setting in which the arterial carbon dioxide tension and pH were held constant. The student can imagine that the ventilatory response to hypoxia would be blunted if the carbon dioxide tension were permitted to decrease.
    TMP12 509

66. **C)** This patient would have increased alveolar ventilation, therefore resulting in a decrease in arterial P_{CO_2}. The effect of this decrease in P_{CO_2} would be an inhibition of the chemosensitive area and a decrease in ventilation until P_{CO_2} was back to normal. Breathing high O_2 does not decrease nerve activity sufficient to decrease respiration. Response of peripheral chemoreceptors to CO_2 and pH are mild, and do not play a major role in the control of respiration.
    TMP12 507–509

67. **E)** It is remarkable that the arterial P_{O_2}, P_{CO_2}, and pH remain almost exactly normal in a healthy athlete during strenuous exercise despite the 20-fold increase in oxygen consumption and carbon dioxide formation. This interesting phenomenon begs the question: What is it during exercise that causes the intense ventilation?
    TMP12 511–512

68. A) Because strenuous exercise does not change significantly the mean arterial P_{O_2}, P_{CO_2}, or pH, it is unlikely that these play an important role in stimulating the immense increase in ventilation. Although the mean venous P_{O_2} decreases during exercise, the venous vasculature does not contain chemoreceptors that can sense P_{O_2}. The brain, on transmitting motor impulses to the contracting muscles, is believed to transmit collateral impulses to the brain stem to excite the respiratory center. Also, the movement of body parts during exercise is believed to excite joint and muscle proprioceptors that then transmit excitatory impulses to the respiratory center.

TMP12 511–512

69. C) Cheyne-Stokes breathing is the most common type of periodic breathing. The person breathes deeply for a short interval and then breathes slightly or not at all for an additional interval. This pattern repeats itself about every minute. Apnea is a transient cessation of respiration so it is true that Cheyne-Stokes breathing is associated with periods of apnea. Biot breathing refers to sequences of uniformly deep gasps, apnea, and then deep gasps. Hyperpnea means increased breathing, usually referring to increased tidal volume with or without increased frequency. Tachypnea means increased frequency of breathing.

TMP12 512–513

70. B) The basic mechanism of Cheyne-Stokes breathing can be attributed to a buildup of carbon dioxide which stimulates overventilation, followed by a depression of the respiratory center due to a low P_{CO_2} of the respiratory neurons. It should be clear that the greatest depth of breathing occurs when the neurons of the respiratory center are exposed to the highest levels of carbon dioxide (point W). This increase in breathing causes carbon dioxide to be blown off and thus the P_{CO_2} of the lung blood is at its lowest value at about point Y on the diagram. The P_{CO_2} of the pulmonary blood gradually increases from point Y to point Z, reaching its maximum value at point V. Thus, it is the phase lag between the P_{CO_2} at the respiratory center and the P_{CO_2} of the pulmonary blood that leads to this type of breathing. The phase-lag often occurs with left heart failure, due to enlargement of the left ventricle which increases the time required for blood to reach the respiratory center. Another cause of Cheyne-Stokes breathing is increased negative feedback gain in the respiratory control areas, which can be caused by head trauma, stroke, and other types of brain damage.

TMP12 512–513

71. D) The forced vital capacity (FVC) is equal to the difference between the total lung capacity (TLC) and the residual volume (RV). The TLC and RV are the points of intersection between the abscissa and flow-volume curve, that is, TLC = 5.5 L and RV = 1.0 L. Therefore, FVC = 5.5 − 1.0 = 4.5 L.

TMP12 516

72. D) The maximum expiratory flow-volume (MEFV) curve is created when a person inhales as much air as possible (point A, total lung capacity = 5.5 L) and then expires the air with a maximum effort until no more air can be expired (point E, residual volume = 1.0 L). The descending portion of the curve indicated by the downward pointing arrow represents the maximum expiratory flow at each lung volume. This descending portion of the curve is sometimes referred to as the "effort-independent" portion of the curve because the patient cannot increase expiratory flow rate to a higher level even when a greater expiratory effort is expended.

TMP12 516

73. B) In obstructive diseases such as emphysema and asthma, the maximum expiratory flow-volume (MEFV) curve begins and ends at abnormally high lung volumes, and the flow rates are lower than normal at any given lung volume. The curve may also have a scooped out appearance, as shown on the diagram. The other diseases listed as answer choices are constricted lung diseases (often called restrictive lung diseases). Lung volumes are lower than normal in constricted lung diseases.

TMP12 516

74. A) Asbestosis is a constricted lung disease characterized by diffuse interstitial fibrosis. In constricted lung disease (more commonly called restrictive lung disease), the MEFV curve begins and ends at abnormally low lung volumes, and the flow rates are often higher than normal at any given lung volume, as shown on the diagram. Lung volumes are expected to be higher than normal in asthma, bronchospasm, emphysema, old age, and other instances in which the airways are narrowed or radial traction of the airways is reduced allowing them to close more easily.

TMP12 516

75. B) The diagram shows that a maximum respiratory effort is needed during resting conditions because the maximum expiratory flow rate is achieved during resting conditions. It should be clear that his ability to exercise is greatly diminished. The man has smoked for 60 years and is likely to have emphysema. Therefore, the student can surmise that the total lung capacity, functional residual capacity, and residual volume are greater than normal. The vital capacity is only about 3.4 L, as shown on the diagram.

TMP12 516–517

76. A) The forced vital capacity (FVC) is the vital capacity measured with a forced expiration. The forced expiratory volume in one second (FEV_1) is the amount of air that can be expelled from the lungs during the first second of a forced expiration. The FEV_1/FVC for the normal individual (curve X) is 4 L/5 L = 80% and 2 L/4 L = 50% for the patient (curve Z). The FEV_1/FVC ratio has diagnostic value for differentiating between normal, obstructive, and constricted patterns of a forced expiration.

TMP12 517

77. **E)** The forced vital capacity (FVC) is the vital capacity measured with a forced expiration. The forced expiratory volume in one second (FEV_1) is the amount of air that can be expelled from the lungs during the first second of a forced expiration. The FEV_1/FVC ratio for the healthy individual (X) is 4 L/5 L = 80%; FEV_1/FVC for patient Z is 3.0/3.5 = 86%. FEV_1/FVC is often increased in silicosis and other diseases characterized by interstitial fibrosis because of increased radial traction of the airways, that is, the airways are held open to a greater extent at any given lung volume, reducing their resistance to air flow. Airway resistance is increased (and therefore FEV_1/FVC is decreased) in asthma, bronchospasm, emphysema, and old age.

TMP12 517

78. **B)** The forced vital capacity (FVC) is the vital capacity measured with a forced expiration (FVC = 4.0 L for patient Z). The forced expiratory volume in one second (FEV_1) is the amount of air that can be expelled from the lungs during the first second of a forced expiration (FVC = 2.0 L for patient Z). FEV_1/FVC is a function of airway resistance. Airway resistance is often increased in emphysematous lungs, which causes FEV_1/FVC to decrease. Note that FEV_1/FVC is 50% in patient Z and 80% in the healthy individual represented by curve X. The FEV_1/FVC ratio is not usually affected in pleural effusion and pneumothorax because airway resistance is normal. FVC is often decreased in asbestosis, fibrotic pleurisy, silicosis, and tuberculosis and the FEV_1/FVC ratio is either normal or slightly increased.

TMP12 517

79. **E)** Prolonged exposure to silica causes interstitial fibrosis, which in turn decreases pulmonary compliance. Compliance is the change in lung volume for a given change in transpulmonary pressure required to inflate the lungs. The volume-pressure curve indicates that the patient has a lower than normal pulmonary compliance, which is consistent with silicosis. The elastic recoil of the lung is increased when fibrous material is deposited in the interstitium and alveolar walls, reducing the distensibility (compliance) of the lung. The pulmonary compliance is increased in emphysema and old age. Asthma and other diseases characterized by bronchospasm also cause the apparent pulmonary compliance to increase.

TMP12 467

80. **B)** The loss of alveolar walls with destruction of associated capillary beds in the emphysematous lung reduces the elastic recoil and increases the compliance. The student should recall that compliance is equal to the change in lung volume for a given change in transpulmonary pressure, that is, compliance is equal to the slopes of the volume-pressure relationships shown in the diagram. Asbestosis, silicosis, and tuberculosis are associated with deposition of fibrous tissue in the lungs, which decreases the compliance. Mitral obstruction and rheumatic heart disease can cause pulmonary edema, which also decreases the pulmonary compliance.

TMP12 467

81. **C)** Curve X represents heavy exercise with a tidal volume of about 3 L. Note that the expiratory flow rate has reached a maximum value of nearly 4.5 L/sec during the heavy exercise. This occurred because a maximum expiratory air flow is required to move the air through the airways with the high ventilatory frequency associated with heavy exercise. Normal breathing at rest is represented by curve Z; note that the tidal volume is less than 1 L during resting conditions. Curve Y was recorded during mild exercise. An asthma attack or aspiration of meat would increase the resistance to air flow from the lungs, making it unlikely that expiratory air flow rate could approach its maximum value at a given lung volume. The tidal volume should not increase greatly with pneumonia or tuberculosis and it should not be possible to achieve a maximum expiratory air flow at a given lung volume with these diseases.

TMP12 516–517

82. **E)** Loss of lung tissue in emphysema leads to an increase in the compliance of the lungs and a decrease in the elastic recoil of the lungs. Pulmonary compliance and elastic recoil always change in opposite directions, that is, compliance is proportional to 1/elastic recoil. The total lung capacity, residual volume, and functional residual capacity are increased in emphysema, but the vital capacity is decreased.

TMP12 467

83. **C)** Asbestosis is associated with deposition of fibrous material in the lungs. This causes the pulmonary compliance (i.e., distensibility) to decrease and the elastic recoil to increase. Pulmonary compliance and elastic recoil change in opposite directions because compliance is proportional to 1/elastic recoil. It is somewhat surprising to learn that the elastic recoil of a rock is greater than the elastic recoil of a rubber band, that is, the more difficult it is to deform an object, the greater the elastic recoil of the object. The total lung capacity, functional residual capacity, residual volume, and vital capacity are decreased in all types of fibrotic lung disease.

TMP12 467

84. **C)** A premature infant with respiratory distress syndrome has absent or reduced levels of surfactant. Loss of surfactant creates a greater surface tension. Since surface tension accounts for a large portion of lung elasticity, increasing surface tension will increase lung elasticity making the lung stiffer and less compliant.

      TMP12 519

85. **C)** Due to destruction of the alveolar walls, there is a decrease in surface/diffusion area. Cardiac output will be normal. Pulmonary artery pressure may be elevated because destruction of alveoli leads to loss of surrounding capillaries which forces blood into remaining capillaries, which tends to increase pulmonary artery pressure. Alveolar P_{CO_2} will tend to increase due to the difficulty expiring.

      TMP12 517–518

86. **D)** Increasing the inspired P_{O_2} will result in an increase in the dissolved amount of oxygen. However, due to the small solubility of oxygen in blood, 0.003 ml O_2/100 ml blood mm Hg O_2, this could end up being about 2 ml O_2/100 ml blood when breathing 100% oxygen. With anemia the hemoglobin is fully saturated and oxygen will have minimal effect. Treatment of the anemia is more beneficial than providing oxygen to an anemic patient. With COPD for a person to have CO_2 retention the person has to have severely damaged lungs. With COPD there will be a decreased P_{O_2}. With CO_2 retention there is a change in the regulation of respiration from being under CO_2 control to being driven by the decrease in O_2. This decrease in O_2 is what is controlling ventilation. Giving supplemental O_2 to a person with CO_2 retention will result in an increase in arterial P_{O_2}, thus decreasing the stimulus to breathe, resulting in the patient stopping breathing. Cyanide poisoning results in a decreased usage by the tissue and additional O_2 would be of no benefit. High altitude has lower barometric pressure, so less P_{O_2} and supplemental oxygen will help.

      TMP12 507–509, 517–518, 521

87. **B)** Total lung capacity and maximum expiratory flow are reduced in restrictive lung disease.

      TMP12 516

Aviation, Space, and Deep-Sea Diving Physiology

1. An aviator is flying at 30,000 ft where the barometric pressure is 226 mm Hg. He is breathing 100% oxygen, his alveolar P_{CO_2} is 40 mm Hg, and his alveolar water vapor pressure is 47 mm Hg. What is the alveolar P_{O_2} of the aviator (in mm Hg)? (Assume that the respiratory quotient is equal to 1.)

   A) 43
   B) 75
   C) 99
   D) 139
   E) 215

2. Which of the following sets of changes best describes a Himalayan native living in the Himalayas, compared to a sea-level native living at sea level?

	Hematocrit	Arterial P_{O_2}	Arterial O_2 content
A)	Decreased	Decreased	Decreased
B)	Decreased	Decreased	No difference
C)	Decreased	Increased	Decreased
D)	Decreased	Increased	No difference
E)	Increased	Decreased	Decreased
F)	Increased	Increased	Decreased
G)	Increased	Increased	No difference
H)	Increased	Decreased	No difference

3. A person is planning to leaving Miami (sea level) and traveling to Colorado to climb Mt. Wilson, at 14,500 ft, barometric pressure = 450 mm Hg. He takes acetazolamide, a carbonic anhydrase inhibitor that forces the kidneys to excrete bicarbonate before his trip. Which of the following would be the expected response before he makes the trip?

   A) Alkalotic blood
   B) Normal ventilation
   C) Elevated ventilation
   D) Normal arterial blood gases

4. A 35-year-old man travels to Mars. His exercise equipment malfunctions so that he is subjected to prolonged weightlessness without appropriate exercise. Which of the following sets of changes best describe the physiologic changes that occur in this man?

	Blood volume	Red cell mass	Maximum cardiac output
A)	Decreased	Decreased	Decreased
B)	Decreased	Increased	Increased
C)	Decreased	No change	Decreased
D)	Increased	Decreased	Decreased
E)	Increased	Increased	Increased
F)	Increased	No change	Decreased

5. A diver carries a 1000-L metal talk-box with an open bottom to a depth of 66 ft so that two divers can insert their heads and talk beneath the water. A person on the surface of the water pumps air into the box until the 1000-L box is completely filled with air. How much air from the surface is required to fill the box (in liters)?

   A) 1000
   B) 2000
   C) 3000
   D) 4000
   E) 5000

6. A diver is breathing 10% O_2 at a pressure of 2000 mm Hg. The diver's body temperature is 37°C, and P_{CO_2} = 32 mm Hg. What is the alveolar P_{O_2}?

   A) 113 mm Hg
   B) 153 mm Hg
   C) 168 mm Hg
   D) 200 mm Hg

7. Regarding a healthy recreational scuba diver at a depth of 66 ft in the Caribbean Sea, which of the following statements is true?

    A) Her lungs are smaller than normal
    B) She has an elevated arterial P_{O_2} and a normal P_{CO_2}.
    C) All gas partial pressures in her blood (oxygen, nitrogen, carbon dioxide, and water vapor) are elevated
    D) There are increases in both fraction of inspired oxygen (F_{IO_2}) and inspired nitrogen (F_{IN_2})

8. A diver has the gaseous pressures in his body fluids indicated in the table. Which of the following best describes the gaseous pressures in his body fluids immediately after sudden decompression (in mm Hg)?

H_2O	47 mm Hg
CO_2	40 mm Hg
O_2	60 mm Hg
N_2	3918 mm Hg

	H_2O	CO_2	O_2	N_2
A)	0	40	100	1428
B)	0	40	60	660
C)	47	40	100	573
D)	47	40	150	523
E)	47	40	60	3918

1. D) The alveolar oxygen tension (P_{AO_2}) can be calculated using the following formula:

$P_{AO_2} = P_{IO_2} - (P_{ACO_2}/R) + F$, where P_{IO_2} is the inspired oxygen tension, P_{ACO_2} is the alveolar carbon dioxide tension, R is the respiratory quotient (R = 1 as indicated in the question), and F is a small correction factor that can be ignored. P_{IO_2} is equal to the barometric pressure minus the water vapor pressure multiplied by the fractional concentration of oxygen in the inspired air, that is, $P_{IO_2} = (226 - 47) \times 1.00 = 179$ mm Hg. Therefore, $P_{AO_2} = 179 - 40/1 = 139$ mm Hg.

TMP12 527

2. H) Acclimatization to hypoxia includes an increase in pulmonary ventilation, an increase in red blood cells, an increase in diffusion capacity of the lungs, an increase in vascularity of the tissues, and an increase in the ability of the cells to use available oxygen. The increase in hematocrit of high-altitude natives allows normal amounts of oxygen (or even greater than normal amounts of oxygen) to be carried in the blood despite lower-than-normal arterial oxygen tension. For example, natives of 15,000 ft have an arterial oxygen tension of only 40 mm Hg, but because of greater amounts of hemoglobin in the blood, the quantity of oxygen carried in the blood is often greater than in the blood of sea-level natives.

TMP12 529–530

3. C) Acetazolamide is a medication that that forces the kidneys to excrete bicarbonate, the base form of carbon dioxide; this reacidifies the blood, balancing the effects of the hyperventilation that occurs at altitude in an attempt to get oxygen. Such reacidification acts as a respiratory stimulant, particularly at night, reducing or eliminating the periodic breathing pattern common at altitude. This would increase ventilation, resulting in a decreased P_{CO_2}.

TMP12 529

4. A) The effects of a prolonged stay in space are similar to those of prolonged bed rest—decrease in blood volume, decrease in red cell mass, decrease in muscle strength and work capacity, decrease in maximum cardiac output, and loss of calcium and phosphate from the bones. Most of these problems can be greatly reduced by extensive exercise programs.

TMP12 533

5. C) Boyle's law states that $P_1V_1 = P_2V_2$, where P_1 and V_1 are the original pressure and volume and P_2 and V_2 are the new volume and pressure. The atmospheric pressure at a depth of 66 ft is three times greater than the atmospheric pressure at the surface of the water, that is, there is 1 atmosphere at the surface plus an additional atmosphere for each 33 ft below the surface. Therefore, it takes three times as much sea level air to fill the box when the box is submerged to a depth of 66 ft because the air is subjected to 3 atmospheres.

TMP12 535

6. A) Alveolar P_{O_2} = Inspired P_{O_2} − (Alveolar P_{CO_2} / Respiratory Quotient). At a pressure of 2000 mm Hg and 10% O_2 the partial pressure is 200 mm Hg. Inspired P_{O_2} = 200 − 47 (water vapor). Alveolar P_{O_2} = 153 − (32/0.8) = 153 − 40 = 113.

TMP12 486–488, 535

7. B) Water vapor pressure and CO_2 remain normal. All other partial pressures are increased. There is a normal tidal volume due to SCUBA gear. The compressed air is normal air 79% N_2 and 21% O_2.

TMP12 535–537

8. E) The pressures of the various gases in the body fluids are identical immediately after sudden decompression. The pressure on the outside of the body becomes 1 atmosphere (760 mm Hg) after sudden decompression, whereas the sum of the pressures of water, carbon dioxide, oxygen, and nitrogen inside the body total 4065 mm Hg. Note that most of the gaseous pressure is caused by nitrogen (e.g., 3918 mm Hg). This difference in gaseous pressure between the inside and outside of the body causes the gases (especially nitrogen) to form bubbles (or cavitate) in the tissues and blood. This leads to a condition called "the bends."

TMP12 538

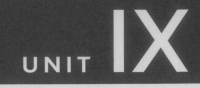

The Nervous System: A. General Principles and Sensory Physiology

1. In a neuron with a resting membrane potential of −65mV, the distribution of which ion across the neuronal membrane represents the greatest potential electromotive force (EMF)?

   A) Potassium
   B) Chloride
   C) Sodium
   D) Calcium

2. Forced rapid breathing results in alkalization of the blood which would lead to which of the following changes in neuronal activity?

   A) Decrease in neuronal activity
   B) Increase in neuronal activity
   C) Initial decrease followed by an increase
   D) No change in neuronal activity

3. The release of neurotransmitter at a chemical synapse in the central nervous system is dependent upon which of the following?

   A) Synthesis of acetylcholinesterase
   B) Hyperpolarization of the synaptic terminal
   C) Opening of ligand-gated ion calcium channels
   D) Influx of calcium into the presynaptic terminal

4. Which of the following is best described as an elongated, encapsulated receptor found in the dermal pegs of glabrous skin and is especially abundant on lips and fingertips?

   A) Merkel's disc
   B) Free nerve endings
   C) Meissner's corpuscle
   D) Ruffini's endings

5. Pain receptors in the skin are typically classified as which of the following?

   A) Encapsulated nerve endings
   B) Single class of morphologically specialized receptors
   C) Same type of receptor that detects position sense
   D) Free nerve endings

6. Which of the following best describes an expanded tip tactile receptor found in the dermis of hairy skin that is specialized to detect continuously applied touch sensation?

   A) Free nerve endings
   B) Merkel's disc
   C) Pacinian corpuscle
   D) Ruffini's endings

7. Hypoventilation has which of the following effects on neuronal activity?

   A) Depresses neuronal activity
   B) Increases neuronal activity
   C) Increases synaptic delay
   D) Increases neurotransmitter release

8. Which of the following best describes the concept of specificity in sensory nerve fibers that transmit only one modality of sensation?

   A) Frequency coding principle
   B) Concept of specific nerve energy
   C) Singularity principle
   D) Labeled line principle

9. Which of the following is an encapsulated receptor found deep in the skin throughout the body as well as in fascial layers where they detect indentation of the skin (pressure) and movement across the surface (vibration)?

   A) Pacinian corpuscle
   B) Meissner's corpuscle
   C) Free nerve endings
   D) Ruffini's endings

10. Which of the following substances enhances the sensitivity of pain receptors but does not directly excite them?

    A) Bradykinin
    B) Serotonin
    C) Potassium ions
    D) Prostaglandins

11. Which of the following is an important functional parameter of pain receptors?

    A) Exhibit little or no adaptation
    B) Not affected by muscle tension
    C) Signal only flexion at joint capsules
    D) Can voluntarily be inhibited

12. The excitatory or inhibitory action of a neurotransmitter is determined by which of the following?

    A) Function of its postsynaptic receptor
    B) Molecular composition
    C) Shape of the synaptic vesicle in which it is contained
    D) Distance between the pre- and post-synaptic membranes

13. Which of the following statements concerning the transmission of pain signals into the central nervous system is correct?

    A) The "fast" pain fibers that conduct at about 6 to 30 m/sec are classified as type C fibers
    B) Type A-delta pain fibers are responsible for the localization of a pain stimulus
    C) Upon entering the spinal cord dorsal horn, the fast and slow pain fibers synapse with the same populations of neurons
    D) The paleospinothalamic tract is specialized to rapidly conduct pain signals to the thalamus

14. Which of the following is the system that transmits somatosensory information with the highest degree of temporal and spatial fidelity?

    A) Anterolateral system
    B) Dorsal column–medial lemniscal system
    C) Corticospinal system
    D) Spinocerebellar system

15. Which of the following pathways crosses in the ventral white commissure of the spinal cord within a few segments of entry and then courses to the thalamus contralateral to the side of the body from which the signal originated?

    A) Anterolateral system
    B) Dorsal column–medial lemniscal system
    C) Corticospinal system
    D) Spinocerebellar system

16. Which of the following statements concerning the mechanoreceptive receptor potential is/are true?

    A) Increase in stimulus energy results in an increase in receptor potential
    B) When receptor potential rises above a certain threshold action potentials will appear in the neuron attached the receptor
    C) Number of action potentials generated in the neuron attached to the receptor is proportional to receptor potential
    D) All of the above are correct

17. In chemical synapses that involve a so-called second messenger, typically a G-protein linked to the postsynaptic receptor is activated when neurotransmitter binds to that receptor. Which of the following represents an activity performed by the activated second messenger?

    A) Closure of a membrane channel for sodium or potassium
    B) Activation of cyclic AMP or cyclic GMP
    C) Inactivation of enzymes that initiate biochemical reactions in the postsynaptic neuron
    D) Inactivation of gene transcription in the postsynaptic neuron

18. Neurons located in which of the following areas release serotonin as their neurotransmitter?

    A) Periaqueductal gray area
    B) Interneurons of the spinal cord
    C) Periventricular area
    D) Nucleus raphe magnus

19. Which of the following systems conveys information concerning highly localized touch sensation and body position (proprioceptive) sensation?

    A) Anterolateral system
    B) Dorsal column–medial lemniscal system
    C) Corticospinal
    D) Spinocerebellar

20. Which of the following explains why individuals in severe pain have difficulty sleeping without sedative medication?

    A) The somatosensory cortical area for pain perception blocks the sleep-generating circuits
    B) Pain fibers entering the dorsal horn and the ascending pain pathways block the sleep-generating circuits
    C) Ascending pain pathways provide excitatory input to brainstem reticular formation areas that are involved in maintenance of the alert, waking state
    D) The neurotransmitters used in the slow pain pathway diffuse to neighboring cell groups and generally raise the excitability of the brain

21. The first-order (primary afferent) cell bodies of the dorsal column–medial lemniscal system are found in which of the following structures?

    A) Spinal cord dorsal horn
    B) Spinal cord ventral horn
    C) Dorsal root ganglia
    D) Nucleus cuneatus

22. Which of the following structures carries axons from the nucleus gracilis to the thalamus?

    A) Fasciculus gracilis
    B) Fasciculus lemniscus
    C) Lateral spinothalamic tract
    D) Medial lemniscus

23. Which of the following represents the basis for trans-duction of a sensory stimulus into nerve impulses?

    A) Change in the ion permeability of the receptor membrane
    B) Generation of an action potential
    C) Inactivation of a G-protein–mediated response
    D) Protein synthesis

24. Which of the following structures carries axons from neurons in the ventral posterolateral nucleus of the thalamus to the primary somatosensory cortex?

    A) Medial lemniscus
    B) External capsule
    C) Internal capsule
    D) Extreme capsule

25. Which of the following is characteristic of the events occurring at an excitatory synapse?

    A) There is a massive efflux of calcium from the pre-synaptic terminal
    B) Synaptic vesicles bind to the postsynaptic membrane
    C) Voltage-gated potassium channels are closed
    D) Ligand-gated channels are opened to allow sodium entry into the postsynaptic neuron

26. In a neuron with a resting membrane potential of −65mV, the distribution of which ion across the neuronal membrane represents the least potential electromotive force (EMF)?

    A) Potassium
    B) Chloride
    C) Sodium
    D) Calcium

27. Stimulation of which brain area can modulate the sensation of pain?

    A) Superior olivary complex
    B) Locus ceruleus
    C) Periaquaductal gray
    D) Amygdala

28. Which of the following body parts is represented supe-riorly and medially within the postcentral gyrus?

    A) Upper limb
    B) Lower limb
    C) Abdomen
    D) Genitalia

29. Which of the following is a group of neurons in the pain suppression pathway that utilizes enkephalin as a neurotransmitter?

    A) Postcentral gyrus
    B) Nucleus raphe magnus
    C) Periaqueductal gray
    D) Type AB sensory fibers

30. As the receptor potential rises higher above threshold, which of the following best characterizes the new frequency of action potentials?

    A) Decrease
    B) Increase
    C) Remain unchanged
    D) Increase only when the receptor potential increases to twice the level of threshold

31. Which of the following is a type of interneuron in this region that utilizes enkephalin to inhibit pain transmission?

    A) Nucleus raphe magnus
    B) Postcentral gyrus
    C) Dorsal horn of spinal cord
    D) Type C sensory fiber

32. The highest degree of pain localization comes from

    A) simultaneous stimulation of free nerve endings and tactile fibers
    B) stimulation of free nerve endings by bradykinin
    C) nerve fibers traveling to the thalamus by way of the paleospinothalamic tract
    D) stimulation of type A delta fibers

33. Inhibition of pain signals by tactile stimulation of a skin surface involves which of the following selections?

    A) Type A alpha fibers in peripheral nerves
    B) Type A beta fibers in peripheral nerves
    C) Type A delta fibers in peripheral nerves
    D) Type C fibers in peripheral nerves

34. Within the primary somatosensory cortex, the various parts of the contralateral body surface are represented in areas of varying size that reflect which of the following?

    A) The relative size of the body parts
    B) The density of the specialized peripheral receptors
    C) The size of the muscles in that body part
    D) The conduction velocity of the primary afferent fibers

35. The gray matter of the primary somatosensory cortex contains six layers of cells. Which of the following layers receives the bulk of incoming signals from the somatosensory nuclei of the thalamus?

    A) Layer I
    B) Layers II and III
    C) Layer III only
    D) Layer IV

36. Which of the following statements concerning the neuronal membrane at rest is correct?

    A) The extracellular sodium concentration is less than its intracellular concentration
    B) The concentration of chloride is greatest inside the cell
    C) If the resting potential is moved to a more negative value, the cell becomes more excitable
    D) The concentration gradient for potassium is such that it tends to move out of the cell

37. Which of the following is the basis for referred pain?

    A) Visceral pain signals and pain signals from the skin synapse with separate populations of neurons in the dorsal horn
    B) Visceral pain transmission and pain transmission from the skin is received by a common set of neurons in the thalamus
    C) Visceral pain signals are rarely of sufficient magnitude to exceed the threshold of activation of dorsal horn neurons
    D) Some visceral pain signals and pain signals from the skin provide convergent input to a common set of neurons in the dorsal horn

38. Post-tetanic facilitation is thought to be the result of

    A) opening voltage-gated sodium channels
    B) opening transmitter gated potassium channels
    C) a buildup of calcium in the presynaptic terminal
    D) electrotonic conduction

39. Pain from the stomach is referred to which area of the body?

    A) upper right shoulder area
    B) abdominal area above the umbilicus
    C) proximal area of the anterior and inner thigh
    D) abdominal area below the umbilicus

40. Which one of the following statements concerning visceral pain signals is correct?

    A) They are transmitted along sensory fibers that course mainly with sympathetic nerves in the abdomen and thorax
    B) They are not stimulated by ischemia in visceral organs
    C) They are transmitted only by the lightly myelinated type A delta sensory fibers
    D) They are typically well localized

Questions 41–43

Each of the disorders in the following three questions is characterized either by the production of excessive pain (hyperalgesia) or the loss of pain sensation.

41. Which disorder is characterized by excessive pain in a skin dermatomal distribution resulting from a viral infection of a dorsal root ganglion?

    A) Tic douloureux
    B) Thalamic pain syndrome
    C) Brown-Séquard syndrome
    D) Herpes zoster

42. Which disorder involves a loss of pain sensation on one side of the body coupled with the loss of proprioception, precise tactile localization, and vibratory sensations on the contralateral side of the body?

    A) Herpes zoster
    B) Thalamic pain syndrome
    C) Lateral medullary syndrome
    D) Brown-Séquard syndrome

43. Which disorder is characterized by the loss of pain sensation throughout one entire side of the body and the opposite side of the face?

    A) Brown-Séquard syndrome
    B) Thalamic pain syndrome
    C) Herpes zoster
    D) Lateral medullary syndrome

44. Which of the following electrical events is characteristic of inhibitory synaptic interactions?

    A) A neurotransmitter agent that selectively opens ligand-gated chloride channels is the basis for an inhibitory postsynaptic potential
    B) Because the Nernst potential for chloride is about −70 mV, chloride ions tend to move out of the cell along its electrochemical gradient
    C) A neurotransmitter that selectively opens potassium channels will allow potassium to move into the cell
    D) An increase in the extracellular sodium concentration usually leads directly to an inhibitory postsynaptic potential

45. Which of the following somatosensory deficits is NOT typically seen following lesions that involve the postcentral gyrus?

    A) Inability to discretely localize touch sensation over the contralateral face and upper limb.
    B) Inability to judge the weight of easily recognizable objects
    C) Inability to accurately assess the texture of common objects by touching them with the fingers
    D) Inability to move the contralateral arm and leg

46. The ability to detect two points simultaneously applied to the skin is based on which of the following physiologic mechanisms?

    A) Presynaptic inhibition
    B) Lateral inhibition
    C) Medial inhibition
    D) Feed-forward inhibition

47. Stimulation by touching or pulling on which of the following structures is least likely to cause a painful sensation?

    A) The postcentral gyrus
    B) The dura overlying the postcentral gyrus
    C) Branches of the middle meningeal artery that lie superficial to the dura over the postcentral gyrus
    D) Branches of the middle cerebral artery that supply the postcentral gyrus

48. Vibratory sensation is dependent on the detection of rapidly changing, repetitive sensations. The high-frequency end of the repetitive stimulation scale is detected by which of the following?

    A) Merkel's discs
    B) Meissner's corpuscles
    C) Pacinian corpuscles
    D) Free nerve endings

49. Prolonged changes in neuronal activity are usually achieved through the activation of

    A) voltage-gated chloride channels
    B) transmitter-gated sodium channels
    C) G-protein–coupled channels
    D) voltage-gated potassium channels

50. Transmission of the electrical signal from the dendrites to the soma of a neuron occurs by which of the following?

    A) Short-circuit current flow
    B) An action potential mechanism
    C) Electrotonic conduction
    D) Capacitive discharge

51. Which one of the following statements concerning sensory neurons or their functional properties is true?

    A) All sensory fibers are unmyelinated
    B) In spatial summation, increasing signal strength is transmitted by using progressively greater numbers of sensory fibers
    C) Increased stimulus intensity is signaled by a progressive decrease in the receptor potential
    D) Continuous subthreshold stimulation of a pool of sensory neurons results in disfacilitation of those neurons
    E) Temporal summation involves signaling of increased stimulus strength by decreasing the frequency of action potentials in the sensory fibers

52. For a sensory nerve fiber that is connected to a Pacinian corpuscle located on palmar surface of the right hand, the synaptic connection with the subsequent neuron in the corresponding sensory pathway is located in

    A) the right dorsal column nucleus
    B) the left dorsal column nucleus
    C) the dorsal horn of the right side of the spinal cord
    D) the dorsal horn of the left side of the spinal cord

53. Migraine headaches typically begin with a prodromal symptom such as nausea, loss of vision, visual aura, or other sensory hallucinations. Which of the following is thought to be the cause of such prodromes?

    A) Increased blood flow to brain tissue in the visual or other sensory cortex
    B) A selective loss of GABA neurons in the various sensory areas of cortex
    C) Constipation
    D) Vasospasm leading to ischemia and a disruption of neuronal activity in the relevant sensory areas of cortex

54. Which statement concerning the generation of an action potential is correct?

    A) When the membrane potential in the soma/axon hillock dips below "threshold," an action potential is initiated
    B) The action potential is initiated in synaptic boutons
    C) The least number of voltage-gated sodium channels in an axon is found near the node of Ranvier
    D) Once an action potential is initiated, it will always run its course to completion

55. Position sense, or more commonly proprioceptive sensation, involves muscle spindles and which of the following selections?

    A) Skin tactile receptors
    B) Deep receptors in joint capsules
    C) Both tactile and joint capsule receptors
    D) Pacinian corpuscles

56. The sensation of temperature is signaled mainly by warm and cold receptors whose sensory fibers travel in association with the sensory fibers carrying pain signals. Which of the following statements best characterizes the transmission of signals from warm receptors?

    A) Warm receptors are well characterized histologically
    B) Signals from warm receptors are mainly transmitted along slow-conducting type C sensory fibers
    C) Warm receptors are located well below the surface of the skin in the subcutaneous connective tissue
    D) There are 3 to 10 times more warm receptors than cold receptors in most areas of the body

57. Like other sensory systems, the somatosensory system has a descending component that functions to regulate the overall sensitivity of the system. Which of the following selections best describes the function of the corticofugal signals transmitted from the somatosensory cortex downward to the thalamus and dorsal column nuclei?

    A) Increase or decrease the perception of signal intensity
    B) Decrease the ability to detect body position sense
    C) Remove the thalamus from the processing of somatosensory signals
    D) Allow ascending information to bypass nucleus cuneatus and gracilis

58. Which of the following statements accurately describes a feature of temperature sensation by the nervous system?

    A) Cold receptors continue to be activated even if skin temperature is lowered well below its freezing point
    B) Both cold and warm receptors each have very specific, nonoverlapping ranges of temperature sensitivity
    C) Warm and cold receptors respond to both steady state temperatures and to changes in temperature
    D) Temperature receptor function is the result of ion conduction changes and not changes in their metabolic rate

59. Which of the following statements concerning synaptic transmission is correct?

    A) When a specific population of synaptic terminals is spread over the considerable surface of a neuron, their collective effects cannot spatially summate and lead to initiation of an action potential
    B) Even if the successive discharges of an excitatory synapse occur sufficiently close in time, they cannot temporally summate and initiate an action potential
    C) A neuron is "facilitated" when its membrane potential is moved in the less negative or depolarizing direction
    D) Even when rapidly stimulated by excitatory synaptic input for a prolonged period of time, neurons typically do not exhibit synaptic fatigue

60. Which of the following statements regarding the processing of sensory signals by a pool of neurons is correct?

    A) Convergence of input signals to individual neurons in the pool, each of which contributes to the same output channel, can lead to amplification of the signal
    B) Divergence of input signals to multiple neurons in the pool, each of which leads to a different output channel, can lead to diffusion of the signal
    C) The combination of multiple input signals from multiple sources onto a single neuron in the pool is an example of divergence
    D) The distribution of multiple input signals from a single source onto many neurons in the pool is an example of convergence

1. **C)** The Nernst potential for sodium is +61 millivolts. A resting membrane potential of +61 millivolts would be required to prevent sodium from moving across the cell membrane. This value is much greater than either the Nernst potential for potassium (−86 millivolts) or that of chloride (−70 millivolts). Therefore the distribution of sodium across the membrane represents the greatest electrochemical potential.
TMP12 552–553

2. **B)** An alkaline pH causes an increase in neuronal activity.
TMP12 557

3. **D)** The release of neurotransmitter is dependent on the influx of calcium through voltage-gated channels. When this occurs, synaptic vesicles fuse with the presynaptic membrane and release the transmitter agent into the synaptic cleft.
TMP12 548

4. **C)** Meissner's corpuscles are found in the dermal pegs.
TMP12 560, 571–572

5. **D)** Pain receptors in the skin are free nerve endings.
TMP12 583

6. **B)** Merkel's discs are found in the dermis of hairy skin and signal continuous touch.
TMP12 572

7. **A)** Hypoventilation results in an acidification of the blood. This will result in a decrease in neuronal activity.
TMP12 557

8. **D)** The association of one sensory modality with one type of nerve fiber is the basis for the labeled line theory.
TMP12 559

9. **A)** Pacinian corpuscles detect pressure and movement across the skin surface and are encapsulated receptors found deep in the skin throughout the body.
TMP12 561,572

10. **D)** Prostaglandins are believed to enhance the sensitivity of pain receptors but do not actually excite them.
TMP12 583

11. **A)** Pain receptors exhibit little or no functional adaptation.
TMP12 583–584

12. **A)** The function of a transmitter agent is solely dependent on the postsynaptic receptor to which it binds.
TMP12 548

13. **B)** Type A-delta and not type C fibers are responsible for pain localization.
TMP12 585

14. **B)** Temporal and spatial fidelity is enhanced in the dorsal column–medial lemniscal system compared with the anterolateral system.
TMP12 574

15. **A)** Fibers in the anterolateral system cross in the anterior white commissure within a few segments of their entry before ascending on the contralateral side. Signals ascending in the dorsal column–medial lemniscal system do not cross until they reach the dorsal column nuclei in the medulla.
TMP12 580–581

16. **D)** The receptor potential is defined as the membrane potential of the neuronal receptor. Once the threshold for activation is reached the number of action potentials generated will increase in proportion to the strength of the stimulus until a plateau is reached.
TMP12 561–562

17. **B)** G-proteins binding can lead to the activation of cyclic AMP or cyclic GMP. Such proteins do not close sodium or potassium channels nor do they inactivate various enzymes, gene transcription, or transmitter agents (see figure on the next page).

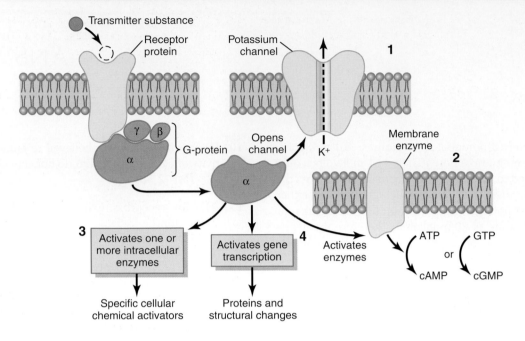

TMP12 548–549

18. **D)** Neurons of the nucleus raphe magnus release serotonin at their nerve endings. In the endogenous pain suppression system, the termination of these neurons is in the spinal cord on interneurons that in turn release enkephalin and block the incoming signals from the pain fibers.

TMP12 587

19. **B)** The sensations of highly localized touch and body position are carried in the dorsal column–medial lemniscal system.

TMP12 574

20. **C)** Individuals experiencing severe chronic pain have difficulty sleeping because the ascending pain pathways provide input to reticular formation elements that comprise the reticular activating system. The latter system maintains the alert, waking state.

TMP12 586

21. **C)** Primary afferent neuronal cell bodies are found in the dorsal root ganglia.

TMP12 573–574

22. **D)** The medial lemniscus conveys axons from the nucleus gracilis and cuneatus to the thalamus (see figure).

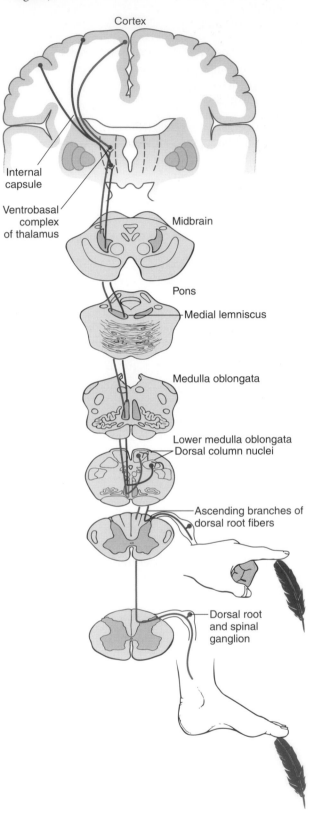

TMP12 574

23. **A)** A central issue in the sensory transduction mechanism is the change (increase) in ion permeability that occurs in the receptor membrane.
    TMP12 549

24. **C)** The internal capsule conveys axons from the ventral posterolateral thalamic nucleus to the primary somatosensory cortex.
    TMP12 574

25. **D)** Ligand-gated channels open and allow sodium entry. This is accompanied by the influx of calcium, binding of synaptic vesicles to the presynaptic membrane, and electrical changes in the postsynaptic membrane.
    TMP12 548

26. **B)** The Nernst potential for chloride is −70 millivolts. This value is closest to the average resting membrane potential of a typical neuron. As such it represents the least electrochemical potential.
    TMP12 552–553

27. **C)** The periaqueductal gray in the midbrain contains neurons that contribute to the descending pain suppression system.
    TMP12 587

28. **B)** The lower limb representation is found in the superior and medial portion of the postcentral gyrus (see figure; from Penfield/Rasmussen. *THE CEREBRAL CORTEX OF MAN.* © 1950 Gale, a part of Cengage Learning, Inc. Reproduced by permission. www.cengage.com/permissions).

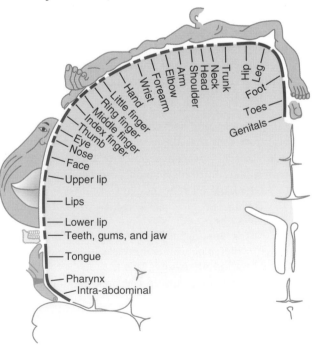

TMP12 576

29. B) Neurons in the nucleus raphe magnus utilize serotonin as a transmitter agent.
TMP12 587

30. B) As the receptor potential increases above threshold, action potential frequency will increase.
TMP12 561

31. C) A spinal cord interneuron in the dorsal horn utilizes enkephalin as a transmitter agent that effectively inhibits pain signaling.
TMP12 587

32. A) In general the sensation of pain is poorly localized. However, when a tactile receptor and a pain receptor are stimulated simultaneously the pain sensation is localized with greater accuracy.
TMP12 586

33. B) Tactile cutaneous stimulation involving type A–beta fibers can lead to pain suppression.
TMP12 585

34. B) The size of the representation of various body parts in the primary somatosensory cortex is correlated with the density of cutaneous receptors in that body part.
TMP12 576

35. D) Layer IV of the somatosensory cortex receives the bulk of the input from the somatosensory nuclei of the thalamus.
TMP12 576

36. D) At rest, intracellular potassium concentration is higher than its extracellular concentration, and potassium tends to move out of the cell. At the same time, extracellular sodium and chloride concentrations are greater than their respective intracellular concentrations.
TMP12 552

37. D) Visceral pain fibers can provide input to anterolateral tract cells that also receive somatic pain from the skin surface. The convergence of these two types of pain signals onto single spinal cord neurons is thought to be the basis for referred pain.
TMP12 588

38. C) Post-tetanic facilitation is the neuronal phenomenon in which a neuron is more easily excited following a brief period of activity. This is thought to be due to the buildup of calcium in the presynaptic membrane caused by the prior neuronal activity. Subsequent neuronal impulses release neurotransmitter more readily as a result of this preplaced calcium from the prior stimulus.
TMP12 555

39. B) Pain from the stomach is referred to the upper abdominal area. In general, it will be above the level of the umbilicus.
TMP12 589

40. A) Visceral pain signals from structures in the abdomen and thorax travel toward the spinal cord in association with fibers of the sympathetic system.
TMP12 589–590

41. D) Herpes zoster is a disorder characterized by excessive pain in a dermatomal distribution that results from a viral infection of a dorsal root ganglion.
TMP12 590

42. D) The Brown-Séquard syndrome is characterized by the loss of pain sensation on one side of the body coupled with a loss of discriminative sensations, such as proprioception and vibratory sensation on the opposite side of the body.
TMP12 590

43. D) The lateral medullary syndrome exhibits one of the most characteristic patterns of sensory loss in clinical neurology—pain sensation is lost over one side of the body from feet to neck and on the opposite side of the face. Moreover, the side of facial pain loss indicates the side of the lesion.
TMP12 590

44. A) Opening of ligand-gated chloride channels and movement of chloride ions into the cell leads to hyperpolarization of the membrane. Neither increasing the extracellular sodium concentration nor the movement of potassium into the cell leads to hyperpolarization of the membrane.
TMP12 554

45. D) Paralysis of the contralateral arm and leg is a motor deficit and such a deficit would not typically be observed following damage to the primary somatosensory cortex.
TMP12 577

46. B) The process of lateral inhibition, illustrated in the figure, underlies the ability to discriminate two points simultaneously applied.

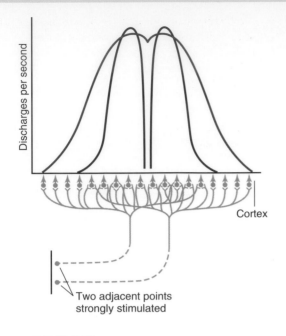

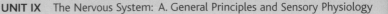

TMP12 567

47. A) Touching or pulling on the postcentral gyrus is least likely to evoke a painful sensation because brain tissue lacks pain receptors.
TMP12 591

48. C) High frequency repetitive stimulation (indentation/pressure) of the skin is sensed by Pacinian corpuscles.
TMP12 572

49. C) Activation of G-proteins usually changes the long-term response characteristics of the neuron.
TMP12 549

50. C) Dendrites have few voltage-gated sodium channels. As such the capability of these structures in generating action potentials is extremely limited. Therefore, the transmission of the electrical signal in the dendrite is via a non action potential mechanism, electrotonic conduction.
TMP12 556

51. B) In spatial summation, increasing signal strength is transmitted by using greater numbers of sensory fibers.
TMP12 564

52. A) The Pacinian corpuscle transmits a modality of sensation (vibration) that is transmitted in the dorsal column–medial lemniscal system. The first synaptic connection in this sensory pathway is in the dorsal column nuclei on the ipsilateral side of the body.
TMP12 574

53. D) Vasospasm and eventually ischemia in a sensory area of cortex is thought to be the basis for the prodromal symptoms experienced by patients with migraines.
TMP12 591

54. D) The action potential is described as an "all or none" process. Once initiated, the action potential runs its course to completion.
TMP12 554

55. C) Proprioceptive sensation is dependent on tactile and joint capsule receptors.
TMP12 590

56. B) Warm receptors mainly transmit signals along relatively slow-conducting type C fibers.
TMP12 592

57. A) Descending cortical modulation of somatosensation involves an increase or decrease in the perception of signal intensity.
TMP12 581–582

58. C) Both warm and cold receptors are able to respond to steady-state temperatures as well as changes in temperature.
TMP12 593

59. C) A facilitated neuron is one whose resting membrane potential is closer to the threshold for activation, that is, less negative or in the depolarizing direction.
TMP12 555

60. D) Divergence occurs when input signals are sent to multiple neurons in a pool, and each neuron then initiates a signal in its own output channel.
TMP12 566

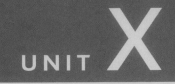

The Nervous System: B. The Special Senses

1. Which of the following statements regarding the lateral geniculate nucleus is correct?

    A) Layer one is called a parvocellular layer
    B) Layer one receives signals from the lateral half of the retina
    C) Layer one receives signals that originate from rods
    D) Layer four receives signals from the ipsilateral retina
    E) Layer four receives signals from Y ganglion cells

2. Which of the following substances will elicit the sensation of sour taste?

    A) Aldehydes
    B) Alkaloids
    C) Amino acids
    D) Hydrogen ions
    E) Ketones

3. Which of the following statements regarding the refraction of light is correct?

    A) Light waves have a longer wavelength in transparent solids than in air
    B) Light waves travel at higher velocity through transparent solids than through air
    C) The refractive index of a transparent solid is the ratio of the velocity of light in air to the velocity of light in the substance
    D) The refractive index of air is zero
    E) When light waves strike a transparent solid, they always reflect away from the solid rather than travel through the solid

4. When comparing the fovea with the periphery of the retina, which of the following statements is correct?

    A) The fovea contains an increased proportion of cones
    B) The fovea contains an increased proportion of ganglion cells
    C) The fovea contains an increased proportion of horizontal cells
    D) The fovea contains an increased proportion of rods
    E) The fovea contains an increased proportion of vasculature

5. Which of the following is the middle ear ossicle that is attached to the tympanic membrane?

    A) Columella
    B) Incus
    C) Malleus
    D) Modiolus
    E) Stapes

6. Light entering the eye passes through which retinal layer first?

    A) Inner nuclear layer
    B) Outer nuclear layer
    C) Outer plexiform layer
    D) Photoreceptor layer
    E) Retinal ganglion layer

7. Ganglion cells attached to photoreceptors located on the temporal portion of the retina project to which of the following structures?

    A) Contralateral lateral geniculate nucleus
    B) Ipsilateral lateral geniculate nucleus
    C) Ipsilateral medial geniculate nucleus
    D) Calcarine fissure
    E) Contralateral medial geniculate nucleus

8. Which of the following best describes the "blind spot" of the eye?

    A) Located 5 degrees lateral to the central point of vision
    B) Exit point of the optic nerve
    C) Contains only rods and thus has monochromatic vision
    D) Contains no blood vessels
    E) Area where chromatic aberration of the lens is the greatest

9. When parallel light rays pass through a concave lens, which of the following will occur?

    A) Rays converge toward each other
    B) Rays diverge away from each other
    C) They maintain parallel relationship
    D) They reflect back in the direction from where they came
    E) Rays refract to one focal point

10. Which of the following regarding the attenuation reflex is correct?

    A) Can increase the intensity of low-frequency sound transmission by 30 to 40 decibels
    B) Increases the rigidity of the ossicular system, thereby reducing conduction of low-frequency sounds
    C) Masks high-frequency sounds in a loud environment so lower frequency sounds are more easily heard
    D) Occurs following a latent period of 4 to 8 seconds after the loud sound
    E) Protects the cochlea from the damaging vibrations of relatively quiet but high-frequency sounds

11. Which of the following substances will elicit the sensation of bitter taste?

    A) Aldehydes
    B) Alkaloids
    C) Amino acids
    D) Hydrogen ions
    E) Ketones

12. Damage to the VIth cranial nerve will produce which of the following deficits in eye movement?

    A) Inability to move the eyes in a vertical up and down motion
    B) Inability to rotate the eyes within the eye socket
    C) Inability to move the eyes laterally towards the midline
    D) Inability to move the eyes laterally away from the midline
    E) Vertical strabismus

13. Which of the following statements is correct regarding the focal length of a convex lens?

    A) Converging light rays passing through a convex lens will converge at a focal point farther away than the focal length of that lens
    B) Diverging light rays passing through a convex lens will converge at a focal point closer than the focal length of that lens
    C) Parallel light rays passing through a convex lens will converge at a focal point equal to the focal length of that lens
    D) The image produced by a convex lens is right side up, but its two lateral sides are reversed with respect to the object
    E) The lens with the greatest convexity will have the longest focal length

14. If a convex lens has a focal length of 1 cm (0.01 m), what is the refractive power of that lens in diopters?

    A) +0.01
    B) +0.10
    C) +1
    D) +10
    E) +100

15. The condition of cataracts is usually the result of which of the following processes or conditions?

    A) Denaturation of the proteins in lens of the eye
    B) Elongated eye globe
    C) Unresponsive and dilated pupil
    D) Coagulation of the proteins in the lens of the eye
    E) Increase in intraocular pressure

16. Which of the following taste sensations is the most sensitive (i.e., has the lowest stimulation threshold)?

    A) Acid
    B) Bitter
    C) Salty
    D) Sour
    E) Sweet

17. Which of the following statements regarding the basilar membrane is correct?

    A) Vibrates best at high frequency near the base of the cochlea, whereas it vibrates best at low frequency at the apex of the cochlea
    B) Spiral ganglion lies on its surface
    C) Contains basilar fibers whose diameter increases from the base of the cochlea to the apex of the cochlea
    D) Contains basilar fibers whose length decreases from the base of the cochlea to the apex of the cochlea
    E) Separates the scala media from the scala vestibuli

18. Which of the following substances is responsible for the umami taste sensation?

    A) Acetic acid
    B) Potassium tartrate
    C) Long-chained organic substances containing nitrogen
    D) Fructose
    E) Glutamate

19. Analysis of visual detail occurs in which secondary visual area?

    A) Brodmann's area 18
    B) Inferior ventral and medial regions of the occipital and temporal cortex
    C) Frontal lobe
    D) Occipitoparietal cortex
    E) Posterior midtemporal area

20. Which of the following statements best describes the role of melanin in the pigment layer of the retina?

    A) Precursor of the light sensitive chemical rhodopsin
    B) Serves as nutritional component for the rods and cones in the retina
    C) Dark pigment that prevents the reflection of light inside the globe of the eye
    D) Responsible for maintaining integrity of the canal of Schlemm
    E) Light reflected off the melanin pigment is a key element used in the process of accommodation of the lens

21. Which of the following pairs of molecules combine to form rhodopsin?

A) Bathorhodopsin and 11-cis-retinal
B) Bathorhodopsin and all-trans-retinal
C) Bathorhodopsin and scotopsin
D) Scotopsin and 11-cis-retinal
E) Scotopsin and all-trans-retinal

22. A deficiency of which vitamin prevents the formation of an adequate quantity of retinal, eventually leading to night blindness?

A) Vitamin A
B) Vitamin C
C) Vitamin D
D) Vitamin E
E) Vitamin K

23. What is the name of the condition whereby the lens of the eye becomes almost totally unaccommodating in persons over 70 years of age?

A) Amblyopia
B) Emmetropia
C) Hyperopia
D) Myopia
E) Presbyopia

24. Which compartment of the cochlea contains the organ of Corti?

A) Ampulla
B) Saccule
C) Scala media
D) Scala tympani
E) Scala vestibuli

25. Which of the following statements regarding the transmission of taste information from the tongue to the cerebral cortex is correct?

A) Majority of thalamic neurons in taste pathway synapse in the occipital lobe
B) Nerve fibers carrying taste information from the tongue have no synapse in the brainstem
C) Nerve fibers carrying taste information from the tongue synapse in the solitary nucleus
D) Thalamic nucleus involved in the taste pathway is the dorsal medial nucleus
E) Thalamic nucleus involved in the taste pathway is the ventral posterolateral nucleus

26. Which cells in layer IV of the primary visual cortex detect orientation of lines and borders?

A) Border cells
B) Complex cells
C) Ganglion cells
D) Hypercomplex cells
E) Simple cells

27. Which of the following best describes when the transmission of sound waves in the cochlea occurs?

A) When the foot of the stapes moves inward against the oval window and the round window bulges outward
B) When the foot of the stapes moves inward against the round window and the oval window bulges outward
C) When the head of the malleus moves inward against the oval window and the round window bulges outward
D) It occurs when the incus moves inward against the oval window and the round window bulges outward
E) It occurs when the incus moves inward against the round window and the oval window bulges outward

28. Under low or reduced light conditions, which of the following chemical compounds is responsible for the inward-directed sodium current in the outer segments of the photoreceptors?

A) Metarhodopsin II
B) Cyclic GMP
C) 11-cis retinal
D) Cyclic AMP
E) 11-trans retinol

29. Which of the following statements regarding the cranial nerve innervation of the tongue is correct?

A) Taste information from the anterior two-thirds of the tongue is transmitted to the solitary nucleus by the glossopharyngeal nerve
B) Taste information from the pharynx is transmitted to the solitary nucleus by the facial nerve
C) Taste information from the posterior third of the tongue is transmitted to the solitary nucleus by the glossopharyngeal nerve
D) Taste information from the posterior third of the tongue initially travels with the lingual nerve
E) Taste information from the posterior third of the tongue initially travels with the chorda tympani nerve

30. Olfactory receptor cells belong to which of the following groups of cells?

A) Bipolar neurons
B) Fibroblasts
C) Modified epithelial cells
D) Multipolar neurons
E) Pseudounipolar neurons

31. Which of the following statements regarding hair cells is correct?

    A) Hair cells depolarize when their stereocilia are bent toward the shortest stereocilium
    B) Nerve fibers stimulated by hair cells have their cell bodies in the cochlear nuclei of the brainstem
    C) The stereocilia of the hair cells are longer on the side of the hair cell nearest the modiolus
    D) There are more inner hair cells than outer hair cells in the organ of Corti
    E) Transmission of auditory signals is performed mainly by inner hair cells rather than outer hair cells

32. Accommodation for far vision (focusing on an object at a distance) requires which of the following processes?

    A) Constriction of the pupil of the eye
    B) Dilation of the pupil of the eye
    C) An increase in the formation of rhodopsin
    D) Causing the lens of the eye to have more curvature (making it fatter)
    E) Causing the lens of the eye to have less curvature (making it thinner)

33. Which of the following events occurs in photoreceptors during phototransduction in response to light?

    A) Phosphodiesterase activity decreases
    B) Transducin activity decreases
    C) Hydrolysis of cGMP increases
    D) Neurotransmitter release increases
    E) Number of open voltage–gated calcium channels increases

34. During photoreception, all of the following increase except

    A) cGMP phosphodiesterase
    B) Transducin
    C) cAMP
    D) Metarhodopsin II
    E) Sodium influx into the outer segment of the rod

35. Which of the following statements is correct regarding astigmatism?

    A) Light rays do not come to a common focal point
    B) Light rays being emitted from distant objects are focused behind the retina
    C) Light rays being emitted from distant objects are focused in front of the retina
    D) Light rays being emitted from distant objects are in sharp focus on the retina
    E) There is a cloudy or opaque area or areas in the lens

36. The stereocilia of hair cells are embedded in which membrane?

    A) Basilar
    B) Reissner's
    C) Tectorial
    D) Tympanic
    E) Vestibular

37. Which of the following cranial nerves is correctly paired with the extraocular muscle it innervates?

    A) Abducens nerve–medial rectus
    B) Oculomotor nerve–inferior oblique
    C) Oculomotor nerve–lateral rectus
    D) Oculomotor nerve–superior oblique
    E) Trochlear nerve–superior rectus

38. After olfactory receptor cells bind odor molecules, a sequence of intracellular events occurs that culminates in the entrance of specific ions that depolarize the olfactory receptor cell. Which of the following ions are involved?

    A) Calcium ions
    B) Chloride ions
    C) Hydrogen ions
    D) Potassium ions
    E) Sodium ions

39. For the eye to adapt to intense light, which of the following may occur?

    A) Bipolar cells will continuously transmit signals at the maximum rate possible
    B) Photochemicals in both rods and cones will be reduced to retinal and opsins
    C) The levels of rhodopsin will be very high
    D) There will be an increase in the size of the pupil
    E) Vitamin A will convert into retinal

40. The condition of myopia is usually corrected by which of the following types of lens?

    A) Compound lens
    B) Convex lens
    C) Spherical lens
    D) Concave lens
    E) Cylindrical lens

41. Which lobe of the cerebral cortex contains the small bilateral cortical area that controls voluntary fixation movements?

    A) Frontal
    B) Limbic
    C) Occipital
    D) Parietal
    E) Temporal

42. Which of the following sensory systems has the smallest range of intensity discrimination?

    A) Auditory
    B) Gustatory
    C) Olfactory
    D) Somatosensory
    E) Visual

43. Which of the following molecules moves from the endolymph into the stereocilia and depolarizes the hair cell?

    A) Calcium ions
    B) Chloride ions
    C) Hydrogen ions
    D) Potassium ions
    E) Sodium ions

44. Which of the following events prompts the auditory system to interpret a sound as loud?

    A) Decreased number of inner hair cells become stimulated
    B) Decreased number of outer hair cells become stimulated
    C) Hair cells excite nerve endings at a diminished rate
    D) Amplitude of vibration of the basilar membrane decreases
    E) Amplitude of vibration of the basilar membrane increases

45. Which of the following statements is correct concerning the elements of the retina?

    A) Total number of cones in the retina is much greater than the total number of rods
    B) Each individual cone responds to all wave lengths of light
    C) Photoreceptors activation (rods and cones) results in hyperpolarization of the receptor
    D) Central fovea contains only rods
    E) Pigment layer of the retina contains the photoreceptors

46. The condition of hyperopia is usually caused by which of the following anomalies of the eye?

    A) Decreased production of melanin
    B) Uneven curvature of the cornea
    C) Eyeball that is shorter than normal
    D) Eyeball that is longer than normal
    E) Lens system that is too powerful and focuses the object in front of the retina

47. In the central auditory pathway which of the following represents the correct sequence of structures in the pathway?

    A) Cochlear nuclei–superior olive–inferior colliculus via the lateral lemniscus - medial geniculate–auditory cortex
    B) Cochlear nuclei–inferior olive–inferior colliculus via the medial lemniscus - medial geniculate–auditory cortex
    C) Cochlear nuclei–superior olive–superior colliculus via the lateral lemniscus - lateral geniculate–auditory cortex
    D) Cochlear nuclei–inferior olive–inferior colliculus via the lateral lemniscus - lateral geniculate–auditory cortex
    E) Cochlear nuclei–trapezoid body–dorsal acoustic stria–inferior colliculus via the lateral lemniscus–medial geniculate–auditory cortex

48. Which of the following statements regarding the transmission of auditory information from the ear to the cerebral cortex is correct?

    A) Inferior colliculus neurons synapse in the cochlear nuclei of the brainstem
    B) Neurons with cell bodies in the spiral ganglion of Corti synapse in the inferior colliculus
    C) The majority of neurons from the cochlear nuclei synapse in the contralateral superior olivary nucleus
    D) There is no crossing-over of information between the right and left auditory pathways in the brainstem
    E) Trapezoid neurons synapse in the cochlear nuclei of the brainstem

49. Which of the following statements regarding color vision is correct?

    A) Green is perceived when only green cones are stimulated
    B) The stimulation ratio of the three types of cones allows specific color perception
    C) The wavelength of light corresponding to white is shorter than that corresponding to blue
    D) When there is no stimulation of red, green, or blue cones, there will be the sensation of seeing white
    E) Yellow is perceived when green and blue cones are stimulated equally

50. The function of the round window can best be described by which of the following?

    A) Provides the connection point for the stapes
    B) Serves to damp out low frequency sounds such as your own voice
    C) Transmits the frequency information into the cochlea from the tympanic membrane
    D) Serves as the pressure relief valve for the cochlea
    E) Transmits amplitude information into the cochlea from the tympanic membrane

51. Which of the following muscles is contracted as part of the pupillary light reflex?

    A) Ciliary muscle
    B) Pupillary dilator muscle
    C) Pupillary sphincter muscle
    D) Radial fibers of the iris
    E) Superior oblique muscle

52. Which of the following allows the visual apparatus to accurately determine the distance of an object from the eye (depth perception)?

    A) Monocular vision
    B) Location of the retinal image on the retina
    C) Phenomenon of stationary parallax
    D) Phenomenon of stereopsis
    E) Size of the retinal image if the object is of unknown size

53. Which of the following is the most common cause of glaucoma?

    A) Drugs that reduce the secretion of aqueous humor
    B) Increased resistance to fluid outflow through trabecular spaces into the canal of Schlemm
    C) Normal function of phagocytes on the surface of trabeculae
    D) Phagocytoses of proteins and small particles by the epithelium of the iris
    E) The activation of reticuloendothelial cells in the interstitial gel outside the canal of Schlemm

54. Which of the following statements regarding the two types of deafness is correct?

    A) An audiogram of a person with conduction deafness would show much greater loss for air conduction than bone conduction of sound
    B) An audiogram of a person with nerve deafness would show much greater loss for bone conduction than air conduction of sound
    C) Conduction deafness occurs when the cochlea or cochlear nerve is impaired
    D) Nerve deafness occurs when the physical structures that conduct the sound into the cochlea are impaired
    E) Prolonged exposure to very loud sounds is more likely to cause deafness for high-frequency sounds than low frequency sounds

55. Consider the situation in which an individual is turning their head to the left about the axis of the neck. The motion begins while the chin is directly over the right shoulder and ends with the chin directly over the left shoulder. Which of the following best describes the eye movements associated with this type of head rotation in a normal individual?

    A) While the head is turning, the eyes will be moving to the right and saccadic eye motion will be to the left
    B) While the head is turning, the eyes will be moving in the same direction as the head rotation and the saccadic eye motion will be to the left
    C) While the head is turning, the eyes will be moving to the right and the saccadic eye motion will be to the right
    D) While the head is turning, the eyes will remain stationary within the orbits and the saccadic eye motion will be to the right
    E) While the head is turning, the eyes will be moving to the left and the saccadic eye motion will be to the right

56. Horner syndrome occurs when sympathetic nerve fibers to the eye are interrupted, leading to which of the following symptoms on the affected side of the face?

    A) Blood vessels of the face become persistently constricted
    B) Profuse sweating occurs
    C) The superior eyelid is maintained in an open position
    D) There is an overproduction of lacrimal gland fluid
    E) There is persistent constriction of the pupil to a smaller diameter than the pupil of the opposite eye

57. Which of the following neurotransmitters is released by both rods and cones at their synapses with bipolar cells?

    A) Acetylcholine
    B) Dopamine
    C) Glutamate
    D) Glycine
    E) Serotonin

58. Olfactory information transmitted to the orbitofrontal cortex passes through which thalamic nucleus?

    A) Dorsomedial
    B) Lateral geniculate
    C) Medial geniculate
    D) Ventral posterolateral
    E) Ventral posteromedial

59. Which of the following provides about two thirds of the 59 diopters of refractive power of the eye?

   A) Anterior surface of the cornea
   B) Anterior surface of the lens
   C) Iris
   D) Posterior surface of the cornea
   E) Posterior surface of the lens

60. Transmission of visual signals to the primary visual cortex from the retina includes a synapse in which structure?

   A) Lateral geniculate nucleus
   B) Medial geniculate nucleus
   C) Pretectal nucleus
   D) Superior colliculus
   E) Suprachiasmatic nucleus

61. Which of the following statements regarding retinal ganglion cells is correct?

   A) One W ganglion cell from the periphery of the retina typically transmits information from one rod
   B) One X ganglion cell from the fovea typically transmits information from as many as 200 cones
   C) W ganglion cells respond best to directional movement or vision under very bright conditions
   D) X ganglion cells respond best to color images and are the most numerous of the three types of ganglion cells
   E) Y ganglion cells respond best to rapid changes in the visual image and are the most numerous of the three types of ganglion cells

62. Auditory information is relayed through which thalamic nucleus?

   A) Dorsomedial nucleus
   B) Lateral geniculate nucleus
   C) Medial geniculate nucleus
   D) Ventral posterolateral nucleus
   E) Ventral posteromedial nucleus

63. The phenomenon of taste preference is

   A) a central nervous system process
   B) the result of neonatal stimulation of circumvallate papilla
   C) a learned behavior in animals
   D) a result of taste bud maturation
   E) a result of taste bud proliferation following exposure to glutamic acid

64. Of the photoreceptors listed below which one responds to the broadest spectrum of wavelengths of light?

   A) Rod receptors
   B) Green cone receptors
   C) Blue cone receptors
   D) Red cone receptors
   E) Cells containing melanin in the pigment layer

65. Which of the following structures secretes the intraocular fluid of the eye?

   A) Ciliary processes
   B) Cornea
   C) Iris
   D) Lens
   E) Trabeculae

66. Which type of papillae is located in the posterior part of the tongue?

   A) Circumvallate
   B) Foliate
   C) Fungiform
   D) Fungiform and circumvallate
   E) Papilla of Vater

67. Which structure functions to ensure that each of the three sets of extraocular muscles is reciprocally innervated so that one muscle of the pair relaxes while the other contracts?

   A) Edinger-Westphal nucleus
   B) Medial longitudinal fasciculus
   C) Pretectal nucleus
   D) Superior colliculus
   E) Suprachiasmatic nucleus

68. Which of the following retinal cells have action potentials?

   A) Amacrine cells
   B) Bipolar cells
   C) Ganglion cells
   D) Horizontal cells
   E) Photoreceptors

69. Which type of papillae is located in the folds along the lateral surfaces of the tongue?

   A) Circumvallate
   B) Foliate
   C) Fungiform
   D) Fungiform and circumvallate
   E) Papilla of Vater

70. The primary auditory cortex lies primarily in which lobe of the cerebral cortex?

   A) Frontal lobe
   B) Limbic lobe
   C) Occipital lobe
   D) Parietal lobe
   E) Temporal lobe

71. The intraocular fluid of the eye flows from the canal of Schlemm into which of the following locations?

   A) Anterior chamber
   B) Aqueous veins
   C) Lens
   D) Posterior chamber
   E) Trabeculae

72. The first central synapse for neurons transmitting the sweet taste sensation is in which of the following structures?

    A) Dorsal sensory nucleus of vagus nerve
    B) Nucleus of solitary tract
    C) Nucleus of olfactory nerve
    D) Nucleus of hypoglossal nerve
    E) Nucleus of facial nerve

73. Which brainstem structure plays a major role in determining the direction from which a sound originates?

    A) Cochlear nucleus
    B) Inferior colliculus
    C) Lateral lemniscus
    D) Superior olivary nucleus
    E) Trapezoid

74. Visual contrast is enhanced due to lateral inhibition by which retinal cells?

    A) Amacrine cells
    B) Bipolar cells
    C) Ganglion cells
    D) Horizontal cells
    E) Photoreceptors

75. Which of the following best describes the underlying basis of the dark current in the outer segment of the photoreceptors?

    A) Dark current results from the influx of sodium ions via c-AMP–dependent sodium channels
    B) Dark current results from the influx of sodium ions via c-GMP–dependent sodium channels
    C) Dark current results from the efflux of potassium ions via c-GMP–dependent potassium channels
    D) Dark current results from the efflux of sodium ions via c-GMP–dependent sodium channels
    E) Dark current results from the efflux of sodium ions via c-AMP–dependent sodium channels

1. **C)** Layers I and II of the lateral geniculate nucleus are called magnocellular layers, and receive rod input from Y retinal ganglion cells. Layers III to VI are called parvocellular layers and receive cone input from X retinal ganglion cells.
   TMP12 623–624

2. **D)** The taste sensation of sour is proportional to the logarithm of the hydrogen ion concentration caused by acids. Sweet is caused by a long list of chemicals, including sugars, alcohols, aldehydes, ketones, and amino acids.
   TMP12 645

3. **C)** Light rays travel through air at a velocity of about 300,000 km/sec, but much slower through transparent solids. Thus, the refractive index of air will be 1.00, and the refractive index of any transparent solid will be >1.00.
   TMP12 597

4. **A)** The fovea is composed almost entirely of cones. Blood vessels, ganglion cells, and other layers of cells are all displaced to one side, which allows light to pass unimpeded to the cones.
   TMP12 609

5. **C)** The malleus is attached to the tympanic membrane, and the stapes is attached to the oval window. The incus has articulations with both of these bones.
   TMP12 633

6. **E)** Light passes through the eye to the retina in the posterior portion of the eye. The most anterior layer of the retina, that which light passes first, is the retinal ganglion layer. Light then passes through the other cell layers of the retina until it reaches the photoreceptors in the posterior region of the retina.
   TMP12 609

7. **B)** The axons of the ganglion cells make up the fibers of the optic nerve. The first synapse in the visual system takes place in the lateral geniculate nucleus. Ganglion cells attached to photoreceptors on the temporal side of the retina project to the same sided or ipsilateral lateral geniculate nucleus. Fibers from the nasal side of the retina cross over to the opposite or contralateral lateral geniculate nucleus in the optic chiasm. The medial geniculate nucleus is a sensory relay for the auditory system.
   TMP12 623

8. **B)** The blind spot is located 15 degrees lateral to the central point of vision. It is the location where fibers that make up the optic nerve exit the globe of the eye. As such there are no photoreceptors in this location.
   TMP12 627

9. **B)** A concave lens diverges light rays; in contrast, a convex lens will converge light rays toward each other. If a convex lens has the appropriate curvature, parallel light rays will be bent so that all pass through a single point called the *focal point*.
   TMP12 598

10. **B)** The tensor tympani muscle pulls the handle of the malleus inward, whereas the stapedius muscle pulls the stapes outward. These two forces oppose each other and thereby cause the entire ossicular system to become more rigid, reducing the intensity of low-frequency sounds by 30 to 40 decibels.
    TMP12 634

11. **B)** The sensation of bitter is caused by many nitrogen-containing organics, as well as by alkaloids.
    TMP12 645

12. **D)** The VIth cranial nerve is also known as the *abducens nerve*. The abducens nerve innervates the lateral rectus muscle which is attached to that lateral surface of the globe of the eye. Contracting the lateral rectus muscle results in moving the eyeball laterally away from the midline of the face in an abducting manner. Thus the name abducens nerve.
    TMP12 627–628

13. **C)** The distance beyond a convex lens at which parallel rays converge to a common focal point is called the focal length of the lens. Thus, the focal point is equal to the focal length for a convex lens. Also, the greater the curvature of the convex lens, the shorter the focal length where these parallel rays will converge.
    TMP12 597–598

14. **E)** The more that a convex lens bends parallel light rays, the greater its refractive power, measured in diopters. By definition, a convex lens with a focal length of 1 m has a refractive power of +1 diopter. If a convex lens can bend parallel light rays twice as much, it is said to have twice the refractive power, or +2 diopters, and a focal length of 0.5 m. Thus, there is an inverse relationship between the focal length and the

refractive power. For this question, the convex lens has a focal length of 1 cm (0.01 m), and therefore has 100 times the refractive power, or 100 diopters.

TMP12 600

15. D) The condition of cataracts causes the lens of the eye to become opaque and resemble the look of water in a waterfall or rapids in a river, thus the name, cataract. A cataract results from the progressive coagulation of the proteins that make up the lens. One can think of this as similar to the white of an egg turning opaque as it is cooked. Heating the egg white results in coagulation of the proteins contained within it.

TMP12 604

16. B) The bitter taste sense is much more sensitive than the other sensations, because it is this sensation that provides an important protective function against many dangerous toxins in food.

TMP12 646

17. A) The basilar membrane (see figure) contains basilar fibers, whose length increases progressively from the base of the cochlea to the apex, whereas the overall stiffness of the basilar fibers decreases. As a result, the stiff fibers near the cochlea vibrate best at high frequency, and the less stiff fibers near the apex vibrate best at low frequency.

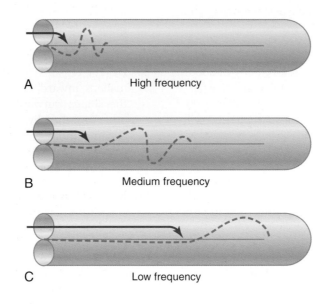

A   High frequency

B   Medium frequency

C   Low frequency

Figure for Answer 17

TMP12 635–636

18. **E)** The term *umami* is derived from the Japanese word for savory or delicious and is often described as similar to the taste of meat. Glutamate is the chemical believed to elicit the umami taste sensation.
TMP12 646

19. **B)** Visual information from the primary visual cortex (Brodmann's area 17) is relayed to Brodmann's area 18, and then into other areas of the cerebral cortex for further processing. Analysis of 3-D position, gross form, and motion of objects occurs in the posterior midtemporal area and occipitoparietal cortex. Analysis of visual detail and color occurs in the inferior ventral and medial regions of the occipital and temporal cortex.
TMP12 624,626

20. **C)** Melanin is the dark pigment that occurs in great abundance in the pigment layer of the retina. The pigment layer functions to limit light scattering inside the globe of the eye and increase contrast and visual acuity.
TMP12 609–611

21. **D)** Rhodopsin is the light-sensitive chemical in rods. Scotopsin and all-trans retinal are the breakdown products of rhodopsin, which has absorbed light energy. The all-trans retinal is converted into 11-cis retinal, which can recombine with scotopsin to form rhodopsin.
TMP12 611

22. **A)** One form of vitamin A is all-trans retinol, which is converted through two different pathways into 11-cis-retinal, which then combines with scotopsin to form rhodopsin. Vitamin A is stored in large quantities in the liver. However, many months of a diet deficient in vitamin A can lead to night blindness, because rhodopsin is crucial for rod function.
TMP12 612

23. **E)** In presbyopia, each eye remains focused permanently at an almost constant distance. The eyes can no longer accommodate for both near and far vision. Hyperopia and myopia refer to farsightedness and nearsightedness, respectively. Emmetropia is normal vision. Amblyopia has several causes that result in either an absence or loss of binocular vision.
TMP12 601

24. **C)** The ampulla and saccule are part of the vestibular apparatus, not the cochlear apparatus. The cochlea has three main compartments, with fluid movement occurring in the scala vestibuli and scala media in response to sound vibrations. The organ of Corti is contained within the scala media.
TMP12 634–635

25. **C)** All taste fibers synapse in the solitary nucleus and send second-order neurons to the ventral posteromedial nucleus of the thalamus. Third order neurons project to the lower tip of the postcentral gyrus in the parietal cortex.
TMP12 648

26. **E)** The simple cells of the primary visual cortex detect orientation of lines and borders, whereas the complex cells detect lines oriented in the same direction but are not position-specific. That is, the line can be displaced moderate distances laterally or vertically, and the same few neurons will be stimulated as long as the line is the same direction.
TMP12 626

27. **A)** The malleus is connected to the tympanic membrane, the incus articulates with the malleus and stapes, and the stapes is connected to the oval window.
TMP12 633

28. **B)** In low light conditions the level of cyclic GMP is high. Cyclic GMP-dependent sodium channels in the outer portions of the rods and cones allow sodium ions to pass from the extracellular space to the intracellular space of the photoreceptor. This results in a membrane potential that is somewhat lower than the resting membrane potential of a typical neuron. The movement of the sodium ions and resulting electrical potential change as a result of this enhanced permeability is known as the *dark current*.
TMP12 612–613

29. **C)** Taste impulses from the anterior two thirds of the tongue pass first into the lingual nerve, then through the chorda tympani into the facial nerve, and finally to the solitary nucleus. Taste sensations from the posterior third of the tongue are transmitted through the glossopharyngeal nerve to the solitary nucleus. Taste signals from the pharyngeal region are transmitted via the vagus nerve.
TMP12 647–648

30. **A)** The receptor cells for the smell sensation are bipolar nerve cells derived originally from the central nervous system itself.
TMP12 649

31. **E)** Although there are three to four times as many outer hair cells as inner hair cells, about 90% of the auditory nerve fibers are stimulated by the inner hair cells.
TMP12 637

32. **E)** Light rays from a distant object do not require as much refraction (bending) as do light rays from an object close at hand. Therefore, the curvature of the lens required to focus these rays on the retina is less.
TMP12 601

33. C) In the dark state, cGMP helps maintain the open state of the sodium channels in the outer membrane of the rod. Hydrolysis of cGMP by light causes these sodium channels to close. Less sodium is able to enter the rod outer segment, thus hyperpolarizing the rod.
TMP12 613–614

34. E) During photoreception the active compound metarhodopsin is formed. This in turn activates a g-protein called transducin. The transducin activates a c-GMP phosphodiesterase which destroys c-GMP. C-GMP dependent sodium channels close and the influx of sodium ions into the outer segment of the photoreceptors decreases.
TMP12 612–614

35. A) Astigmatism most often results when there is too great a curvature of the cornea in one of its planes. Because the curvature of the astigmatic lens along one plane is less than the curvature along the other plane, light rays striking the two planes will be bent to different degrees. Thus, light rays passing through an astigmatic lens do not come to a common focal point.
TMP12 603

36. C) The scala media is bordered by the basilar membrane and Reissner's membrane, and contains a tectorial membrane. The apical border of hair cells has stereocilia that are embedded in the tectorial membrane.
TMP12 637

37. B) The abducens nerve innervates the lateral rectus muscle. The trochlear nerve innervates the superior oblique muscle. The oculomotor nerve innervates the medial rectus, inferior oblique, superior rectus, and inferior rectus muscles.
TMP12 628

38. E) Even the minutest concentration of a specific odorant initiates a cascading effect that opens extremely large numbers of sodium channels. This accounts for the exquisite sensitivity of the olfactory neurons to even the slightest amount of odorant.
TMP12 650

39. B) The reduction of rhodopsin and cone pigments by light reduces the concentrations of photosensitive chemicals in rods and cones. Thus, the sensitivity of the eye to light is correspondingly reduced. This is called light adaptation.
TMP12 614–615

40. D) In myopia the focal point of the lens system of the eye is in front of the retina. A concave lens will diverge light rays. By placing the proper concave lens in front of the eye the divergence of light rays will move the focal point from in front of the retina to a position on the retina.
TMP12 603

41. A) A bilateral premotor cortical region of the frontal lobes controls voluntary fixation movements. A lesion of this region makes it difficult for a person to "unlock" their eyes from one point of fixation and then move them to another point.
TMP12 628–629

42. C) Concentrations that are only 10 to 50 times above threshold values will evoke maximum intensity of smell, which is in contrast to most other sensory systems of the body, where the range of intensity discrimination may reach 1 trillion to 1. This, perhaps, can be explained by the fact that smell is concerned more with detecting the presence or absence of odors than with quantitative detection of their intensities.
TMP12 650

43. D) Although most cells in the nervous system depolarize in response to sodium entry, hair cells are one group of cells that depolarize in response to potassium entry.
TMP12 637

44. E) There are at least three ways that the auditory system determines loudness. First, the amplitude of vibration of the basilar membrane increases so that hair cells excite nerve endings at more rapid rates. Second, more and more hair cells on the fringes of the resonating portion of the basilar membrane become stimulated. Third, outer hair cells become recruited at a significant rate.
TMP12 636, 638

45. C) Unlike most other sensory receptors that depolarize when activated, the photoreceptors produce the opposite response, which is hyperpolarization. The total number of rods is much greater than the number of cones. Cones respond to a very specific range of wavelengths of light. The pigment layer is posterior to the retinal layer that contains the photoreceptors.
TMP12 612

46. D) In hyperopia the focal point of the eye's lens system is behind the retina. This is usually the result of an eyeball that is too short in the anterior to posterior direction.
TMP12 602

47. A) Auditory fibers enter the cochlear nucleus. Fibers from the cochlear nucleus pass to the inferior colliculus via the lateral lemniscus. Fibers from the inferior colliculus travel to the medial geniculate nucleus and from there to the primary auditory cortex.
TMP12 639

48. C) Neurons with cell bodies in the spiral ganglion of Corti synapse in the cochlear nuclei. The majority of the cochlear nuclei neurons synapse in the contralateral superior olivary nucleus. Crossing over occurs in at least three places in the pathway, and a preponderance of auditory transmission is in the contralateral pathway. From the superior olivary nucleus, the auditory pathway then passes upward through the lateral lemniscus, with most auditory fibers terminating at the inferior colliculus. From there, the pathway continues on to the medial geniculate nucleus and then the primary auditory cortex.

TMP12 639

49. B) Research showed that the nervous system perceives the sensation of a specific color by interpreting the set of ratios of stimulation of the three types of cones. Investigators used only red, green, and blue monochromatic lights mixed in different combinations. All gradations of colors the human eye can detect were detected using just these three colors.

TMP12 615–616

50. D) The cochlea is a structure of tubes and chambers that is filled with fluid. The fluid is non compressible. As the stapes moves back and forth against the oval window the increase and decrease in pressure caused by that in and out movement of the oval window is relieved by the opposite back and forth movement of the round window.

TMP12 635

51. C) In a normal individual, shining a light in either eye will result in both pupils constricting due to contraction of the pupillary sphincter muscles. In contrast, the pupillary dilator muscle dilates the pupil. The ciliary muscle is involved in focusing the eye (accommodation).

TMP12 632

52. D) Because one eye is a little more than 2 inches to the side of the other eye, the images on the two retinae differ from one another. This binocular parallax (stereopsis) allows a person with two eyes far greater ability to judge relative distances when objects are nearby than a person with only one eye.

TMP12 605

53. B) Glaucoma is a disease of the eye in which the intraocular pressure becomes pathologically high, sometimes rising acutely to 60 to 70 mm Hg. Pressures above 30 mm Hg for long periods of time can lead to loss of vision. The most common cause of this higher intraocular pressure is when fluid outflow into the canal of Schlemm is obstructed.

TMP12 607–608

54. A) With nerve deafness, there is damage to the cochlea, auditory nerve, or the neural pathway. The ability to hear sound as tested by both air conduction and bone conduction is greatly reduced or lost with nerve deafness. However, with conduction deafness, the person retains the ability to hear sound by bone conduction, but not by air conduction.

TMP12 642

55. A) In the situation described the eyes will fix on an object in the visual field and remain on that object while the head is turning to the left. This will result in eye movement to the right as the head is turned to the left. When the object is no longer in the central field of vision the eyes will exhibit a quick jumping movement to the left (i.e., in the direction of the head rotation) and fix on a new object in the visual field. This jump is called a saccade. This process will repeat until the head has turned all the way to the left. During saccadic eye movement vision is suppressed.

TMP12 629–630

56. E) Horner syndrome typically occurs when the sympathetic nerve fibers that originated from thoracic spinal cord are interrupted in the cervical sympathetic chain on their way to the eye.

TMP12 632

57. C) At least eight types of neurotransmitter substances have been identified for amacrine cells. The neurotransmitters used for bipolar and horizontal cells are unclear, but it is well established that rods and cones release glutamate at their synapses with bipolar cells (pictured here).

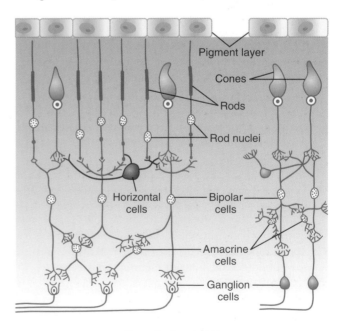

Figure for Answer 57

TMP12 617

58. A) A newer olfactory pathway has been found that projects to the dorsomedial thalamic nucleus and then to the orbitofrontal cortex. However, the older olfactory pathways bypass the thalamus to reach the cortex, in contrast to other sensory systems, which have thalamic relays.
TMP12 651

59. A) The principal reason why the anterior surface of the cornea provides most of the refractive power of the eye is that the refractive index of the cornea is markedly different from that of air.
TMP12 600

60. A) Retinal ganglion cells synapse in several locations, but those conveying information that will ultimately end up in the primary visual cortex synapse in the lateral geniculate nucleus. From there, neurons project to the primary visual cortex.
TMP12 623–624

61. D) There are three distinct groups of retinal ganglion cells, designated as W, X, and Y cells. W cells transmit rod visual signals. Y cells are the least numerous and transmit information about rapid changes in the visual image. X cells are the most numerous and receive input from cones regarding the visual image and color vision.
TMP12 619

62. C) The medial geniculate nucleus is the thalamic nucleus that conveys auditory information from the brainstem to the primary auditory cortex.
TMP12 639

63. A) Taste preference, while not completely understood, is believed to involve a central process.
TMP12 648

64. D) Intuitively one would guess that the rod photoreceptor would have the greatest range of spectral sensitivity. However, it is the red cone that has the broadest spectral sensitivity followed by the rods, the green cones, and finally the blue cones, which have the narrowest range of spectral sensitivity.
TMP12 614

65. A) Ciliary processes secrete all of the aqueous humor of the intraocular fluid, at an average rate of 2 to 3 μl/min. These processes are linear folds that project from the ciliary muscle into the space behind the iris. The intraocular fluid flows from behind the iris through the pupil into the anterior chamber of the eye.
TMP12 606

66. A) Circumvallate papillae are located in the posterior part of the tongue, fungiform papillae in the anterior part of the tongue, and foliate papillae on the lateral part of the tongue. The papilla of Vater empties pancreatic secretions and bile into the duodenum.
TMP12 647

67. B) The medial longitudinal fasciculus is a pathway for nerve fibers entering and leaving the oculomotor, trochlear, and abducens nuclei of the brainstem. This allows communication to coordinate the contraction of the various extraocular eye muscles.
TMP12 628

68. C) Only ganglion cells have action potentials. Photoreceptors, bipolar cells, amacrine cells, and horizontal cells all appear to operate through graded potentials.
TMP12 617

69. A) Foliate papillae are located in the folds along the lateral surfaces of the tongue, fungiform papillae are located in the anterior part of the tongue, and circumvallate papillae are located in the posterior part of the tongue. The papilla of Vater empties pancreatic secretions and bile into the duodenum.
TMP12 647

70. E) Most of the primary auditory cortex is in the temporal lobe, but the association auditory cortices extend over much of the insular lobe and even onto the lateral portion of the parietal lobe.
TMP12 640

71. B) Intraocular fluid flows from the anterior chamber of the eye, between the cornea and the iris through a meshwork of trabeculae into the canal of Schlemm, which empties into extraocular aqueous veins (see figure).

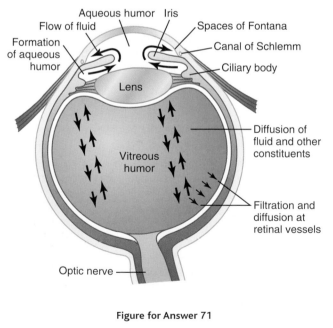

Figure for Answer 71

TMP12 607

72. B) The termination of taste fibers for all taste sensations is in the nucleus of the solitary tract in the medulla.
TMP12 647–648

73. D) The superior olivary nuclei (see figure) receive auditory information from both ears and begin the process of detecting the direction from which a sound comes. The lateral part of the superior olivary nucleus does so by comparing the difference in intensities of sound reaching the two ears, whereas the medial part of the superior olivary nucleus detects time lag between signals entering both ears.

74. D) There appear to be many types of amacrine cells and at least six types of functions. In a sense, amacrine cells begin the analysis of visual signals before they leave the retina. However, horizontal cells, which are always inhibitory, have lateral connections between photoreceptors and bipolar cells. This lateral connection provides the same phenomenon of lateral inhibition that is important in all other sensory systems, helping to ensure transmission of visual contrast.

> TMP12 618

75. B) Cyclic GMP–dependent sodium channels in the outer portions of the rods and cones allow sodium ions to pass from the extracellular space to the intracellular space of the photoreceptor. This results in a membrane potential that is somewhat lower than the resting membrane potential of a typical neuron. The movement of the sodium ions and resulting electrical potential change as a result of this enhanced permeability is known as the *dark current*.

> TMP12 612

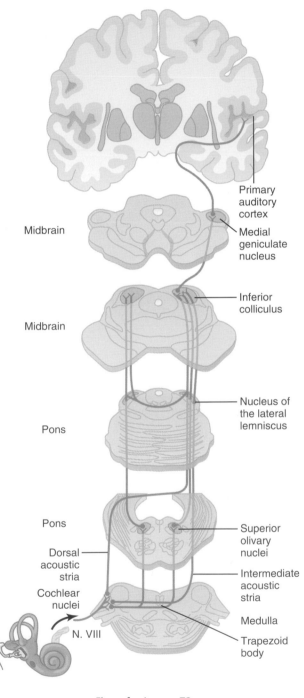

Figure for Answer 73

TMP12 641

The Nervous System: C. Motor and Integrative Neurophysiology

1. The phylogenetically new cerebral cortex, the neocortex, is composed of six layers tangential to the pial surface of the hemisphere. Which of the following statements concerning the organization of these six layers is correct?
   A) The neurons in layers I, I, and III perform most of the thalamocortical connections within the same hemisphere
   B) The neurons in layers II and III form connections with the basal ganglia
   C) Specific incoming signals from the cerebellum terminate primarily in layer IV
   D) The neurons in layer V have axons that extend beyond layer V to subcortical regions and the spinal cord
   E) The neurons in layer VI send their axons to the hippocampus

2. As they leave the spinal cord and course peripherally to skeletal muscle, the axons of motor neurons must pass through which of the following structures?
   A) Posterior column
   B) Posterior root
   C) Ventral white commissure
   D) Posterior horn
   E) Anterior root

3. Which of the following items is the type of neuron whose axon forms synaptic junctions with the skeletal muscle cells (extrafusal fibers) that comprise the major part of a muscle?
   A) Alpha motor neurons
   B) Pyramidal neurons
   C) Gamma motor neurons
   D) Granule cells
   E) Purkinje cells

4. Ascending fibers from the excitatory elements of the reticular activating system reach the intralaminar nuclei of the thalamus and from there they are distributed to which of the following locations?

   A) They project to the somatosensory nuclei of the thalamus
   B) They extend widely throughout many areas of cortex
   C) They reach the motor nuclei of the thalamus
   D) They course primarily to the precentral gyrus
   E) They extend primarily to the postcentral gyrus

5. Which of the following statements concerning the general functional role of the cerebellum is correct?
   A) The cerebellum directly stimulates motor neurons required to make a movement
   B) The cerebellum is unable to make corrective adjustments to the movement once it is performed
   C) The cerebellum does not receive feedback from muscles that execute the actual movement
   D) The cerebellum is not involved in the planning of a movement, only its execution
   E) The cerebellum plays an active role in the coordination of the muscles required to make a movement

6. Which of the following spinal cord levels contains the entire population of preganglionic sympathetic neurons?
   A) C5-T1
   B) C3-C5
   C) S2-S4
   D) T1-L2
   E) T6-L1

7. Which of the following statements best describes a functional role for the lateral hemispheres of the cerebellum?
   A) Controls and coordinates movements of the axial muscles as well as the shoulder and hip
   B) Controls movements that involve distal limb musculature
   C) Functions with the cerebral cortex to plan movements
   D) Stimulates motor neurons through its connections to the spinal cord

8. Which of the following items would produce an increase in cerebral blood flow?

    A) Increase in carbon dioxide concentration
    B) Increase in oxygen concentration
    C) Decrease in the activity of cerebral cortex neurons
    D) Decrease in carbon dioxide concentration
    E) Decrease in arterial blood pressure from 120 mm Hg to 90 mm Hg

9. Which of the following is the correct Brodmann number designation for the primary motor cortex?

    A) 6
    B) 5
    C) 4
    D) 3
    E) 1

10. Which of the following body parts is represented most laterally and inferiorly within the primary motor cortex?

    A) Face
    B) Hand
    C) Neck
    D) Abdomen
    E) Lower limb

11. Which of the following items is the type of neuron whose axon forms synaptic junctions with skeletal muscle cells (intrafusal fibers) within the muscle spindles?

    A) Alpha motor neurons
    B) Pyramidal neurons
    C) Gamma motor neurons
    D) Granule cells
    E) Purkinje cells

12. Preganglionic sympathetic axons pass through which of the following structures?

    A) Dorsal root
    B) Dorsal primary rami
    C) White rami
    D) Gray rami
    E) Ventral primary rami

13. Which of the following statements best describes a functional role for the cerebellar vermis?

    A) Controls and coordinates movements of the axial muscles as well as the shoulder and hip
    B) Controls movements that involve distal limb musculature
    C) Functions with the cerebral cortex to plan movements
    D) Stimulates motor neurons through its connections to the spinal cord

14. Which of the following statements about sleep is correct?

    A) Although fast-wave sleep is frequently referred to as "dreamless sleep," dreams and sometimes nightmares do occur at this time
    B) Individuals rarely will awaken spontaneously from rapid eye movement (REM) sleep
    C) Muscle tone throughout the body is markedly suppressed during REM sleep
    D) Heart rate and respiratory rate typically become very regular during REM sleep

15. Which of the following statements concerning intrinsic spinal cord circuitry is correct?

    A) Motor neurons greatly outnumber spinal cord interneurons
    B) Most incoming sensory fibers from the periphery synapse with motor neurons and not interneurons
    C) Most descending supraspinal motor system axons synapse directly with motor neurons
    D) Spinal cord interneurons are localized solely within the anterior horn
    E) Both excitatory and inhibitory interneurons are found in the spinal cord

16. Which of the following statements best describes a functional role for the intermediate zone of the cerebellum?

    A) Controls and coordinates movements of the axial muscles as well as the shoulder and hip
    B) Controls movements that involve distal limb musculature
    C) Functions with the cerebral cortex to plan movements
    D) Stimulates motor neurons through its connections to the spinal cord

17. The gigantocellular neurons of the reticular formation release which of the following neurotransmitters?

    A) Norepinephrine
    B) Serotonin
    C) Dopamine
    D) Acetylcholine
    E) Glutamate

18. A large portion of the cerebral cortex does not fit into the conventional definition of motor or sensory cortex. Which of the terms below is used to refer to the type of cortex that receives input primarily from several other regions of the cerebral cortex?

    A) Cortex that is agranular
    B) Secondary somatosensory cortex
    C) Association cortex
    D) Supplementary motor cortex
    E) Secondary visual cortex

19. Which statement concerning the premotor cortex is correct?

    A) The premotor cortex is located just posterior to the primary motor cortex
    B) The lateral to medial sequence in the somatotopic organization of the premotor cortex is just the reverse of that seen in the primary motor cortex
    C) Stimulation of a small discrete group of neurons in premotor cortex will produce contraction of an individual muscle
    D) Stimulation of premotor cortex does not lead to any muscle activation
    E) The premotor cortex sets the specific posture required for the limb to produce the desired movement

20. Which of the following features is characteristic of the supplementary motor cortex?

    A) It has no somatotopic representation of the body
    B) Stimulation of the supplementary motor cortex leads to bilateral movements, typically involving both hands
    C) It is located just anterior to the premotor cortex on the lateral surface of the hemisphere
    D) Like the premotor cortex, stimulation in the supplementary motor cortex leads to discrete movement of individual muscles
    E) The supplementary cortex functions totally independent of the premotor and primary motor cortex

21. Administration of a drug that blocks serotonin production will have which of the following effects on sleep?

    A) Sleep induction will be almost immediate
    B) Rapid eye movement (REM) sleep will be blocked
    C) Sleep induction will be significantly prolonged or blocked
    D) REM sleep will be immediately induced

22. Which brain structure serves as the major controller of the limbic system?

    A) Hypothalamus
    B) Hippocampus
    C) Amygdala
    D) Mammillary body
    E) Fornix

23. Which of the following projection systems is contained in the superior cerebellar peduncle?

    A) Pontocerebellar
    B) Cerebellothalamic
    C) Posterior spinocerebellar
    D) Corticospinal

24. Which of the following terms applies to the combination of a motor neuron and all the skeletal muscle fibers contacted by that motor neuron?

    A) Golgi tendon organ
    B) Motor unit
    C) Propriospinal neurons
    D) Skeletal muscle fibers

25. The creation of memory can be interrupted by which of the following activities?

    A) Phosphorylation of a potassium channel to block activity
    B) Activation of adenylate cyclase
    C) Unnatural loss of consciousness
    D) Increase in protein synthesis
    E) Activation of cGMP phosphodiesterase

26. The condition of prosopagnosia usually results from dysfunction or damage to which area of the cerebral cortex?

    A) Prefrontal area
    B) Junction of parietal and temporal lobe on non-dominant side of the brain
    C) Frontal eye fields
    D) Underside of medial occipital and temporal lobes
    E) Limbic association areas of frontal and anterior temporal lobes

27. Lesions of which of the following areas of the brain would have the most devastating effect on verbal and symbolic intelligence?

    A) Hippocampus
    B) Amygdala
    C) Wernicke's area on the non-dominant side of the brain
    D) Broca's area
    E) Wernicke's area on the dominant side of the brain

28. The two hemispheres of the brain are connected by which nerve fibers or pathways?

    A) Lateral lemniscus
    B) Corticofugal fibers
    C) Corpus callosum
    D) Arcuate fasciculus
    E) Medial longitudinal fasciculus

29. Broca's area is a specialized portion of motor cortex. Which of the following conditions best describes the deficit resulting from damage to Broca's area?

    A) Spastic paralysis of the contralateral hand
    B) Paralysis of the muscles of the larynx and pharynx
    C) Inability to use the two hands to grasp an object
    D) Inability to direct the two eyes to the contralateral side
    E) Inability to speak whole words correctly

30. A stroke involving the middle cerebral artery on the left side is likely to cause which of the following symptoms?

    A) Paralysis of left side of face and left upper extremity
    B) Paralysis of left lower extremity
    C) Complete loss of vision in both eyes
    D) Loss of ability to comprehend speech
    E) Loss of vision in left half of both eyes

31. The fibers of the corticospinal tract pass through which one of the following structures?

    A) Medial lemniscus
    B) Medullary pyramid
    C) Posterior funiculus
    D) Medial longitudinal fasciculus
    E) Anterior roots

32. Which of the following structures serves to connect Wernicke's area to Broca's area in the cerebral cortex?

    A) Arcuate fasciculus
    B) Lateral lemniscus
    C) Medial longitudinal fasciculus
    D) Anterior commissure
    E) Internal capsule

33. Which of the following maneuvers will attenuate the stretch reflex in skeletal muscle?

    A) Sectioning the dorsal root of a spinal nerve
    B) Disruption of the spinocerebellar tract
    C) Disruption of the corticospinal tract
    D) Sectioning the medial lemniscus on the contralateral side of the skeletal muscle in question
    E) Creating a lesion in the contralateral globus pallidus

34. The peripheral sensory input that activates the ascending excitatory elements of the reticular formation comes mainly from which of the following?

    A) Pain signals
    B) Proprioceptive sensory information
    C) Corticospinal system
    D) Medial lemniscus
    E) Input from Pacinian corpuscles

35. Signals from motor areas of the cortex reach the contralateral cerebellum after first passing through which one of the following structures?

    A) Thalamus
    B) Caudate nucleus
    C) Red nucleus
    D) Basilar pontine nuclei
    E) Dorsal column nuclei

36. Cells of the adrenal medulla receive synaptic input from which of the following types of neurons?

    A) Preganglionic sympathetic neurons
    B) Postganglionic sympathetic neurons
    C) Preganglionic parasympathetic neurons
    D) Postsynaptic parasympathetic neurons
    E) Presynaptic parasympathetic neurons

37. Which of the following statements about muscle and passive stretch of muscle spindles is true?

    A) Primary (Ia) sensory fibers increase their firing rate
    B) Secondary sensory fibers decrease their firing rate
    C) Alpha motor neurons are inhibited
    D) Gamma motor neurons are stimulated
    E) Muscle spindles go completely slack

38. Which of the following statements concerning electro-encephalogram activity is correct?

    A) Beta waves occur in normal adults who are awake but in a quiet, resting state
    B) Alpha waves occur at 14 to 80 cycles per second during periods of heightened excited activity or high tension
    C) Theta waves are commonly seen in children but also occur in adults during emotional disappointment or in degenerative brain states
    D) Delta waves are characteristic of slow wave sleep
    E) Both C and D are correct

39. Which of the following projection systems is contained in the middle cerebellar peduncle?

    A) Pontocerebellar projections
    B) Cerebellothalamic projections
    C) Posterior spinocerebellar projections
    D) Corticospinal projections
    E) Ventrospinocerebellar projections

40. Which of the following projection systems is contained in the inferior cerebellar peduncle?

    A) Pontocerebellar projections
    B) Cerebellothalamic projections
    C) Posterior spinocerebellar projections
    D) Corticospinal projections
    E) Dorsospinocerebellar projections

41. Cerebrospinal fluid (CSF) provides a cushioning effect both inside and outside the brain. Which of the following spaces lies outside the brain or spinal cord and contains CSF?

    A) Lateral ventricle
    B) Third ventricle
    C) Cisterna magna
    D) Epidural space
    E) Aqueduct of Sylvius

42. In a muscle spindle receptor, which type of muscle fiber is responsible for the dynamic response?

A) Extrafusal muscle fiber
B) Static nuclear bag fiber
C) Nuclear chain fiber
D) Dynamic nuclear bag fiber
E) Smooth muscle fibers

43. Neurological disease associated with the cerebellum produces which of the following types of symptoms?

A) Resting tremor
B) Athetosis
C) Rigidity
D) Ataxia
E) Akinesia

44. Preganglionic parasympathetic neurons that contribute to the innervation of the descending colon and rectum are found in which of the following structures?

A) Superior cervical ganglion
B) Dorsal motor nucleus of the vagus
C) Superior mesenteric ganglion
D) Ciliary ganglion
E) Spinal cord levels S2 and S3

45. A complex spike pattern in the Purkinje cells of the cerebellum can be initiated by stimulation of which of the following brain areas?

A) Inferior olivary complex
B) Brainstem reticular nuclei
C) Neurons in red nucleus
D) Superior olivary complex
E) Dorsal vestibular nucleus

46. Which of the following activities will increase the sensitivity of the stretch reflex?

A) Cutting the dorsal root fibers associated with the muscle in which the stretch reflex is being examined
B) Increasing the activity of the medullary reticular nuclei
C) Bending the head forward
D) Enhanced activity in the fusimotor (gamma motor neuron) system
E) Stimulating the lateral hemispheres of the cerebellum

47. Which of the following structures serves as an "alternative pathway" for signals from the motor cortex to the spinal cord?

A) Red nucleus
B) Basilar pontine nuclei
C) Caudate nucleus
D) Thalamus
E) Dorsal column nuclei

48. The phenomenon of decerebrate rigidity can be explained, at least in part, by which of the following?

A) Stimulation of type 1b sensory neurons
B) Loss of cerebellar inputs to the red nucleus
C) Overactivity of the medullary reticular nuclei involved in motor control
D) Unopposed activity of the pontine reticular nuclei
E) Degeneration of the nigrostriatal pathway

49. Like the primary visual cortex, the primary motor cortex is organized into vertical columns composed of cells linked together throughout the six layers of the cortex. The cells that contribute axons to the corticospinal tract are concentrated in which cortical layer?

A) Layer I
B) Layer II
C) Layer III
D) Layer IV
E) Layer V

50. When a muscle is suddenly stretched, a signal is transmitted over Ia sensory fibers from muscle spindles. Which of the following statements best describes the response elicited by these spindle afferent signals?

A) Contraction of the muscle in which the active spindles are located
B) Relaxation of the muscle in which the active spindles are located
C) Contraction of muscles antagonistic to those in which the active spindles are located
D) Relaxation of intrafusal fibers in the active spindles
E) Direct synaptic activation of gamma motor neurons

51. Which of the following foramina allows cerebrospinal fluid to pass directly from the ventricular system into the subarachnoid space?

A) Foramen of Magendie
B) Aqueduct of Sylvius
C) Third ventricle
D) Lateral ventricle
E) Arachnoid villi

52. There is an area in the dominant hemisphere, which when damaged, might leave the sense of hearing intact but not allow words to be arranged into a comprehensive thought. Which of the following terms is used to identify this portion of the cortex?

A) Primary auditory cortex
B) Wernicke's area
C) Broca's area
D) Angular gyrus
E) Limbic association cortex

53. Efferent fibers from the cerebellum originate in

    A) Deep cerebellar nuclei
    B) Purkinje cell layer of cerebellar cortex
    C) Granular cell layer of cerebellar cortex
    D) Molecular cell layer of cerebellar cortex
    E) Floccular cortex of cerebellum

54. Afferent signals from the periphery of the body travel to the cerebellum in which of the following nerve tracts?

    A) Ventral spinocerebellar tract
    B) Fastigioreticular tract
    C) Vestibulocerebellar tract
    D) Reticulocerebellar tract
    E) Dorsal spinocerebellar tract

55. Motor cortex neurons receive feedback from muscles activated by the corticospinal system. This feedback arises from which of the following structures?

    A) Red nucleus
    B) Spinocerebellar tracts
    C) Skin surface of fingers used to grasp an object
    D) Muscle spindles in muscles antagonistic to those used to make the movement
    E) Vestibular nuclei

56. Which epileptic condition involves a postictal depression period lasting from several minutes to perhaps as long as several hours?

    A) Grand mal seizure
    B) Petit mal seizure
    C) Jacksonian seizure
    D) Phase-out clonic seizure
    E) Temporal lobe seizure

57. The sweat glands and piloerector muscles of hairy skin are innervated by which of the following fiber types?

    A) Cholinergic postganglionic parasympathetic fibers
    B) Cholinergic postganglionic sympathetic fibers
    C) Adrenergic preganglionic parasympathetic fibers
    D) Adrenergic postganglionic sympathetic fibers
    E) Adrenergic preganglionic sympathetic fibers

58. In controlling the fine muscles of the hands and fingers, corticospinal axons can synapse primarily with which of the following?

    A) Posterior horn neurons
    B) Spinal cord interneurons
    C) Spinal cord motor neurons
    D) Purkinje cells
    E) Renshaw cells

59. Which of the following statements concerning spinal cord motor circuits is correct?

    A) Dynamic gamma motor neurons innervate static nuclear bag fibers
    B) Descending supraspinal axons will synapse with either alpha or gamma motor neurons
    C) Clonus is caused by a hyperactive stretch reflex
    D) The contractile elements of intrafusal fibers are found at the central (nuclear) region of the fiber
    E) Both types of sensory fibers in a muscle spindle are mechanoreceptors that signal stretch of the two polar, noncontractile ends of the intrafusal fiber

60. Which of the following cells receives direct synaptic input from Golgi tendon organs?

    A) Type Ia inhibitory interneurons
    B) Dynamic gamma motor neurons
    C) Alpha motor neurons
    D) Type Ib inhibitory interneurons
    E) Type II excitatory interneurons

61. Which of the following neurotransmitters is used by the axons of locus ceruleus neurons that distribute throughout much of the brain?

    A) Norepinephrine
    B) Dopamine
    C) Serotonin
    D) Acetylcholine

62. Which of the following statements concerning mossy and climbing fibers is correct?

    A) Mossy fibers provide direct excitatory input to Purkinje cells
    B) Climbing fibers evoke simple spikes in Purkinje cells
    C) All spinocerebellar axons terminate as mossy fibers in the cerebellar cortex
    D) All pontocerebellar axons terminate as climbing fibers in the cerebellar cortex
    E) All climbing fibers originate in the red nucleus

63. Fine motor movement of the index finger can be elicited by stimulation of which of the following brain areas?

    A) Primary motor cortex
    B) Lateral cerebellar hemisphere
    C) Premotor cortex
    D) Supplemental motor area
    E) Red nucleus

64. The perivascular space (Virchow-Robin space) in the brain is formed between the wall of small penetrating vessels and which of the following structures?

A) Dura mater
B) Arachnoid membrane
C) Pia mater
D) Choroid plexus
E) Ependymal cells

65. Which of the following types of seizures is associated with a spike and dome EEG pattern during the seizure activity?

A) Grand mal seizures
B) Temporal lobe seizures
C) Jacksonian seizures
D) Petit mal seizures
E) Apoplectic seizures

66. The excitatory or inhibitory effect of a postganglionic sympathetic fiber is determined by which of the following features or structures?

A) Function of the postsynaptic receptor to which it binds
B) Specific organ innervated
C) Ganglion where the postganglionic fiber originates
D) Ganglion containing the preganglionic fiber
E) Emotional state of the individual

67. Which of the following neurotransmitters is used by the axons of substantia nigra neurons that project to the caudate and putamen?

A) Norepinephrine
B) Dopamine
C) Serotonin
D) Acetylcholine
E) GABA

68. Which of the following statements concerning the function of cerebellar neurons is correct?

A) Basket cells evoke excitatory responses in Purkinje cells
B) Granule cells evoke excitatory responses in Purkinje cells
C) Golgi cells evoke excitatory responses in basket cells
D) Purkinje cells evoke excitatory responses in cerebellar nuclear cells
E) Stellate cells evoke excitatory responses in basket cells

69. Which of the following items correctly describes the relationship of cerebrospinal fluid pressure to the venous pressure in the superior sagittal sinus?

A) A few millimeters higher
B) A few millimeters lower
C) Equal to
D) Twice the value
E) One-half the value

70. A vascular lesion that causes degeneration of corticospinal axons in the basilar pons will most likely lead to which of the following conditions?

A) Paralysis primarily involving muscles around the contralateral should and hip joints
B) Paralysis of the muscles of mastication
C) Loss of voluntary control of discrete movements of the contralateral hand and fingers
D) Inability to speak clearly
E) Inability to convert short-term memory to long-term memory

71. Which statement best describes a characteristic functional difference between a Golgi tendon organ and a muscle spindle?

A) The output signals of a Golgi tendon organ lead to inactivation of the muscle associated with the active tendon organ
B) Golgi tendon organs do not function in the course of voluntary movements that require a normal level of tension development in the associated muscle
C) Signals arising from Golgi tendon organs do not contribute to conscious proprioception
D) Signals arising from Golgi tendon organs are synaptically linked directly to an alpha motor neuron
E) The signals from a Golgi tendon organ are conducted along sensory fibers that conduct more rapidly than those of the muscle spindle

72. The cerebellum is sometimes described as a "timing device." Which of the following statements best describes the basis for this function?

A) The cerebellum receives visual input that enables it to determine any point in the 24-hour light-dark cycle
B) The cerebellum computes the exact time used to excite adjacent Purkinje cells
C) The cerebellar circuitry determines only the duration or end-point of each movement
D) The cerebellar circuitry enhances the turn-on and turn-off times for each movement by delivering an excitatory signal followed by a precisely timed inhibitory signal
E) The cerebellar circuitry determines only the precise timing of the turn-on signal, and the turn-off signal begins when the cerebellum ceases to function

73. Output signals from Golgi tendon organs are transmitted to which of the following higher centers?

A) Inferior colliculus
B) Globus pallidus
C) Cerebellum
D) Red nucleus
E) Substantia nigra

74. Which type of cholinergic receptor is found at synapses between preganglionic and postganglionic neurons of the sympathetic system?

A) Muscarinic
B) Nicotinic
C) Alpha
D) Beta$_1$
E) Beta$_2$

75. Damage limited to the primary motor cortex (area 4) is thought to cause hypotonia in the affected muscles. However, most cortical lesions, particularly those caused by vascular infarcts, generally involve primary motor cortex in addition to surrounding areas of cortex or cortical efferent axons. The latter type of cortical lesion will cause which of the following?

A) Spastic muscle paralysis
B) Flaccid muscle paralysis
C) No paralysis, only jerky, fast movements
D) Complete blindness in the contralateral eye
E) Loss of sensation in the contralateral foot

76. The term limbic cortex includes the orbitofrontal cortex, subcallosal gyrus, cingulate gyrus, and which one of the following areas?

A) Supplementary motor cortex
B) Postcentral gyrus
C) Lingual gyrus
D) Parahippocampal gyrus
E) Paracentral lobule

77. The cerebellum participates in the learning of motor skills, and the climbing fiber input to Purkinje cells is thought to be most important to this process. Which of the following statements concerning this process is correct?

A) Under resting conditions, climbing fibers evoke complex spikes in Purkinje cells at a very rapid rate
B) When a novel movement is performed, the actual movement may not match the intended movement, which tends to decrease the firing rate of climbing fiber-initiated simple spikes
C) The decrease in climbing fiber input decreases the overall sensitivity (excitability) of the Purkinje cells
D) On the very first trial of the new movement, the Purkinje cell adopts a new, relatively long-term level of excitability
E) Neurons in the inferior olivary complex and their axons projecting to the cerebellum are important contributors to the process

78. Occlusion of which of the following structures would lead to communicating hydrocephalus?

A) Aqueduct of Sylvius
B) Lateral ventricle
C) Foramen of Luschka
D) Foramen of Magendie
E) Arachnoid villi

79. Evaluation of a patient reveals the following deficits: (1) decreased aggressiveness and ambition, and inappropriate social responses; (2) inability to process sequential thoughts in order to solve a problem; and (3) inability to process multiple bits of information that could then be recalled instantaneously to complete a thought or solve a problem. Damage to which of the following brain regions might be responsible for such deficits?

A) Premotor cortex
B) Parieto-occipital cortex in nondominant hemisphere
C) Broca's area
D) Limbic association cortex
E) Prefrontal association cortex

80. The withdrawal reflex is initiated by stimulation delivered to which of the following receptors?

A) Muscle spindle
B) Joint capsule receptor
C) Cutaneous free nerve ending
D) Golgi tendon organ
E) Pacinian corpuscle

81. Which substance activates adrenergic alpha and beta receptors equally well?

A) Acetylcholine
B) Norepinephrine
C) Epinephrine
D) Serotonin
E) Dopamine

82. The posterior and lateral hypothalamus, in combination with the preoptic area, are involved in the control of which of the following functions?

A) Cardiovascular functions involving blood pressure and heart rate
B) Regulation of thirst and water intake
C) Stimulation of uterine contractility and milk ejection from the breast
D) Signaling that food intake is sufficient (satiety)
E) Secretion of hormones from the anterior lobe of the pituitary gland

83. Which statement concerning the reticulospinal system is correct?

A) Reticulospinal neurons do not receive input from motor areas of the cerebral cortex
B) Medullary reticulospinal fibers excite motor neurons that activate extensor muscles
C) Pontine reticulospinal fibers course in the spinal cord posterior funiculus
D) Medullary reticulospinal fibers course in the medial part of the ventral funiculus of the spinal cord
E) Pontine reticulospinal fibers excite spinal cord motor neurons that activate limb extensor muscles

84. The neurons located in the locus ceruleus release which of the following neurotransmitters at their synaptic terminals?

    A) Norepinephrine
    B) Dopamine
    C) GABA
    D) Acetylcholine
    E) Serotonin

85. In the patellar tendon reflex, which of the following items will synapse directly on alpha motor neurons that innervate the muscle being stretched?

    A) Ia sensory fiber
    B) Ib sensory fiber
    C) Excitatory interneurons
    D) Gamma motor neurons
    E) Inhibitory interneurons

86. Which of the following statements best describes the functional role played by the pontine reticulospinal fibers in comparison to the medullary reticulospinal system?

    A) The pontine system works in concert with the medullary system with each providing excitatory influence to extensor muscles
    B) The pontine system essentially functions in an opposing manner relative to the medullary system
    C) The pontine system provides an initial slow excitatory influence, which is then followed by rapid excitation from the medullary system
    D) The medullary system provides slow excitation to extensor motor neurons, whereas the pontine system provides slow excitation of flexor motor neurons
    E) The medullary system provides excitation to upper limb extensor motor neurons, whereas the pontine system provides excitation for lower limb extensor motor neurons

87. Which of the following reflexes is correctly paired with the sensory structure that mediates the reflex?

    A) Autogenic inhibition—muscle spindle
    B) Reciprocal inhibition—Golgi tendon organ
    C) Reciprocal inhibition—Pacinian corpuscle
    D) Stretch reflex—muscle spindle
    E) Golgi tendon reflex—Meissner corpuscle

88. Which of the following items represents the structural basis of the blood–cerebrospinal fluid barrier?

    A) Tight junctions between the ependymal cells forming the ventricular walls
    B) Arachnoid villi
    C) Tight junctions between adjacent choroid plexus cells
    D) Astrocyte foot processes
    E) Tight junctions between adjacent endothelial cells of brain capillaries

89. Damage to which of the following brain areas leads to the inability to comprehend the written or the spoken word?

    A) Insular cortex on the dominate side of the brain
    B) Anterior occipital lobe
    C) Junction of the parietal, temporal, and occipital lobes
    D) Medial portion of the precentral gyrus
    E) Most anterior portion of the temporal lobe

90. In an otherwise normal individual, dysfunction of which brain area will lead to behavior which is not appropriate for the given social occasion?

    A) Ventromedial nuclei of hypothalamus
    B) Amygdala
    C) Corpus callosum
    D) Fornix
    E) Uncus

91. Nasal, lacrimal, salivary, and gastrointestinal glands are stimulated by which of the following substances?

    A) Acetylcholine
    B) Norepinephrine
    C) Epinephrine
    D) Serotonin
    E) Dopamine

92. Which of the following reflexes best describes incoming pain signals that elicit movements performed by antagonistic muscle groups on either side of the body?

    A) Crossed extensor reflex
    B) Withdrawal reflex
    C) Reciprocal inhibition
    D) Autogenic inhibition

93. The spinocerebellum is involved in the control of ballistic movements. This type of movement is entirely preplanned in that the initiation, trajectory, and endpoint are programmed by the cerebellum. Which of the following statements is correct concerning the symptoms observed in patients with cerebellar lesions that interfere with ballistic movements?

    A) Movements are slow to be initiated
    B) The speed of the movement is faster than desired
    C) The movement turn-off is reached more quickly
    D) Spastic paralysis appears in the affected muscle group
    E) A resting tremor develops in the affected limbs

94. Decerebrate rigidity results from which of the following situations?

    A) Damage to the brainstem systems that control flexor motor neurons
    B) Overactivity in the medullary reticulospinal system leads to hyperactivity in limb extensor muscles
    C) An imbalance in the activity of medullary and pontine reticulospinal systems such that excitation of extensor motor neurons is the end result
    D) Interruption of the medullary reticulospinal axons
    E) Interruption of the pontine reticulospinal axons

95. Brain edema is a serious complication of altered fluid dynamics in the brain. Continued progression of brain edema may lead to which of the following situations?

    A) Relaxation of the vasculature smooth muscle and decreased blood flow
    B) Increased blood flow leading to increased oxygen concentration
    C) Vasoconstriction and decreased edema
    D) Relaxation of the vasculature smooth muscle and increased blood flow
    E) Compression of blood vessels leading to ischemia and compensatory capillary dilation

96. Which portion of the cerebellum functions in the planning of sequential movement?

    A) Vermis and fastigial nucleus
    B) Intermediate zone and fastigial nucleus
    C) Lateral hemisphere and interposed nucleus
    D) Cerebrocerebellum and dentate nucleus
    E) Spinocerebellum and interposed nucleus

97. Bilateral lesions involving the ventromedial hypothalamus will lead to which of the following deficits?

    A) Decreased eating and drinking
    B) Loss of sexual drive
    C) Excessive eating, rage and aggression, hyperactivity
    D) Uterine contractility, mammary gland enlargement
    E) Obsessive compulsive disorder

98. Which structure is an important pathway for communication between the limbic system and the brainstem?

    A) Mamillothalamic tract
    B) Fornix
    C) Anterior commissure
    D) Indusium griseum
    E) Medial forebrain bundle

99. Which of the following terms best describes the cerebellar deficit in which there is a failure to perform rapid alternating movements indicating a failure of "progression" from one part of the movement to the next?

    A) Past-pointing
    B) Intention tremor
    C) Dysarthria
    D) Cerebellar nystagmus
    E) Dysdiadochokinesia

100. The function of which of the following organs or systems is dominated by the sympathetic nervous system?

    A) Systemic blood vessels
    B) Heart
    C) Gastrointestinal gland secretion
    D) Salivary glands
    E) Gastrointestinal motility

101. Which of the following structures in the vestibular apparatus is responsible for the detection of angular acceleration?

    A) Statoconia
    B) Macula
    C) Semicircular canals
    D) Saccule
    E) Ampullae

102. A person who has had a traumatic brain injury seems to be able to understand the written and spoken word but cannot create the correct sounds to be able to speak a word that is recognizable. This person most likely has damage to which area of the brain?

    A) Wernicke's area
    B) Broca's area
    C) Angular gyrus
    D) Dentate nucleus
    E) Prefrontal lobe

103. Schizophrenia is thought to be caused in part by excessive production and release of which of the following neurotransmitter agents?

    A) Norepinephrine
    B) Serotonin
    C) Acetylcholine
    D) Substance P
    E) Dopamine

104. Which of the following structures **is not** considered to be part of the basal ganglia?

    A) Caudate nucleus
    B) Dentate nucleus
    C) Substantia nigra
    D) Putamen
    E) Globus pallidus

105. Stimulation of which of the following subcortical areas can lead to contraction of a single muscle or small groups of muscles?

    A) Dentate nucleus of the cerebellum
    B) Ventrobasalar complex of the thalamus
    C) Red nucleus
    D) Subthalamic nucleus
    E) Nucleus accumbens

106. Under awake, resting conditions, brain metabolism accounts for about 15% of the total metabolism of the body, and this is among the highest metabolic rates of all tissues in the body. Which of the following cellular populations of the nervous system contributes most substantially to this high rate of metabolism?

    A) Astrocytes
    B) Neurons
    C) Ependymal cells
    D) Choroid plexus cells
    E) Brain endothelial cells

107. The concept of "autonomic tone" is quite advantageous because it allows the nervous system to have much finer control over the function of an organ or organ system. This is exemplified in the control of systemic arterioles. Which of the following actions would lead to vasodilation of systemic arterioles?

    A) Increased activity of preganglionic parasympathetic neurons
    B) Decreased activity of postganglionic parasympathetic neurons
    C) Increased activity of postganglionic sympathetic neurons
    D) Decreased activity of postganglionic sympathetic neurons
    E) Increased activity of preganglionic sympathetic neurons

108. Which structures in the cerebellum have a topographical representation of the body?

    A) The dentate nucleus
    B) The lateral hemispheres
    C) The flocculonodular lobe
    D) The vermis and intermediate hemisphere
    E) The cerebellar peduncles

109. Which statement concerning memory processing in the brain is correct?

    A) The brain forms positive memory through facilitation of synaptic circuits, but is unable to form negative memory by learning to ignore irrelevant information
    B) Short-term memory is considered to be a list of 7–10 discrete facts that can be recalled within a period of a several hours
    C) It appears that rehearsal and repetition of information is not advantageous in converting short-term memory to long-term memory
    D) Lesions involving the hippocampus cause a profound deficit in short-term memory
    E) No morphologic or structural changes occur in the process of long-term memory formation

110. Which of the following structures is maximally sensitive to linear head movement in the vertical plane?

    A) Macula of the utricle
    B) Macula of the saccule
    C) Crista ampullaris of the anterior semicircular duct
    D) Crista ampullaris of the horizontal semicircular duct

111. Retrograde amnesia is the inability to recall long-term memories from the past. When damaged, which of the following brain regions leads to retrograde amnesia?

    A) Hippocampus
    B) Dentate gyrus
    C) Amygdaloid complex
    D) Thalamus
    E) Mammillary nuclei of hypothalamus

112. Hemiballismus, the sudden flailing movements of an entire limb, results when damage occurs to which area of the brain?

    A) The subthalamic nucleus
    B) The ventral basal complex of the thalamus
    C) The globus pallidus
    D) The red nucleus
    E) The lateral hypothalamus

113. Although the sympathetic nervous system is often activated in such a way that it leads to mass activation of sympathetic responses throughout the body, it can also be activated to produce relatively discrete responses. Which of the following is an example of a local or discrete sympathetic action?

    A) Heating of a patch of skin causes a relatively restricted vasodilation in the heated region
    B) Food in the mouth causes salivation
    C) Emptying of the bladder may cause reflexive emptying of the bowel
    D) Dust particle in the eye causes increased tear fluid release
    E) Bright light introduced into one eye

114. Which statement concerning the transduction mechanism in vestibular hair cells is correct?

    A) Movement that bends the stereocilia away from the kinocilium has a depolarizing influence on the hair cell
    B) The attachment of the stereocilia to the kinocilium is such that it activates voltage-gated sodium channels in the membrane of the kinocilium
    C) Depolarization of the hair cell is achieved by inward movement of sodium from the endolymph
    D) Deflection of the cupula such that stereocilia move toward the kinocilium causes the hair cell to depolarize
    E) Inward movement of potassium through voltage-gated potassium channels in the stereocilia membrane has a depolarizing influence on the hair cell

115. Which structure connects the hippocampus to the limbic system?

   A) Mamillothalamic tract
   B) Fornix
   C) Anterior commissure
   D) Medial forebrain bundle
   E) Arcuate fasciculus

116. The condition of athetosis results when which area of the brain is dysfunctional?

   A) Globus pallidus
   B) Substantia nigra
   C) Ventral anterior complex of the thalamus
   D) Putamen
   E) Purkinje cell layer of the cerebellum

117. Which component of the basal ganglia plays the major role in the control of cognitive (memory-guided) motor activity?

   A) Globus pallidus
   B) Substantia nigra
   C) Caudate nucleus
   D) Putamen
   E) Subthalamic nucleus

118. The brain's use of energy is among the highest of any organ in the body, but unfortunately the storage of glycogen in the brain is minimal and thus anaerobic glycolysis is not a significant source of energy. Considering this information about brain metabolism, which of the following statements is correct?

   A) The brain is dependent on glucose delivery via the vascular system
   B) Glucose delivered to the brain via the vascular system can be stored in neurons for several hours
   C) Cessation of blood flow to the brain can be safely tolerated for up to about 10 minutes due to the considerable capacity for oxygen storage in brain tissue
   D) Glucose delivery to neurons is vitally dependent on insulin
   E) An overdose of insulin causes glucose to be rapidly transported into the brain at the expense of other insulin-dependent tissues

119. All the hair cells in the crista ampullaris of the horizontal semicircular duct have their stereocilia and kinocilium oriented according to which of the following patterns?

   A) Same pattern with progressive increase in length of stereocilia from shortest to tallest with the tallest located adjacent to the kinocilium
   B) Random pattern with progression from short to tall stereocilia such that the shortest is adjacent to the kinocilium
   C) Same pattern with progressive decrease in length of stereocilia from tallest to shortest, with the shortest located adjacent to the kinocilium
   D) Random pattern with progression from tallest to shortest stereocilia, with the shortest adjacent to the kinocilium
   E) Random pattern with random distribution of stereocilia of various lengths

120. Stimulation of the punishment center can inhibit the reward center, demonstrating that fear and punishment can take precedence over pleasure and reward. Which of the following cell groups is considered the punishment center?

   A) Lateral and ventromedial hypothalamic nuclei
   B) Periventricular hypothalamus and midbrain central gray
   C) Supraoptic nuclei of hypothalamus
   D) Anterior hypothalamic nucleus

121. A wide variety of neurotransmitters have been identified in the cell bodies and afferent synaptic terminals in the basal ganglia. A deficiency of which of the following transmitters is typically associated with Parkinson disease?

   A) Norepinephrine
   B) Dopamine
   C) Serotonin
   D) GABA
   E) Substance P

122. Drugs that stimulate specific adrenergic receptors are called sympathomimetic drugs. Which of the following is a sympathomimetic drug?

   A) Reserpine
   B) Phentolamine
   C) Propranolol
   D) L-dopa
   E) Phenylephrine

1. **D)** Neurons in layer V project into the subcortical white matter and from there to a wide variety of subcortical locations, including the basal ganglia, brainstem, and spinal cord. The cells in layer VI project to the thalamus. Cells in layers I, II, and III form intracortical connections of various types, and those in layer IV receive thalamocortical projections.
   TMP12 697–698

2. **E)** Axons of motor neurons in the anterior horn exit the spinal cord through the anterior root. The posterior root serves as the entry point for sensory fibers coming into the posterior horn region of the spinal cord. The posterior column and ventral white commissure are fiber tracts located solely within the spinal cord.
   TMP12 655–656

3. **A)** Alpha motor neurons form direct synaptic contact with skeletal extrafusal muscle fibers, whereas gamma motor neurons form synaptic junctions with intrafusal muscle fibers. Pyramidal, granule, and Purkinje neurons are located in the central nervous system and have no direct contact with skeletal muscle.
   TMP12 656

4. **B)** A characteristic feature of the reticular activating system is that it produces widespread activation of many cortical regions. This is achieved through diffuse projections from the intralaminar nuclei of the thalamus.
   TMP12 711

5. **E)** The output of the cerebellum is quite removed from motor neurons and the activation of muscle, particularly in the case of limb or paraxial musculature. Although the output of the cerebellum clearly influences muscle activity, it does so by very indirect means. The cerebellar nuclei project to the motor nuclei of the thalamus and to the red nucleus, and thus can influence activity in the corticospinal and rubrospinal tracts.
   TMP12 681

6. **D)** All preganglionic sympathetic neurons are located in the intermediolateral cell column (lateral horn); and this cell group extends from T1 to L2.
   TMP12 730

7. **C)** The lateral cerebellar hemispheres function with the cerebral cortex in the planning of complex movements.
   TMP12 682

8. **A)** The most potent stimulator of cerebral blood flow is a local increase in carbon dioxide concentration, followed in order by a decrease in oxygen concentration and an increase in local neuronal activity.
   TMP12 744

9. **C)** The primary motor cortex corresponds to Brodmann's area 4 and is located within the precentral gyrus. Area 6 is the premotor cortex, area 5 is part of the superior parietal lobule, and areas 3 and 1 form part of the primary somatosensory cortex in the postcentral gyrus.
   TMP12 667

10. **A)** The face region of the motor cortex is most inferior and lateral in the territory of the middle cerebral artery, whereas the lower limb is in the paracentral lobule in the territory of the anterior cerebral artery.
    TMP12 668

11. **C)** Gamma motor neurons form direct synaptic contact with the skeletal muscle fibers known as intrafusal fibers. Extrafusal muscle fibers are innervated by alpha motor neurons, whereas Purkinje, granule, and pyramidal neurons have no synaptic contact with muscles in the periphery.
    TMP12 656

12. **C)** Preganglionic sympathetic axons pass through the white communicating rami to enter the sympathetic trunk. Postganglionic sympathetic axons course through gray rami and might be found in dorsal and ventral primary rami.
    TMP12 729

13. **A)** The cerebellar vermis is involved with the control of axial muscles as well as proximal limb muscles in the shoulder and hip.
    TMP12 682

14. **C)** Although some bodily movements, in addition to eye movements, may occur during rapid eye movement (REM) sleep, there is a significant overall reduction in muscle tone during the REM period. A slow-wave sleep sometimes includes dreaming. Individuals will often awake spontaneously from REM sleep. Heart and respiratory rates become irregular during REM sleep.
    TMP12 721–722

15. **E)** There are two populations of spinal cord interneurons, one capable of producing excitation and the other producing inhibition in their postsynaptic target neurons. All other statements are false.
    TMP12 656

16. **B)** The intermediate zone of the cerebellum influences the function of distal limb muscles.
    TMP12 682

17. **D)** The gigantocellular neurons of the reticular formation reside in the pons and mesencephalon. These neurons release acetylcholine which functions as an excitatory neurotransmitter in most brain areas.
    TMP12 713

18. **C)** The association cortex is defined by the fact that it receives multiple inputs from a wide variety of sensory areas of cortex. It is the true multimodal cortex.
    TMP12 699–700

19. **E)** The postural set necessary to initiate limb movements is controlled by the premotor cortex.
    TMP12 668

20. **B)** A characteristic feature of the supplementary motor cortex is that stimulation on one side produces bilateral limb movements, usually involving both hands.
    TMP12 668

21. **C)** Stimulation of the raphe nuclei in the caudal pons and medulla causes a very strong induction of sleep.
    TMP12 722

22. **A)** The hypothalamus, despite its small size, is the most important control center for the limbic system. It controls most of the vegetative and endocrine functions of the body and many aspects of behavior.
    TMP12 715

23. **B)** Cerebellothalamic projections are contained in the superior cerebellar peduncle.
    TMP12 684

24. **B)** The combination of a motor neuron and all the muscle fibers innervated by that motor neuron is called a motor unit.
    TMP12 656

25. **E)** For an event or sensory experience to be remembered it must first be consolidated. The consolidation of memory takes time. A disruption of consciousness during the process of consolidation will prevent the development of memory for the event or sensory experience.
    TMP 708

26. **D)** Prosopagnosia is the inability to recognize faces. This occurs in people who have extensive damage on the medial undersides of both occipital lobes and along the medioventral surfaces of the temporal lobes.
    TMP12 700

27. **E)** The somatic, visual, and auditory association areas all meet one another at the junction of the parietal, temporal, and occipital lobes. This area is known as Wernicke's area. This area on the dominant side of the brain plays the single greatest role for the highest comprehension levels we call intelligence.
    TMP12 700–701

28. **C)** The corpus callosum is the main fiber pathway for communication between the two hemispheres of the brain.
    TMP12 701–702

29. **E)** Broca's aphasia typically involves an inability to speak words correctly in the absence of any true paralysis of the laryngeal or pharyngeal musculature.
    TMP12 668–669

30. **D)** A stroke involving the left middle cerebral artery is likely to cause an aphasic syndrome that might involve the loss of speech comprehension and/or the loss of the ability to produce speech sounds. Any paralysis resulting from the lesion would affect the right side of the body and similarly any visual field deficits would affect the right visual field of each eye.
    TMP12 701

31. **B)** Corticospinal fibers pass through the medullary pyramid.
    TMP12 669–670

32. **A)** The connection between Wernicke's area and Broca's area in made by the arcuate fasciculus.
    TMP12 703–704

33. **A)** Type 1a sensory fibers that innervate the stretch receptors of the muscle spindle travel in the appropriate spinal nerve that provides both the sensory and motor innervation of the muscle. The spinal nerves carry both afferent and efferent fibers. The afferent fibers (which contain the sensory fibers innervating the muscle spindle) pass through the dorsal root. Cutting the dorsal root will remove the afferent limb of the stretch reflex arc.
    TMP12 656, 658–659

34. **A)** Pain signals traveling through the anterolateral system, but not any of the discriminative sensations coursing through the medial lemniscal system, provide input to the cells in the reticular formation that give rise to ascending projections to the intralaminar nuclei of the thalamus.
    TMP12 711–712

35. **D)** The main pathway linking the cerebral cortex and the cerebellum involves cortical projections to the ipsilateral basilar pontine nuclei, the cells of which then project to the contralateral cerebellum.
    TMP12 682–683

36. **A)** Preganglionic sympathetic axons synapse on cells in the adrenal medulla that function as postganglionic sympathetic neurons.
    TMP12 730

37. **A)** When a muscle and its spindles are passively stretched, the Ia sensory fibers increase their firing rate. The firing of type II sensory fibers is largely unaffected, whereas alpha motor neurons can be stimulated and gamma motor neurons are unaffected.
    TMP12 657–658

38. **E)** Delta waves exhibit the highest voltage and lowest frequency among the commonly described electroencephalogram waves. They occur during very deep sleep. They occur in the cortex of animals whose subcortical connections to the thalamus have been removed. They are thought to represent the activity of the cortex independent of stimulation by lower brain areas. Alpha waves are seen in the quiet waking state; beta waves are seen in a heightened state of alertness. Theta occur normally in the parietal and temporal region in children and during stress in adults, particularly during disappointment or frustration.
    TMP12 724

39. **A)** Pontocerebellar axons are contained in the middle cerebellar peduncle.
    TMP12 682–683

40. **C)** Posterior spinocerebellar fibers pass through the inferior cerebellar peduncle.
    TMP12 683

41. **C)** The cerebrospinal fluid outside the brain and spinal cord is located within the subarachnoid space. Dilated regions of the subarachnoid space are identified as cisterns. The cisterna magna is one of the largest cisterns and is positioned at the caudal end of the fourth ventricle between the cerebellum and posterior surface of the medulla.
    TMP12 746

42. **D)** The dynamic nuclear bag fiber responds to the rate of change of length of the muscle spindle receptor. It is this fiber that is responsible for the dynamic response of the muscle spindle.
    TMP12 658

43. **D)** The cerebellum is responsible for coordinating and timing motor activity. Disorders of the cerebellum are associated with lack of coordination of motor activity. An example of this is ataxia, which is an unsteady gait.
    TMP12 689

44. **E)** Preganglionic parasympathetic neurons that contribute to the innervation of the descending colon and rectum are found at S2 and S3 levels of the spinal cord.
    TMP12 731

45. **A)** Complex spike output from the Purkinje cells of the cerebellum is a response to activation of climbing fibers in cerebellar neural circuitry. All climbing fibers originate in the inferior olivary nucleus
    TMP12 684

46. **D)** Gamma motor neurons innervate the contractile ends of the muscle spindle receptor. Stimulation of gamma motor neurons will cause the ends of the spindle to contract which in turn will stretch the center of the spindle receptor is the muscle in which the spindle receptor is imbedded does not shorten. The activity of the gamma motor neurons is influenced by the fusimotor system. Enhanced activity of this system will lead to an increase in gamma motor tone and increase the sensitivity of the muscle spindle as a stretch receptor.
    TMP12 659–660

47. **A)** Cortical projections to the red nucleus provide an alternative pathway for the cerebral cortex to control flexor muscles through the rubrospinal tract.
    TMP12 670–671

48. **D)** The pontine reticular nuclei are tonically active. These nuclei have a stimulatory effect on the antigravity muscles of the body. The pontine nuclei are normally apposed by the medullary reticular nuclei. The medullary nuclei are not tonically active and require stimulation from higher brain centers to counterbalance the signal from the pontine nuclei. Decerebrate rigidity results when the stimulatory signal from higher brain areas to the medullary nuclei is absent. This allows an unopposed and vigorous activation of the antigravity muscles resulting in extension of the arms and legs and contraction of the axial muscles of the spinal column.
    TMP12 674

49. **E)** Corticospinal axons originate from cell bodies (pyramidal neurons) in layer V of the motor areas of the cortex.
    TMP12 669–670

50. **A)** When a muscle is stretched, signals traveling over Ia sensory fibers will lead to contraction of the muscle in which the active spindles are located. At the same time, the antagonist muscles will be inactivated. The intrafusal fibers in the spindle do not go slack due to the tonic activation of gamma motor neurons by supraspinal systems. They are not influenced by signals carried on Ia sensory fibers.
    TMP12 658–659

51. **A)** The foramen of Magendie and the two lateral foramina of Luschka form the communication channels between the ventricular system within the brain and the subarachnoid space that lies outside the brain and spinal cord.
    TMP12 746–747

52. **B)** Wernicke's area in the dominant hemisphere is responsible for interpreting spoken language. Damage to Wernicke's area will eliminate comprehension of spoken language.
    TMP12 700–701

53. **A)** All output from the cerebellum originates in the deep cerebellar nuclei.
    TMP12 683–684

54. **E)** Afferent signals to the cerebellum travel primarily in the dorsal and ventral spinocerebellar tracts. The dorsal spinocerebellar tract carries signals from the muscle spindle receptors, and Golgi tendon receptors, as well as large tactile receptors of the skin and joint proprioceptors. The ventral spinocerebellar tract carries information from the anterior portion of the spinal cord. This tract relays information on which motor signals from the motor areas of the brain have arrived at the level of the spinal cord.
    TMP12 683

55. **C)** The palmar (volar) surfaces of the skin contain receptors that project through the medial lemniscal system to the primary somatosensory cortex. When these fingers are flexed and grasp an object, the cutaneous receptors send signals to the primary somatosensory cortex. These cortical neurons then project to the adjacent motor cortex and the pyramidal neurons that sent the original message down the corticospinal tract to cause contraction of the finger flexors. The motor cortex neurons are then said to be "informed of the muscle contractions" that they originally specified.
    TMP12 671–672

56. **A)** A grand mal epileptic seizure is associated with the sudden onset of unconsciousness, an overall steady but uncoordinated contracture of many muscles of the body followed by alternating contractions of flexor and extensor muscles, that is, tonic, clonic activity. This is the result of widespread and uncontrolled activity in many parts of the brain. It takes the brain from a few minutes to a few hours to recover from this vigorous activity.
    TMP12 725–726

57. **B)** Sweat glands and the piloerector smooth muscle of hairy skin are innervated by the population of cholinergic postganglionic sympathetic neurons.
    TMP12 731

58. **C)** Although the majority of corticospinal axons synapse with the pool of spinal cord interneurons, some will synapse directly with the motor neurons that innervate muscles controlling the wrist and finger flexors.
    TMP12 672

59. **C)** Clonus is caused by hyperactive stretch reflexes. All the other statements are incorrect.
    TMP12 660

60. **D)** Golgi tendon organs provide direct synaptic input to type Ib inhibitory interneurons. Type Ia interneurons and alpha motor neurons receive input from muscle spindle afferents, whereas dynamic gamma motor neurons and excitatory interneurons receive their input from supraspinal systems.
    TMP12 661

61. **A)** Neurons in the locus ceruleus utilize the neurotransmitter norepinephrine in their widespread projections throughout the brain.
    TMP12 712–713

62. **C)** All spinocerebellar axons terminate as mossy fibers; only the axons that arise in the inferior olivary nucleus form climbing fibers.
    TMP12 684–685

63. **A)** A large area of the primary motor cortex is dedicated to activating the muscles that control the movement of the fingers. Stimulation of the primary motor cortex usually results in very discrete contractions of small groups of muscles. Stimulation of the premotor cortex results in the contraction of large groups of muscles and stimulation of the supplemental motor area results in bilateral movements.
    TMP12 667–668

64. **C)** The perivascular space (also known as the Virchow-Robin space) is formed between the outer wall of small vessels penetrating into the brain and the pia mater, which lines the outer surface of the brain and is only loosely attached to the brain.
    TMP12 747

65. **D)** The spike and dome pattern is characteristic of a petit mal seizure.
    TMP12 726

66. **A)** The excitatory or inhibitory effect of a postganglionic sympathetic fiber is determined solely by the type of receptor to which it binds.
    TMP12 732–733

67. **B)** Cells in the pars compacta portion of the substantia nigra utilize the neurotransmitter dopamine in their projections to the caudate and putamen.
    TMP12 692–693

68. **B)** Granule cell axons have branches that form the parallel fiber system in the molecular layer, where they provide excitatory input to Purkinje cell dendrites.
    TMP12 684

69. **A)** Cerebrospinal fluid (CSF) will flow across the valve-like arachnoid villi when the CSF pressure is only a few millimeters higher than the pressure within the superior sagittal sinus.
    TMP12 747–748

70. **C)** The most characteristic deficit following damage to corticospinal tract neurons involves discrete voluntary movement of the contralateral hand and fingers.
TMP12 673

71. **A)** Signals from Golgi tendon organs lead to inhibition of the associated muscle, whereas muscle spindle activity leads to excitation of the muscles associated with the active spindle. Golgi tendon organs, similar to muscle spindles, function in the course of normal movement. Golgi tendon organ afferents conduct more slowly than spindle afferents, and tendon organs provide input to interneurons and not motor neurons, similar to the muscle spindles.
TMP12 661

72. **D)** Cerebellar circuitry enhances the turn-on and turn-off times for each movement. This provides the precise timing for the start and end of each movement.
TMP12 688

73. **C)** Golgi tendon organs provide input to the cerebellum. They do not provide input to the inferior colliculus, globus pallidus, red nucleus, or substantia nigra.
TMP12 661

74. **B)** Nicotinic cholinergic receptors are found at synapses between preganglionic and postganglionic sympathetic neurons.
TMP12 733

75. **A)** Lesions that damage primary motor cortex and other surrounding motor cortical areas lead to spastic paralysis in the affected muscles.
TMP12 673

76. **D)** The parahippocampal gyrus is an important component of the "limbic cortex" or limbic lobe.
TMP12 714–715

77. **E)** The climbing fiber (inferior olive) input to a Purkinje cell is thought to alter the excitability of the Purkinje cell, making it more or less responsive to granule cell input.
TMP12 686

78. **E)** Noncommunicating hydrocephalus results when a blockage of cerebrospinal fluid flow occurs within the ventricular system or at the sites of communication between the ventricular system and the subarachnoid space. Communicating hydrocephalus occurs when a blockage occurs either within the subarachnoid space or at the arachnoid villi, thus preventing communication between the subarachnoid space and the superior sagittal sinus.
TMP12 748

79. **E)** Behavioral deficits, changes in personality, and diminished problem-solving ability are all signs of damage to the prefrontal association cortex.
TMP12 702–701

80. **C)** The withdrawal reflex is activated by stimuli from free nerve endings. Muscle spindles provide the afferent signals for the stretch reflex, and Golgi tendon organs are the source of stimuli for the inverse myotatic reflex.
TMP12 661–662

81. **C)** Epinephrine activates alpha and beta adrenergic receptors equally well. Norepinephrine excites both types of receptors, but has a markedly greater effect on alpha receptors.
TMP12 733

82. **A)** The posterior and lateral hypothalamus, in combination with the preoptic hypothalamus, form an important group of cells controlling cardiovascular functions such as heart rate and blood pressure.
TMP12 715–716

83. **E)** Pontine reticulospinal fibers excite motor neurons supplying extensor muscles. In contrast, medullary reticulospinal fibers will lead to inhibition of extensor motor neurons.
TMP12 673–674

84. **A)** The neurons located in the locus ceruleus release norepinephrine at their nerve terminals.
TMP12 712–713

85. **A)** Ia sensory fibers synapse directly with alpha motor neurons, whereas Ib sensory fibers synapse with inhibitory interneurons. Excitatory interneurons play an important role in the withdrawal reflex. Gamma motor neurons receive input primarily from supraspinal systems.
TMP12 658–660

86. **B)** The pontine reticulospinal and medullary reticulospinal systems function in an opposing manner to influence the motor neurons that control axial and limb extensor muscles.
TMP12 674

87. **D)** The stretch reflex is mediated by muscle spindles. Autogenic inhibition involves Golgi tendon organs. Reciprocal inhibition is also related to muscle spindles.
TMP12 658–659

88. **C)** The tight junctions formed between adjacent choroid epithelial cells represent the structural basis of the blood-cerebrospinal fluid barrier. The blood-brain barrier is formed by the tight junctions between adjacent endothelial cells of brain capillaries.
TMP12 748–749

89. **C)** The junction of the parietal, temporal and occipital lobe is commonly referred to as Wernicke's area. This area of the brain is responsible for the ability to comprehend both the written and spoken word.
TMP12 699

90. **B)** The amygdala seems to function in behavioral awareness at a semiconscious level. The amygdala also is thought to project into the limbic system the individual's current status with respect to their surroundings. Therefore, the amygdala is believed to help pattern behavior appropriate for each occasion.
TMP12 719–720

91. **A)** The nasal, lacrimal, salivary and gastrointestinal glands are stimulated by cholinergic postganglionic parasympathetic neurons.
TMP12 735

92. **A)** The crossed extensor reflex is dependent on incoming pain signals distributed to both sides of the spinal cord via excitatory interneurons.
TMP12 663

93. **A)** Both the initiation and execution of ballistic-type movements are slowed very dramatically with lesions that involve the spinocerebellum.
TMP12 688

94. **C)** In decerebrate rigidity, the cortical projections that normally activate the inhibitory reticulospinal system are lost. Although cortical activation of the excitatory pontine reticulospinal system is also lost, the latter system continues to be activated by intact ascending somatosensory (pain) pathways. This leads to activation of extensor motor neurons without the inhibitory influence of the medullary reticulospinal fibers.
TMP12 674

95. **E)** Brain edema leads to compression of brain vasculature, decreased blood flow, ischemia, and compensatory vasodilation. This ultimately leads to an even further increase in edema.
TMP12 749

96. **D)** The cerebrocerebellum and the dentate nucleus are involved with the thalamus and cortex in the planning of complex movements.
TMP12 682

97. **C)** Lesions involving the ventromedial hypothalamus lead to excessive eating (hyperphagia), excessive drinking, rage and aggression, and hyperactivity.
TMP12 717

98. **E)** The medial forebrain bundle extends from the septal and orbitofrontal regions of the cerebral cortex downward through the center of the hypothalamus to the brainstem reticular area. This structure serves as an important communication system between the limbic system and the brainstem.
TMP12 715

99. **E)** Dysdiadochokinesia is a cerebellar deficit that involves a failure of progression from one part of a movement to the next. Consequently, movements that

include rapid alternation between flexion and extension are most severely affected.
TMP12 689

100. **A)** The innervation and function of systemic blood vessels is influenced primarily, if not exclusively, by the sympathetic nervous system.
TMP12 735

101. **C)** Linear acceleration is in a straight line; angular acceleration is that which occurs by turning about a point. The semicircular canals respond to the turning motions of the head and body.
TMP12 677

102. **B)** Damage to Broca's area leads to motor aphasia, the inability to form words correctly.
TMP12 704

103. **E)** Schizophrenia is thought to be caused in part by excessive release of dopamine. Occasionally, patients with Parkinson's disease exhibit schizophrenic symptoms due to an inability to control L-dopa therapy and the subsequent production of dopamine.
TMP12 727

104. **B)** The basal ganglia consist of the striatum (caudate nucleus and putamen), the globus pallidus, the substantia nigra, and the subthalamic nucleus.
TMP12 690

105. **C)** The magnocellular portion of the red nucleus has a somatographic representation of all the muscles of the body. This is similar to the motor cortex. Stimulation of this area in the red nucleus results in contraction of a single muscle or small groups of muscles.
TMP12 671

106. **B)** The high metabolic rate in the nervous system is primarily due to the high metabolic activity in neurons, even in the resting state.
TMP12 749

107. **D)** Decreased activity of postganglionic sympathetic neurons leads to vasodilation of systemic arterioles. In contrast, increased activity in postganglionic sympathetics results in vasoconstriction.
TMP12 737

108. **D)** The vermis and the intermediate zone of the cerebellar hemisphere have a distinct topographic representation of the body. These areas are responsible for coordinating the contraction of the muscles of the body for intended motion.
TMP12 682

109. **D)** Hippocampal lesions interfere with the formation and conversion of short-term memory to long-term memory. These patients retain previously formed long-term memory but are unable to form

new long-term memory and are said to exhibit anterograde amnesia. The brain is able to form both positive and negative memories. The duration of short-term memory is a matter of seconds to minutes. Rehearsal and repetition are helpful in forming long-term memories. Certain structural changes in neurons and synaptic boutons may contribute to long-term memory formation and storage.

TMP12 707–709

110. **B)** Hair cells in the macula of the saccule are maximally sensitive to linear head movement in the vertical plane.

TMP12 676

111. **D)** Lesions involving the thalamus lead to retrograde amnesia, because they are believed to interfere with the process of retrieving long-term memory stored in other portions of the brain.

TMP12 709

112. **A)** Hemiballismus is the result of damage to the subthalamic nucleus of the basal ganglia.

TMP12 691

113. **A)** An example of a relatively restricted or local sympathetic action is the vasodilation or vasoconstriction of blood vessels that occurs upon warming or cooling of a patch of skin.

TMP12 738

114. **D)** When cupula deflection moves the stereocilia toward the kinocilium, mechanically gated potassium channels are opened in the kinocilium membrane, and potassium in the endolymph moves into the hair cell and causes it to be depolarized.

TMP12 676

115. **B)** The fornix connects the hippocampus to the anterior thalamus, hypothalamus, and the limbic system.

TMP12 718

116. **A)** Athetosis is a slow and continuous writhing movement of the arm, neck, or the face. It results from damage or dysfunction of the globus pallidus.

TMP12 691

117. **C)** The caudate nucleus is involved in the basal ganglia circuits that control memory-guided motor activity.

TMP12 691–692

118. **A)** The brain is totally dependent on a minute-to-minute supply of glucose delivered by the vascular system, since there is no substantial storage of either glucose or glycogen by the brain. The delivery of glucose to the brain is not at all dependent on the availability of insulin.

TMP12 749

119. **A)** All the hair cells in the crista ampullaris of the horizontal semicircular duct have the same orientation. The stereocilia proceed in sequence from shortest to tallest, with the tallest stereocilium located adjacent to the kinocilium.

TMP12 675–676

120. **B)** The punishment center is primarily localized to the periventricular hypothalamus and the midbrain central gray.

TMP12 717–718

121. **B)** Degeneration of the dopaminergic cells in the pars compacta of the substantia nigra is thought to be the primary defect in Parkinson's disease.

TMP12 692–693

122. **E)** Phenylephrine is a sympathomimetic drug that stimulates adrenergic receptors. Reserpine, phentolamine, and propranolol are sympathetic antagonists.

TMP12 740

Gastrointestinal Physiology

1. Which of the following food substances requires chewing for digestion?

   A) Cheese
   B) Eggs
   C) Vegetables
   D) Meat

2. Which of the following is the main digestible carbohydrate normally consumed in the human diet?

   A) Amylose
   B) Cellulose
   C) Maltose
   D) Starch

3. Which of the following is not normally found in abundance in the portal blood?

   A) Amino acids
   B) Glucose
   C) Short-chain fatty acids
   D) Triglycerides

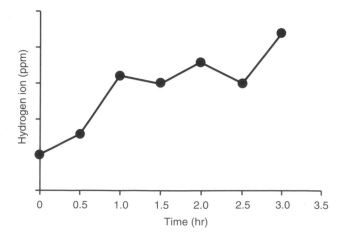

4. A 19-year-old woman visits her physician because of nausea, diarrhea, light headedness, and flatulence. The physician administers 50 g of oral lactose at time zero, and measures breath hydrogen every 30 min for 3 hr using a hand-held monitor. The results are shown above. Which of the following best describes this patient's condition?

   A) Brush border lactase deficiency
   B) Brush border lactase excess
   C) Decreased pancreatic lactase
   D) Increased pancreatic lactase
   E) No digestive abnormality

5. Digestion of which of the following foodstuffs is impaired to the greatest extent in patients with achlorhydria?

   A) Carbohydrate
   B) Fat
   C) Protein

6. The proenzyme pepsinogen is secreted mainly from which of the following structures?

   A) Acinar cells of the pancreas
   B) Ductal cells of the pancreas
   C) Epithelial cells of the duodenum
   D) Gastric glands of the stomach

7. Compared to plasma, saliva has the highest relative concentration of which of the following ions under basal conditions?

   A) Bicarbonate
   B) Chloride
   C) Potassium
   D) Sodium

8. Which of the following ions has the highest concentration in saliva under basal conditions?

   A) Bicarbonate
   B) Chloride
   C) Potassium
   D) Sodium

9. A 33-year-old man comes to the physician because his chest hurts when he eats, especially when he eats meat. He also belches excessively and has heartburn. His wife complains about bad breath. X-ray shows a dilated esophagus. Which one of the pressure tracings was most likely taken at the lower esophageal sphincter of this patient before and after swallowing (indicated by arrow)? The dashed line represents a pressure of 0 mm Hg.

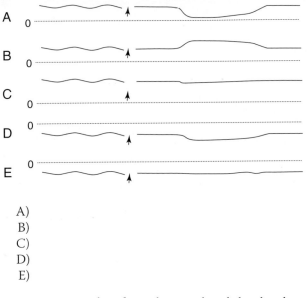

    A)
    B)
    C)
    D)
    E)

10. Biopsies are taken from the antral and duodenal mucosa of a 65-year-old woman. Which of the following hormones can be found in tissue homogenates from both locations?

    A) Cholecystokinin (CCK)
    B) Glucose-dependent insulinotropic peptide (GLIP)
    C) Gastrin
    D) Motilin
    E) Secretin

11. A 10-year-old boy consumes a cheeseburger, fries, and chocolate shake. The meal stimulates the release of several gastrointestinal hormones. The presence of fat, carbohydrate, or protein in the duodenum stimulates the release of which of the following hormones from the duodenal mucosa?

    A) Cholecystokinin (CCK)
    B) Glucose-dependent insulinotropic peptide (GLIP)
    C) Gastrin
    D) Motilin
    E) Secretin

12. Which of the following hormones is released by the presence of fat and protein in the small intestine and has a major effect to decrease gastric emptying?

    A) Cholecystokinin (CCK)
    B) Glucose-dependent insulinotropic peptide (GLIP)
    C) Gastrin
    D) Motilin
    E) Secretin

13. A clinical experiment is conducted in which one group of subjects is given 50 g of glucose intravenously and another group is given 50 g of glucose orally. Which of the following factors can explain why the oral glucose load is cleared from the blood at a faster rate compared to the intravenous glucose load? (CCK, cholecystokinin; GLIP, glucose-dependent insulinotropic peptide; VIP, vasoactive intestinal peptide)

    A) CCK-induced insulin release
    B) CCK-induced VIP release
    C) GLIP-induced glucagon release
    D) GLIP-induced insulin release
    E) VIP-induced GLIP release

14. Which of the following factors can inhibit gastric acid secretion? (GLIP, glucose-dependent insulinotropic peptide)

	Somatostatin	Secretin	GLIP	Enterogastrones	Nervous reflexes
A)	No	No	Yes	No	Yes
B)	No	Yes	No	No	No
C)	No	Yes	No	Yes	No
D)	Yes	No	No	Yes	Yes
E)	Yes	No	Yes	No	No
F)	Yes	Yes	Yes	Yes	Yes

15. The gastrointestinal hormones have physiological effects that can be elicited at normal concentrations as well as pharmacological effects that require higher than normal concentrations. What is the direct physiological effect of the various hormones on gastric acid secretion? (GLIP, glucose-dependent insulinotropic peptide)

	Gastrin	Secretin	Cholecystokinin	GLIP	Motilin
A)	No effect	Stimulate	Stimulate	No effect	No effect
B)	Stimulate	Inhibit	No effect	Inhibit	No effect
C)	Stimulate	Inhibit	No effect	No effect	No effect
D)	Stimulate	Inhibit	Inhibit	Stimulate	Stimulate
E)	Stimulate	Stimulate	Inhibit	Inhibit	No effect

16. The cephalic phase of gastric secretion accounts for about 30% of the acid response to a meal. Which of the following can totally eliminate the cephalic phase of gastric secretion?

    A) Antacids (e.g., Rolaids)
    B) Anti-gastrin antibody
    C) Atropine
    D) Histamine H_2 blocker
    E) Vagotomy
    F) Sympathectomy

17. A newborn boy does not pass meconium in the first 24 hr. His abdomen is distended and he begins vomiting. Various tests lead to a diagnosis of Hirschsprung disease. An obstruction is most likely found in which portion of the gut?

    A) Ascending colon
    B) Ileocecal sphincter
    C) Lower esophageal sphincter
    D) Pylorus
    E) Sigmoid colon

18. Migrating motility complexes (MMC) occur about every 90 min between meals and are thought to be stimulated by the gastrointestinal hormone, motilin. An absence of MMCs causes an increase in which of the following?

    A) Duodenal motility
    B) Gastric emptying
    C) Intestinal bacteria
    D) Mass movements
    E) Swallowing

19. Which one of the following manometric recordings illustrate normal function of the esophagus at midthoracic level before and after swallowing (indicated by arrow)? The dashed lines represent a pressure of 0 mm Hg.

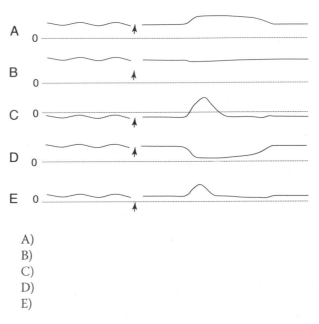

    A)
    B)
    C)
    D)
    E)

20. Gastric emptying is tightly regulated to ensure that chyme enters the duodenum at an appropriate rate. Which of the following events promotes gastric emptying under normal physiological conditions in a healthy person?

	Tone of orad stomach	Segmentation contractions in small intestine	Tone of pyloric sphincter
A)	Decrease	Decrease	Decrease
B)	Decrease	Increase	Decrease
C)	Increase	Decrease	Decrease
D)	Increase	Decrease	Increase
E)	Increase	Increase	Increase

21. Parasympathetic stimulation increases gastrointestinal motility and sympathetic stimulation decreases motility. The autonomic nervous system controls gut motility by changing which of the following?

    A) Gastrin secretion
    B) Pacemaker discharge frequency
    C) Secretin secretion
    D) Slow wave frequency
    E) Spike potential frequency

22. Swallowing is a complex process that involves signaling between the pharynx and swallowing center in the brainstem. Which of the following structures is critical for determining whether a bolus of food is small enough to be swallowed?

    A) Epiglottis
    B) Larynx
    C) Palatopharyngeal folds
    D) Soft palate
    E) Upper esophageal sphincter

23. A 54-year-old woman eats a healthy meal. Approximately 20 min later the woman feels the urge to defecate. Which of the following reflexes results in the urge to defecate when the stomach is stretched?

    A) Duodenocolic reflex
    B) Enterogastric reflex
    C) Gastrocolic reflex
    D) Intestino-intestinal reflex
    E) Rectosphincteric

24. A 60-year-old woman severs her spinal cord at T6 in an automobile accident. She devises a method to distend the rectum to initiate the rectosphincteric reflex. Rectal distension causes which of the following in this woman?

	Relaxation of internal anal sphincter	Contraction of external anal sphincter	Contraction of rectum
A)	No	No	No
B)	No	No	Yes
C)	No	Yes	Yes
D)	Yes	No	Yes
E)	Yes	Yes	No
F)	Yes	Yes	Yes

25. The gastrointestinal hormones have physiological effects that can be elicited at normal concentrations as well as pharmacological effects that require higher than normal concentrations. What is the physiological effect of the various hormones on gastric emptying?

26. A 48-year-old woman consumes a healthy meal. At which location are smooth muscle contractions most likely to have the highest frequency in the diagrams shown?

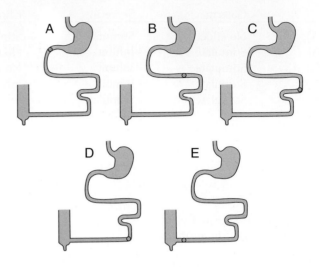

27. Cholecystokinin (CCK) and gastrin share multiple effects at pharmacological concentrations. Which of the following effects do CCK and gastrin share (or not share) at physiological concentrations?

	Stimulation of acid secretion	Inhibition of gastric emptying	Stimulation of gastric mucosal growth	Stimulation of pancreatic growth
A)	Not shared	Not shared	Not shared	Not shared
B)	Not shared	Not shared	Shared	Not shared
C)	Not shared	Shared	Not shared	Not shared
D)	Shared	Shared	Not shared	Not shared
E)	Shared	Shared	Shared	Shared

Answer Choices for Question 25

	Gastrin	Secretin	Cholecystokinin	GLIP	Motilin
A)	Decrease	Decrease	Decrease	Decrease	Increase
B)	Increase	Decrease	None	Decrease	Increase
C)	Increase	None	None	Increase	Increase
D)	None	None	Decrease	Increase	Increase
E)	None	None	Decrease	None	None
F)	None	None	Increase	None	None

28. Vomiting is a complex process that requires coordination of numerous components by the vomiting center located in the medulla. Which of the following occurs during the vomiting act?

	Lower esophageal sphincter	Upper esophageal sphincter	Abdominal muscles	Diaphragm
A)	Contract	Contract	Contract	Contract
B)	Contract	Contract	Relax	Relax
C)	Relax	Contract	Contract	Relax
D)	Relax	Relax	Contract	Contract
E)	Relax	Relax	Relax	Relax

29. Various proteolytic enzymes are secreted in an inactive form into the lumen of the gastrointestinal tract. Which of the following substances is/are important for activating one or more proteolytic enzymes, converting them to an active form?

	Trypsin	Enterokinase	Pepsin
A)	No	No	No
B)	No	No	Yes
C)	No	Yes	No
D)	Yes	Yes	No
E)	Yes	Yes	Yes

30. Mass movements constitute an important intestinal event that lead to bowel movements. Mass movements cause which of the following?

A) Contraction of internal anal sphincter
B) Duodenal peristalsis
C) Gastric retropulsion
D) Hunger sensations
E) Rectal distension

31. An 82-year-old woman with upper abdominal pain and blood in the stool has been taking NSAIDS for arthritis. Endoscopy revealed patchy gastritis throughout the stomach. Biopsies were negative for *Helicobacter pylori*. Pentagastrin administered intravenously would lead to a less than expected (i.e., less than normal) increase in which of the following?

A) Duodenal mucosal growth
B) Gastric acid secretion
C) Gastrin secretion
D) Pancreatic enzyme secretion
E) Pancreatic growth

32. Which of the following is a likely consequence of ileal resection?

A) Achalasia
B) Atrophic gastritis
C) Constipation
D) Peptic ulcer
E) Vitamin B12 deficiency

33. Which of the following factors have a physiologic role to stimulate the release of hormones or stimulate nervous reflexes, which in turn can inhibit gastric acid secretion?

	Acid	Fatty acids	Hyperosmotic solutions	Isotonic solutions
A)	No	No	Yes	No
B)	No	No	Yes	Yes
C)	Yes	Yes	No	Yes
D)	Yes	Yes	Yes	Yes
E)	Yes	Yes	Yes	No

34. A 23-year-old medical student consumes a cheeseburger, fries, and chocolate shake. Which of the following hormones produce physiological effects at some point over the next several hours?

	Gastrin	Secretin	Cholecystokinin	GLIP
A)	No	Yes	Yes	Yes
B)	Yes	No	Yes	Yes
C)	Yes	Yes	No	Yes
D)	Yes	Yes	Yes	Yes
E)	Yes	Yes	Yes	Yes

35. A 68-year-old woman with hematemesis has heartburn and stomach pain. Endoscopy shows inflammation involving the gastric body and antrum as well as a small gastric ulcer. Biopsies were positive for *Helicobacter pylori*. *H. pylori* damages the gastric mucosa primarily by increasing mucosal levels of which substance?

A) Ammonium
B) Bile salts
C) Gastrin
D) NSAIDS
E) Pepsin

36. A 71-year-old man with hematemesis and melena has a cresenteric ulcer in the duodenum. Lavage dislodged the clot, revealing an underlying raised blood vessel, which was successfully eradicated via cautery with a bipolar gold probe. Which of the following factors are diagnostic for duodenal ulcer?

	Endoscopy	Plasma gastrin levels	Rate of acid secretion
A)	No	No	No
B)	Yes	No	No
C)	Yes	No	Yes
D)	Yes	Yes	No
E)	Yes	Yes	Yes

Questions 37 and 38

The following diagram shows manometric recordings from a patient before and after pelvic floor training. A balloon placed in the rectum was blown up (arrows) and deflated repeatedly. Tracing Z is a manometric recording obtained from the external anal sphincter before and after pelvic floor training.

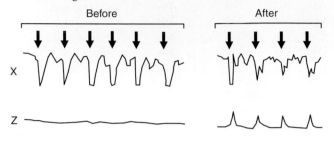

37. Which of the following best describes the origin of tracing X shown in the upper panel?

    A) Distal rectum
    B) Ileocecal valve
    C) Internal anal sphincter
    D) Lower esophageal sphincter
    E) Proximal rectum

38. Which of the following best describes the condition for which the patient received pelvic floor training?

    A) Anal fissure (i.e., tear or superficial laceration)
    B) Chronic diarrhea
    C) Fecal incontinence (i.e., no control over defecation)
    D) Hemorrhoids
    E) Hirschsprung disease

39. A clinical study is conducted in which gastric acid secretion is stimulated using pentagastrin before and after treatment with a histamine H_2 blocker. Which of the following rates of gastric acid secretion (in mEq/hr) is most likely to have occurred in this experiment?

	Pentagastrin alone	Pentagastrin + H_2 blocker
A)	15	15
B)	25	25
C)	25	15
D)	26	28
E)	40	45

40. A tsunami tidal wave hits the east coast of South America and the people living there are forced to drink unclean water. Within the next several days, a large number of people develop severe diarrhea and about half of these people expire. Samples of drinking water are positive for *Vibrio cholerae*. Which of the following types of ion channels is most likely to be irreversibly opened in the epithelial cells of the crypts of Lieberkühn in these people with severe diarrhea?

    A) Calcium channels
    B) Chloride channels
    C) Magnesium channels
    D) Potassium channels
    E) Sodium channels

41. One of the following hormones can stimulate growth of the intestinal mucosa and two other hormones can stimulate pancreatic growth. Which three hormones are these?

	Gastrin	Secretin	Cholecystokinin	GLIP	Motilin
A)	No	Yes	Yes	Yes	No
B)	Yes	No	Yes	No	Yes
C)	Yes	No	Yes	Yes	No
D)	Yes	No	Yes	Yes	No
E)	Yes	Yes	Yes	No	No

42. Which of the following structures undergoes receptive relaxation when a bolus of food is swallowed?

    A) Orad stomach
    B) Palatopharyngeal folds
    C) Pharynx
    D) Thoracic esophagus
    E) Upper esophageal sphincter

43. A 65-year-old man eats a healthy meal. Approximately 40 min later the ileocecal sphincter relaxes and chyme moves into the cecum. Gastric distention leads to relaxation of the ileocecal sphincter by way of which reflex?

    A) Enterogastric reflex
    B) Gastroileal reflex
    C) Gastrocolic reflex
    D) Intestino-intestinal reflex
    E) Rectosphincteric reflex

44. A healthy, 21-year-old woman eats a big meal and then takes a 3-hr ride on a bus that does not have a bathroom. Twenty minutes after eating, the woman feels a strong urge to defecate, but manages to hold it. Which of the following have occurred in this woman?

	Relaxation of internal anal sphincter	Contraction of external anal sphincter	Contraction of rectum
A)	No	No	No
B)	No	Yes	Yes
C)	Yes	No	Yes
D)	Yes	No	No
E)	Yes	Yes	Yes

45. The gastric mucosal barrier has a physiological and an anatomical basis to prevent back-leak of hydrogen ions into the mucosa. Some factors are known to strengthen the integrity of the gastric mucosal barrier, whereas other factors can weaken the barrier. Which of the following factors strengthen or weaken the barrier?

	Bile salts	Mucous	Aspirin	NSAIDS	Gastrin	Ethanol
A)	Strengthen	Strengthen	Weaken	Weaken	Strengthen	Strengthen
B)	Strengthen	Strengthen	Weaken	Weaken	Weaken	Strengthen
C)	Weaken	Strengthen	Strengthen	Weaken	Strengthen	Weaken
D)	Weaken	Strengthen	Weaken	Weaken	Strengthen	Weaken
E)	Weaken	Weaken	Weaken	Strengthen	Strengthen	Weaken

46. A 48-year-old man consumes a healthy meal. At which of the following locations is vitamin B12 most likely to be absorbed?

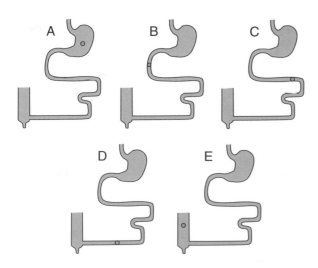

47. A 45-year-old man presents with abdominal pain and hematemesis. An abdominal exam was relatively benign, and abdominal x-rays were suggestive of a perforated viscus. Endoscopy revealed a chronically perforated gastric ulcer, through which the liver was visible. Which of the following is a forerunner to gastric ulcer formation?

A) Back-leak of hydrogen ions
B) Mucus secretion
C) Proton pump inhibition
D) Tight junctions between cells
E) Vagotomy

48. A 19-year-old man is fed intravenously for several weeks following a severe automobile accident. The intravenous feeding leads to atrophy of the gastrointestinal mucosa most likely because the blood level of which of the following hormones is reduced?

A) Cholecystokinin only
B) Gastrin only
C) Secretin only
D) Gastrin and cholecystokinin
E) Gastrin and secretin
F) Secretin and cholecystokinin

49. A 62-year-old man with dyspepsia and a history of chronic gastric ulcer has abdominal pain. Endoscopy shows a large ulcer in the proximal gastric body. Biopsies were positive for *Helicobacter pylori*. Which of the following are used clinically for treatment of gastric ulcers of various etiologies?

	Antibiotics	NSAIDS	H$_2$ blockers	Proton pump inhibitors
A)	No	No	Yes	Yes
B)	Yes	No	No	Yes
C)	Yes	No	Yes	Yes
D)	Yes	Yes	Yes	Yes
E)	No	Yes	Yes	Yes

50. Eating a meal leads to a large increase in gastric acid secretion that peaks within about 5 min and returns to normal about 4 hr after a meal is taken. How long after a meal does the pH of the gastric contents reach its lowest level (in hours)?

A) 1.0
B) 1.5
C) 2.0
D) 2.5
E) 3.0
F) 4.0

51. Cystic fibrosis (CF) is an inherited disorder of the exocrine glands, affecting children and young people. Mucus in the exocrine glands becomes thick and sticky and eventually blocks the ducts of these glands (especially in the pancreas, lungs, and liver), forming cysts. A primary disruption in the transfer of which ion across cell membranes occurs in CF leading to decreased secretion of fluid?

    A) Calcium
    B) Chloride
    C) Phosphate
    D) Potassium
    E) Sodium

52. Which of the following stimulus-mediator pairs normally inhibit gastrin release? (CCK, cholecystokinin; GLIP, glucose-dependent insulinotropic peptide)

	Stimulus	Mediator
A)	Acid	CCK
B)	Acid	GLIP
C)	Acid	Somatostatin
D)	Fatty acid	Motilin
E)	Fatty acid	Somatostatin

53. A newborn boy has a distended abdomen, fails to pass meconium within the first 48 hr of life, and vomits repeatedly. Analysis of a rectal biopsy provides a definitive diagnosis of Hirschsprung disease. The absence of which type of cell is diagnostic for Hirschsprung disease?

    A) Lymphatic endothelial cells
    B) Capillary endothelial cells
    C) Parasympathetic ganglion cells
    D) Red blood cells
    E) Smooth muscle cells

54. Mass movements are often stimulated after a meal by distention of the stomach (gastrocolic reflex) and distention of the duodenum (duodenocolic reflex). Mass movements often lead to which of the following?

    A) Bowel movements
    B) Gastric movements
    C) Haustrations
    D) Esophageal contractions
    E) Pharyngeal peristalsis

55. A 45-year-old man adds lots of high-fiber wheat and bran foods to his diet to reduce his cholesterol. He loses 30 lb on the new diet, but has undesirable side effects such as stomach cramps, flatulence, and diarrhea. His gastroenterologist diagnoses a syndrome called gluten-enteropathy or celiac sprue. Which of the following is decreased in this man?

    A) Absorption of nutrients
    B) Digestion of fat
    C) Stool carbohydrates
    D) Stool fat
    E) Stool nitrogen

56. A 57-year-old man is admitted as an emergency for upper GI bleeding. Endoscopy reveals multiple ulcers in the duodenum. Serum gastrin levels are eight-fold higher compared to normal. Zollinger-Ellison syndrome (ZES, gastrinoma) is suspected. Administration of which of the following substances is useful in confirming the diagnosis?

    A) Cholecystokinin (CCK)
    B) Glucose-dependent insulinotropic peptide (GLIP)
    C) Motilin
    D) Pentagastrin
    E) Secretin

57. A 71-year-old man with upper abdominal pain and blood in the stool takes NSAIDS for the pain and washes it down with whiskey. Pentagastrin administration produced lower than predicted levels of gastric acid secretion. Secretion of which of the following substances is most likely to be diminished in this patient with gastritis?

    A) Intrinsic factor
    B) Ptyalin
    C) Rennin
    D) Saliva
    E) Trypsin

58. Gastric acid is secreted when a meal is consumed. Which of the following factors have a direct action on the parietal cell to stimulate acid secretion?

	Gastrin	Somatostatin	Acetylcholine	Histamine
A)	No	No	Yes	Yes
B)	Yes	No	No	Yes
C)	Yes	No	Yes	Yes
D)	Yes	Yes	Yes	Yes
E)	Yes	Yes	No	Yes

59. An 84-year-old man with hematemesis and melena is diagnosed with a duodenal ulcer. A patient diagnosed with a duodenal ulcer is likely to exhibit which of the following?

	Parietal cell density	Acid secretion	Plasma gastrin
A)	Decreased	Decreased	Decreased
B)	Decreased	Increased	Decreased
C)	Increased	Decreased	Increased
D)	Increased	Increased	Decreased
E)	Increased	Increased	Increased

60. The gastric phase of gastric secretion accounts for about 60% of the acid response to a meal. Which of the following can virtually eliminate the secretion of acid during the gastric phase?

   A) Antiacids (e.g., Rolaids)
   B) Antigastrin antibodies
   C) Atropine
   D) Histamine H_2 blocker
   E) Proton pump inhibitor

61. A 53-year-old man with a recurrent history of ulcer disease associated with diarrhea and a strong family history of duodenal ulcer disease is suspected of having Zollinger-Ellison syndrome (gastrinoma). Secretin (2 units/kg) was given as a rapid intravenous injection to test for gastrinoma. Which of the following results would support the existence of gastrinoma following secretin administration?

   A) Decreased serum gastrin
   B) Increased serum gastrin
   C) Inhibition of gastric acid secretion
   D) Inhibition of gastric emptying
   E) Stimulation of pancreatic $HCO3^-$ secretion

62. Damage to the gastric mucosal barrier is a forerunner of gastric ulcer. Which of the following can both damage the gastric mucosal barrier and stimulate gastric acid secretion?

   A) Bile salts
   B) Epidermal growth factor
   C) Gastrin
   D) *Helicobacter pylori*
   E) Mucous

63. Gastric emptying is regulated to ensure the chyme enters the duodenum at an appropriate rate. Which of the following factors promotes gastric emptying?

   A) Anorexia nervosa
   B) Antral peristalsis
   C) Bulimia nervosa
   D) Obesity
   E) Scleroderma
   F) Type I diabetes

64. Cystic fibrosis is the most common cause of pancreatitis in children. Which of the following best explains the mechanism of cystic fibrosis–induced pancreatitis?

   A) Activation of enterokinase
   B) Activation of trypsin inhibitor
   C) Autodigestion of pancreas
   D) Excessive secretion of CCK
   E) Gallstone obstruction

65. Vagal stimulation plays an essential role during the cephalic and gastric phases of gastric secretion. Vagal stimulation tends to cause which of the following changes in the release of gastric releasing peptide (GRP) and somatostatin?

	GRP	Somatostatin
A)	↑	↑
B)	↓	↓
C)	↑	↓
D)	↓	↑
E)	↔	↓

66. The control of gastric acid secretion in response to a meal involves several events that take place over a 4- or 5-hr period following the meal. These events include (1) a decrease in the pH of the gastric contents, (2) an increase in the rate of acid secretion, (3) a decrease in the rate of acid secretion, and (4) an increase in the pH of the gastric contents. Which of the following best describes the correct temporal order of events over a 4- or 5-hr period following a meal?

   A) 4, 3, 2, 1
   B) 3, 1, 4, 2
   C) 3, 4, 1, 2
   D) 2, 1, 4, 3
   E) 4, 2, 1, 3
   F) 1, 2, 3, 4
   G) 2, 3, 1, 4
   H) 1, 3, 2, 4

67. A 43-year-old obese woman with a history of gallstones is admitted to the emergency department because of excruciating pain in the upper right quadrant. The woman is jaundiced and x-ray suggests obstruction of the common bile duct. Which of the following values of direct and indirect bilirubin are most likely to be present in the plasma of this woman (in milligrams per deciliter)?

	Direct	Indirect
A)	1.0	1.3
B)	2.3	2.4
C)	5.0	1.7
D)	1.8	6.4
E)	6.8	7.5

1. C) Chewing is important for the digestion of all solid foods. It is especially important for most fruits and vegetables because these foods have an indigestible cellulose membrane surrounding the nutrient portion that must be broken to allow contact with digestive enzymes.
  TMP12 763

2. D) The three major sources of carbohydrates in the normal human diet include sucrose mainly from sugar-cane and sugar beets, lactose from milk, and a wide variety of large polysaccharides collectively known as starches. Although some diets may contain a large quantity of cellulose, this substance cannot be digested by the human gut and is not considered a food. Maltose is a product of the digestion of starch but is not consumed in large quantities in the human diet.
  TMP12 790

3. D) Triglycerides are digested within the intestinal lumen to monoglycerides and free fatty acids, which are then absorbed directly through the membrane of the intestinal epithelial cells. After entering the epithelial cell, the fatty acids and monoglycerides are taken up by the cell's smooth endoplasmic reticulum where they are mainly used to form new triglycerides that are subsequently released in the form of chylomicrons through the base of the epithelial cell. The chylomicrons are absorbed by the central lacteal in the villus and transported in lymph through the thoracic lymph duct to the circulating blood. Thus, most triglycerides bypass the portal circulation.
  TMP12 792

4. A) Patients with a lactase deficiency cannot digest milk products containing lactose (milk sugar). The operons of gut bacteria quickly switch over to lactose metabolism, which results in fermentation that produces copious amounts of gas (a mixture of hydrogen, carbon dioxide, and methane). This gas, in turn, may cause a range of abdominal symptoms, including stomach cramps, bloating, and flatulence. The gas is absorbed by blood (especially in the colon), and exhaled from the lungs.
  TMP12 790

5. C) Achlorhydria means simply that the stomach fails to secrete hydrochloric acid; it is diagnosed when the pH of the gastric secretions fails to decrease below 4 after stimulation by pentagastrin. When acid is not secreted, pepsin also usually is not secreted; even when it is, the lack of acid prevents it from functioning because pepsin requires an acid medium for activity. Thus, protein digestion is impaired.
  TMP12 800

6. D) Pepsinogen is the precursor of the enzyme pepsin. Pepsinogen is secreted from the peptic or chief cells of the gastric gland (also called the oxyntic gland). To be converted from the precursor form to the active form (pepsin), pepsinogen must come in contact with hydrochloric acid or pepsin itself. Pepsin is a proteolytic enzyme that digests collagen and other types of connective tissue in meats.
  TMP12 777

7. C) Under basal conditions, saliva contains high concentrations of potassium and bicarbonate ions and low concentrations of sodium and chloride ions. The primary secretion of saliva by acini has an ionic composition similar to that of plasma. As the saliva flows through the ducts, sodium ions are actively reabsorbed and potassium ions are actively secreted in exchange for sodium. Because sodium is absorbed in excess, chloride ions follow the electrical gradient causing chloride levels in saliva to decrease greatly. Bicarbonate ions are secreted by an active transport process causing an elevation of bicarbonate concentration in saliva. The net result is that, under basal conditions, sodium and chloride concentrations in saliva are about 10% to 15% of that of plasma, bicarbonate concentration is about three-fold greater than that of plasma, and potassium concentration is about seven times greater than that of plasma.
  TMP12 775

8. A) Although the potassium concentration in saliva is about seven times greater than that of plasma, and the bicarbonate concentration in saliva is only about three times greater than that of plasma, the actual concentration of bicarbonate in saliva is 50 to 70 mEq/L, whereas the concentration of potassium is about 30 mEq/L, under basal conditions.
  TMP12 775

9. **C)** Achalasia is a condition in which the lower esophageal sphincter (LES) fails to relax during swallowing. As a result, food swallowed into the esophagus then fails to pass from the esophagus into the stomach. Trace C shows a high, positive pressure that fails to decrease after swallowing, which is indicative of achalasia. Trace A shows a normal pressure tracing at the level of the LES reflecting typical receptive relaxation in response to the food bolus. Trace E is similar to trace C, but the pressures are subatmospheric. Subatmospheric pressures occur only in the esophagus where it passes through the chest cavity.

   TMP12 799

10. **C)** The gastrointestinal hormones are secreted from endocrine cells located in the mucosa. The endocrine cells are not clumped together but are dispersed among the epithelial cells, making it virtually impossible to remove surgically the source of any one gastrointestinal hormone. Gastrin is the only listed hormone found in the antrum, but it is also found in the duodenal and to a lesser extent the jejunal mucosa. CCK and secretin secreting endocrine cells are found in the duodenum, jejunum, and ileum. Motilin and GLIP secreting cells are found in the duodenum and jejunum.

    TMP12 758

11. **B)** GLIP is the only gastrointestinal hormone released by all three major foodstuffs (fats, proteins, and carbohydrates). The presence of fat and protein in the small intestine stimulates the release of CCK, but carbohydrates do not stimulate its release. The presence of protein in the antrum of the stomach stimulates the release of gastrin, but fat and carbohydrates do not stimulate its release. Fat has a minor effect to stimulate the release of motilin and secretin, but neither hormone is released by the presence of protein or carbohydrate in the gastrointestinal tract.

    TMP12 758

12. **A)** CCK is the only gastrointestinal hormone that inhibits gastric emptying under physiological conditions. This inhibition of gastric emptying keeps the stomach full for a prolonged time, which is one reason why a breakfast containing fat and protein "sticks with you" better than breakfast meals containing mostly carbohydrates. CCK also has a direct effect on the feeding centers of the brain to reduce further eating. Although CCK is the only gastrointestinal hormone that inhibits gastric emptying, all of the gastrointestinal hormones with the exception of gastrin are released to some extent by the presence of fat in the intestine.

    TMP 758

13. **D)** GLIP is released by the presence of fat, carbohydrate, or protein in the gastrointestinal tract. GLIP is a strong stimulator of insulin release and is responsible for the observation that an oral glucose load releases more insulin and is metabolized more rapidly than an equal amount of glucose administered intravenously. Intravenously administered glucose does not stimulate the release of GLIP. Neither CCK nor VIP stimulates the release of insulin. GLIP does not stimulate glucagon release, and glucagon has the opposite effect of insulin, that is, it would decrease the rate of glucose clearance from the blood. VIP does not stimulate GLIP release.

    TMP12 758

14. **F)** All of these factors can inhibit gastric acid secretion under normal physiological conditions. Gastric acid stimulates the release of somatostatin (a paracrine factor), which has a direct effect on the parietal cell to inhibit acid secretion as well as an indirect effect mediated by suppression of gastrin secretion. Secretin and GLIP inhibit acid secretion through a direct action on parietal cells as well as indirectly through suppression of gastrin secretion. Enterogastrones are unidentified substances released from the duodenum and jejunum that directly inhibit acid secretion. When acid or hypertonic solutions enter the duodenum, a neurally mediated decrease in gastric acid secretion follows.

    TMP12 758, 780

15. **B)** Gastrin stimulates gastric acid secretion, and secretin and GLIP inhibit gastric acid secretion under normal, physiological conditions. It is important to differentiate the physiological effects of the gastrointestinal hormones from their pharmacological actions. For example, gastrin and cholecystokinin (CCK) have identical actions on gastrointestinal function when large, pharmacological doses are administered, but they do not share any actions at normal, physiological concentrations. Likewise, GLIP and secretin share multiple actions when pharmacological doses are administered, but only one action is shared at physiological concentrations: inhibition of gastric acid secretion.

    TMP12 758

16. **E)** The cephalic phase of gastric secretion occurs before food enters the stomach. Seeing, smelling, chewing, and anticipating food is perceived by the brain, which, in essence, tells the stomach to prepare for a meal. Stimuli for the cephalic phase thus include mechanoreceptors in the mouth, chemoreceptors (smell and taste), thought of food, and hypoglycemia. Because the cephalic phase of gastric secretion is mediated entirely by way of the vagus nerve, vagotomy can abolish the response. Antacids neutralize gastric acid, but they do not inhibit gastric secretion. An anti-gastrin antibody would attenuate (but not abolish) the cephalic phase because this would have no effect on histamine and acetylcholine stimulation of acid secretion. Atropine would attenuate the cephalic phase by blocking acetylcholine receptors on parietal cells; however, atropine does not abolish acetylcholine

stimulation of gastrin secretion. A histamine H₂ blocker would attenuate the cephalic phase of gastric secretion, but would not abolish it.
    TMP12 779

17. **E)** Hirschsprung disease is characterized by a congenital absence of ganglion cells in the distal colon resulting in a functional obstruction. Most cases of Hirschsprung disease are diagnosed in the newborn period. Hirschsprung disease should be considered in any newborn who fails to pass meconium within 24 to 48 hr after birth. Although contrast enema is useful in establishing the diagnosis, rectal biopsy remains the criterion standard. Aganglionosis begins with the anus, which is nearly always involved, and continues proximally for a variable distance. Both the myenteric (Auerbach) and submucosal (Meissner) plexus are absent, resulting in reduced bowel peristalsis and function. The precise mechanism underlying the development of Hirschsprung disease is poorly understood.
    TMP12 802

18. **C)** Migrating motility complexes (sometimes called interdigestive myoelectric complexes) are peristaltic waves of contraction that begin in the stomach and slowly migrate in an aboral direction along the entire small intestine to the colon. By sweeping undigested food residue from the stomach, through the small intestine, and into the colon, MMCs function to maintain low bacterial counts in the upper intestine. Bacterial overgrowth syndrome can occur when the normally low bacterial colonization in the upper gastrointestinal tract increases significantly. It should be clear that an absence of MMCs would decrease duodenal motility and gastric emptying. MMCs do not have a direct effect on mass movements and swallowing.
    TMP12 758–759

19. **C)** Trace C shows a basal subatmospheric pressure with a positive pressure wave cause by passage of the food bolus. Trace A does not correspond to any normal event in the esophagus. Trace B could represent the lower esophageal sphincter (LES) in a patient with achalasia. Trace D depicts normal operation of the LES. Trace E show a basal positive pressure trace, which does not occur where the esophagus passes through the chest cavity.
    TMP12 764

20. **C)** Gastric emptying is accomplished by coordinated activities of the stomach, pylorus, and small intestine. Conditions that favor gastric emptying include (a) increased tone of the orad stomach because this helps to push chyme toward the pylorus, (b) forceful peristaltic contractions in the stomach that move chyme toward the pylorus, (c) relaxation of the pylorus which allows chyme to pass into the duodenum, and (d) absence of segmentation contractions in the intestine, which can otherwise impede the entry of chyme into the intestine.
    TMP12 768

21. **E)** Gastrointestinal smooth muscle undergoes rhythmical changes in membrane potential called slow waves. The slow waves are thought to be caused by variations in the sodium conductance of specialized pacemaker cells, called interstitial cells of Cajal. The discharge frequency of the pacemaker cells and hence the frequency of slow waves is fixed (i.e., does not change) in various parts of the gut. Slow-wave frequency averages about 3 per minute in the stomach, 12 per minute in the duodenum, 10 per minute in the jejunum, and 8 per minute in the ileum. When a slow wave depolarizes sufficiently, it elicits spike potentials which are true action potentials. In the small intestine, slow waves cannot initiate smooth muscle contraction in the absence of spike potentials; however, slow waves themselves can initiate the contraction of smooth muscle in the stomach. The number of spike potentials associated with a given slow wave is increased by parasympathetic stimulation and decreased by sympathetic stimulation. Therefore, the autonomic nervous system controls gut motility by changing the frequency of spike potentials. Neither gastrin nor secretin has significant effects on gut motility at physiological concentrations.
    TMP12 755

22. **C)** The palatopharyngeal folds located on each side of the pharynx are pulled medially forming a sagittal slit through which the bolus of food must pass. This slit performs a selective function, allowing food that has been masticated sufficiently to pass by but impeding the passage of larger objects. The soft palate is pulled upward to close the posterior nares, which prevents food from passing into the nasal cavities. The vocal cords of the larynx are strongly approximated during swallowing, and the larynx is pulled upward and anteriorly by the neck muscles. The epiglottis then swings backward over the opening of the larynx. The upper esophageal sphincter relaxes, allowing food to move from the posterior pharynx into the upper esophagus.
    TMP12 764

23. **C)** The gastrocolic reflex occurs when distension of the stomach (gastro) stimulates mass movements in the colon (colic). All of the gut reflexes are named with the anatomical origin of the reflex as the prefix followed by the name of the gut segment in which the outcome of the reflex is observed, that is, the gastrocolic reflex begins in the stomach and ends in the colon. The duodenocolic reflex has a similar function to the gastrocolic reflex. When the duodenum is distended, nervous signals are transmitted to the colon, which stimulates mass movements. The enterogastric reflex occurs when signals originating in the intestines inhibit gastric motility and gastric secretion. The intestino-intestinal reflex occurs when overdistension or injury to a bowel segment signals the bowel to relax. The rectosphincteric reflex, also called the defecation

reflex, is initiated when feces enters the rectum and stimulates the urge to defecate.

TMP12 757

24. **D)** When feces enters the rectum, distention of the rectal wall initiates signals that spread through the myenteric plexus to initiate peristaltic waves in the descending colon, sigmoid colon, and rectum all of which force feces toward the anus. At the same time the internal anal sphincter relaxes allowing the feces to pass. In people with transected spinal cords, the defecation reflexes can cause automatic emptying of the bowel because the external anal sphincter is normally controlled by the conscious brain through signals transmitted in the spinal cord.

TMP12 771–772

25. **E)** Cholecystokinin (CCK) is the only gastrointestinal hormone that inhibits gastric emptying under normal, physiological conditions. CCK inhibits gastric emptying by relaxing the orad stomach, which increases its compliance. When the compliance of the stomach is increased, the stomach can hold a larger volume of food without excess build up of pressure in the lumen. None of the gastrointestinal hormones increase gastric emptying under physiological conditions; however, gastrin, secretin, and GLIP can inhibit gastric emptying when pharmacological doses are administered experimentally.

TMP12 758

26. **A)** The frequency of slow waves is fixed in various parts of the gut. The maximum frequency of smooth muscle contractions cannot exceed the slow wave frequency. The slow wave frequency averages about 3 per minute in the stomach, 12 per minute in the duodenum, 10 per minute in the jejunum, and 8 per minute in the ileum. Therefore, the duodenum is most likely to have the highest frequency of smooth muscle contractions.

TMP12 754

27. **A)** Gastrin and CCK do not share any effects on gastrointestinal function at normal, physiological conditions; however, they have identical actions on gastrointestinal function when pharmacological doses are administered. Gastrin stimulates gastric acid secretion and mucosal growth throughout the stomach and intestines under physiological conditions. CCK stimulates growth of the exocrine pancreas and inhibits gastric emptying under normal conditions. CCK also stimulates gallbladder contraction, relaxation of the sphincter of Oddi, and secretion of bicarbonate and enzymes from the exocrine pancreas.

TMP12 758

28. **D)** The act of vomiting is preceded by antiperistalsis that may begin as far down in the gastrointestinal tract as the ileum. Distension of the upper portions of the gastrointestinal tract (especially the duodenum) becomes the exciting factor that initiates the actual act of vomiting. At the onset of vomiting, strong contractions occur in the duodenum and stomach along with partial relaxation of the lower esophageal sphincter. From then on, a specific vomiting act ensues that involves (a) a deep breath, (b) relaxation of the upper esophageal sphincter, (c) closure of the glottis, and (d) strong contractions of the abdominal muscles and diaphragm.

TMP12 803

29. **E)** Essentially all proteolytic enzymes are secreted in an inactive form, which prevents autodigestion of the secreting organ. Enterokinase is physically attached to the brush border of the enterocytes which line the inner surface of the small intestine. Enterokinase activates trypsinogen to become trypsin in the gut lumen. The trypsin then catalyzes the formation of additional trypsin from trypsinogen as well as several other proenzymes (e.g., chymotrypsinogen, procarboxypeptidase, proelastase, and others). Pepsin is first secreted as pepsinogen, which has no proteolytic activity. However, as soon as it comes into contact with hydrochloric acid, and especially in contact with previously formed pepsin plus hydrochloride acid, it is activated to form pepsin.

TMP12 778, 781

30. **E)** The rectum is empty of feces most of the time. When a mass movement forces feces into the rectum, the desire to defecate is initiated immediately. Reflex contraction of the rectum and relaxation of the internal anal sphincter follows. If a person is in a place where defecation is possible (like a bathroom), the external anal sphincter is consciously relaxed and the feces is expelled. It should be clear that mass movements do not cause duodenal peristalsis, gastric retropulsion, or hunger sensations.

TMP12 770–771

31. **B)** The use of nonsteroidal anti-inflammatory drugs (NSAIDs) may result in NSAID-associated gastritis or peptic ulceration. Chronic gastritis, by definition, is a histopathological entity characterized by chronic inflammation of the stomach mucosa. When inflammation affects the gastric corpus, parietal cells are inhibited, leading to reduced acid secretion. Although diagnosis of chronic gastritis can only be ascertained histologically, the administration of pentagastrin should produce a less than expected increase in gastric acid secretion. Pentagastrin is a synthetic gastrin composed of the terminal four amino acids of natural gastrin plus the amino acid alanine. It has all the same physiologic properties of natural gastrin. Although gastrin and pentagastrin can both stimulate growth of the duodenal mucosa, it should be clear that intravenous pentagastrin would not cause substantial growth in the context of a clinical test. In any case, chronic

administration of pentagastrin would not lead to a less than expected growth of the duodenal mucosa. Pentagastrin is not expected to increase gastrin secretion, pancreatic enzyme secretion, or pancreatic growth.

   TMP12 800

32. **E)** Vitamin B12 absorption requires intrinsic factor, which is a glycoprotein secreted by parietal cells in the stomach. Binding of intrinsic factor to dietary vitamin B12 is necessary for attachment to specific receptors located in the brush border of the ileum. Therefore, ileal resection can lead to vitamin B12 deficiency. Achalasia is a neuromuscular failure of relaxation at the lower end of the esophagus with progressive dilation, tortuosity, incoordination of peristalsis, and often hypertrophy of the proximal esophagus. Atrophic gastritis is a type of autoimmune gastritis that is mainly confined to the acid-secreting corpus mucosa. The gastritis is diffuse and eventually severe atrophy develops. Ileal resection is likely to cause diarrhea, but not constipation. Benign gastric and duodenal ulcers are best classified together as peptic ulcers even though their etiology is different. In both types of ulcer it is acid and pepsin which causes the mucosal damage. Duodenal ulcers are more common.

   TMP12 778

33. **E)** The presence of acid, fatty acids, and hyperosmotic solutions in the duodenum and jejunum lead to suppression of acid secretion through a variety of mechanisms. Acid stimulates the secretion of secretin from the small intestine, which in turn inhibits acid secretion from parietal cells. Acidification of the antrum and oxyntic gland area of the stomach stimulates the release of somatostatin, which in turn inhibits acid secretion by a direct action on the parietal cells and an indirect action mediated by suppression of gastrin secretion. The presence of fatty acids in the small intestine stimulates the release of GLIP (glucose-dependent insulinotropic peptide), which inhibits acid secretion both directly (parietal cell inhibition) and indirectly (by decreasing gastrin secretion). Hyperosmotic solutions in the small intestine cause the release of unidentified enterogastrones, which directly inhibit acid secretion from parietal cells. Isotonic solutions have no effect on acid secretion.

   TMP12 758, 780

34. **E)** All of the GI hormones are released following a meal and all have physiological effects.

   TMP12 758

35. **A)** *H. pylori* is a bacterium that accounts for 95% of patients with duodenal ulcer and virtually 100% of patients with gastric ulcer when chronic use of aspirin or other non-steroidal anti-inflammatory drugs (NSAIDS) are eliminated. *H. pylori* is characterized by high urease activity, which metabolizes urea to NH_3 (ammonia). Ammonia reacts with H^+ to become ammonium (NH_4^+). This reaction allows the bacterium to withstand the acid environment of the stomach. The ammonium production is believed to be the major cause of cytotoxicity because the ammonium directly damages epithelial cells, increasing the permeability of the gastric mucosal barrier. Bile salts and NSAIDS can also damage the gastric mucosal barrier, but these are not directly related to *H. pylori* infection. Pepsin can exacerbate the mucosal lesions cause by *H. pylori* infection, but pepsin levels are not increased by *H. pylori*. It should be clear that gastrin does not mediate the mucosal damage caused by *H. pylori*.

   TMP12 801

36. **B)** Neither plasma gastrin levels nor the rate of acid secretion are diagnostic for duodenal ulcer. However, when duodenal ulcer patients are pooled together they exhibit a statistically significant increase in the rate of acid secretion and a statistically significant decrease in plasma gastrin levels. How is this possible? The basal and maximal acid secretion rates of normal subjects range from 1 to 5 mEq/hr and from 6 to 40 mEq/hr, respectively, which overlaps with the basal (2–10 mEq/hr) and maximal (30–80 mEq/hr) acid secretion rates of duodenal ulcer patients. The increase in acid secretion of the average duodenal ulcer patient suppresses the secretion of gastrin from the antrum of the stomach. It should be obvious that endoscopy is diagnostic for duodenal ulcer.

   TMP12 801

37. **C)** The internal anal sphincter relaxes when the rectum is stretched, as indicated by repeated decreases in pressure following inflation of the rectal balloon. Pressures in the distal and proximal rectum are expected to increase following inflation of the rectal balloon. Inflation of a rectal balloon should not affect pressures at the lower esophageal sphincter or ileocecal valve.

   TMP12 771–772

38. **C)** Prior to pelvic floor training, the pressure at the external anal sphincter was unchanged following inflation of the rectal balloon. This failure of the external anal sphincter to contract is expected to result in defecation. After pelvic floor training, the external anal sphincter contracts when the rectal balloon is inflated, which prevents inappropriate defecation.

   TMP12 771–772

39. **C)** The various secretagogues, which include acetylcholine, gastrin, and histamine, have a multiplicative or synergistic effect on gastric acid secretion. This means that histamine potentiates the effects of gastrin and acetylcholine, and that H_2 blockers attenuate the secretory responses to both acetylcholine and gastrin. Likewise, acetylcholine potentiates the effects of gastrin and histamine, and atropine attenuates the secretory effects of histamine and gastrin. Therefore, in the experiment described, the stimulation of acid secretion by pentagastrin is attenuated by the H_2

blocker because of this multiplicative effect of the secretagogues.

   TMP12 780–781

40. B) Cholera toxin causes an irreversible increase in cAMP levels in enterocytes, which leads to an irreversible opening of chloride channels on the luminal surface. Movement of chloride into the gut lumen causes a secondary movement of sodium ions through paracellular pathways into the gut lumen. Water follows the osmotic gradient causing a tremendous increase in fluid loss into the gut lumen, which results in severe diarrhea.

   TMP12 796

41. E) One of the most critical actions of gastrointestinal hormones is their trophic activity. Gastrin can stimulate mucosal growth throughout the gastrointestinal tract as well as growth of the exocrine pancreas. If most of the endogenous gastrin is removed by antrectomy, the gastrointestinal tract atrophies. Exogenous gastrin prevents the atrophy. Partial resection of the small intestine for tumor removal, morbid obesity, or other reasons results in hypertrophy of the remaining mucosa. The mechanism for this adaptive response is poorly understood. Both cholecystokinin and secretin stimulate growth of the exocrine pancreas. GLIP (glucose-dependent insulinotropic peptide) and motilin do not appear to have trophic actions on the gastrointestinal tract.

   TMP12 758

42. A) During a swallow, the orad portion of the stomach and lower esophageal sphincter relax at about the same time. Intraluminal pressures in both regions decrease before the arrival of the swallowed bolus. This phenomenon is called receptive relaxation. Because the orad stomach relaxes with each swallow, the stomach can accept a large volume of food with only a few mm Hg rise in intragastric pressure. Receptive relaxation is mediated by afferent and efferent pathways in the vagus. Receptive relaxation and gastric distensibility are impaired following vagotomy. The palatopharyngeal folds are important for determining whether a bolus of food is small enough to be swallowed. The pharynx and thoracic esophagus undergo peristaltic contractions during swallowing, but they do not undergo receptive relaxation. The upper esophageal sphincter opens during a swallow, but this is not considered to be receptive relaxation.

   TMP12 765

43. B) Relaxation of the ileocecal sphincter occurs with or shortly after eating. This reflex has been termed the gastroileal reflex. It is not clear whether the reflex is mediated by gastrointestinal hormones (gastrin and cholecystokinin) or extrinsic autonomic nerves to the intestine. Note that the gastroileal reflex is named with the origin of the reflex first (gastro) and the target of the reflex named second (ileal). This method of naming is characteristic of all the gastrointestinal reflexes. The enterogastric reflex involves signals from the colon and small intestine that inhibit gastric motility and gastric secretion. The gastrocolic reflex causes the colon to evacuate when the stomach is stretched. The intestino-intestinal reflex causes a bowel segment to relax when it is overstretched. The rectosphincteric reflex is also called the defecation reflex.

   TMP12 769, 772

44. E) The defecation reflex (also called the rectosphincteric reflex) occurs when a mass movement forces feces into the rectum. When the rectum is stretched, the internal anal sphincter relaxes and the rectum contracts pushing the feces toward the anus. The external anal sphincter is controlled voluntarily and can be contracted when defecation is not possible. Therefore, when a person feels the urge to defecate, the internal anal sphincter is relaxed, the rectum is contracting, and the external anal sphincter is either contracted or relaxed depending on the circumstances.

   TMP12 771–772

45. D) Damage to the gastric mucosal barrier allows hydrogen ions to back-leak into the mucosa in exchange for sodium ions. A low pH in the mucosa causes mast cells to leak histamine, which damages the vasculature causing ischemia. The ischemic mucosa allows a greater leakage of hydrogen ions—more cell injury and death—resulting in a vicious cycle. Factors that normally strengthen the gastric mucosal barrier include mucus (which impedes the influx of hydrogen ions), gastrin (which stimulates mucosal growth), certain prostaglandins (which can stimulate mucus secretion), and various growth factors that can stimulate growth of blood vessels, gastric mucosa, and other tissues. Factors that weaken the gastric mucosal barrier include *Helicobacter pylori* (a bacterium that produces toxic levels of ammonium) as well as aspirin, NSAIDS, ethanol, and bile salts.

   TMP12 779–780

46. D) Vitamin B12 is absorbed primarily by the ileum.

   TMP12 778

47. A) Hydrogen ions leak into the mucosa when it is damaged. As the hydrogen ions accumulate in the mucosa, the intracellular buffers become saturated, and the pH of the cells decreases resulting in injury and cell death. The hydrogen ions also damage mast cells causing them to secrete excess amounts of histamine. The histamine exacerbates the condition by damaging blood capillaries within the mucosa. The result is focal ischemia, hypoxia, and vascular stasis. The mucosal lesion is a forerunner of gastric ulcer. Mucus secretion helps to strengthen the gastric mucosal barrier because mucus impedes the leakage of hydrogen ions into the mucosa. Various proton pump inhibitors are used as a treatment modality for gastric ulcer because these can decrease the secretion of hydrogen ions (protons). The tight junctions between cells within the mucosa help to prevent the back-leak of hydrogen ions. Vagotomy was once used to treat gastric ulcer disease because severing or crushing the vagus nerve decreases gastric acid secretion.

    TMP12 779–800

48. **B)** Gastrin has a critical role to stimulate mucosal growth throughout the gastrointestinal system.

    TMP12 758

49. **C)** The medical treatment of gastric ulcers is aimed at restoring the balance between acid secretion and mucosal protective factors. Proton pump inhibitors are drugs that covalently bind and irreversibly inhibit the H^+/K^+ adenosine triphosphatase (ATPase) pump, effectively inhibiting acid release. Therapy can also be directed toward histamine release, that is, H_2 blockers, such as cimetidine (Tagamet), ranitidine (Zantac), famotidine (Pepcid), and nizatidine (Axid). These agents selectively block the H_2 receptors in the parietal cells. Antibiotic therapy is used to eradicate the *H. pylori* infection. NSAIDS (nonsteroidal anti-inflammatory agents) can cause damage to the gastric mucosal barrier, which is a forerunner of gastric ulcer.

    TMP12 801

50. **F)** It is a common misconception that the pH of the gastric contents is lowest (most acidic) following a meal when acid secretion is highest. Before a meal, when the stomach is empty, the pH of the gastric contents is the lowest and acid secretion is suppressed. Acid secretion is low because (a) the acid stimulates somatostatin release (which has a direct action to decrease secretion of both gastrin and acid), and (b) acid has a direct effect to suppress parietal cell secretions. When a meal is taken, the buffering effects of the food cause the gastric pH to increase, which allows the various secretagogues to stimulate acid secretion.

    TMP12 779

51. **B)** Movement of chloride ions out of cells leads to secretion of fluid by cells. Cystic fibrosis (CF) is caused by abnormal chloride ion transport on the apical surface of epithelial cells in exocrine gland tissues. The CF transmembrane regulator (CFTR) protein functions both as a cyclic AMP-regulated Cl^- channel and, as its name implies, a regulator of other ion channels. The fully processed form of CFTR is found in the plasma membrane of normal epithelia. Absence of CFTR at appropriate cellular sites is often part of the pathophysiology of CF. However, other mutations in the CF gene produce CFTR proteins that are fully processed but are nonfunctional or only partially functional at the appropriate cellular sites.

    TMP12 775, 787, 796

52. **C)** Acid acts directly on somatostatin cells to stimulate the release of somatostatin. The somatostatin decreases acid secretion by directly inhibiting the acid secreting parietal cells and indirectly by inhibiting gastrin secretion from G cells in the antrum. Acid is a weak stimulus for CCK release, but CCK does not inhibit (or stimulate) gastrin release. Acid does not stimulate GLIP release. Fatty acids are a weak stimulus for motilin, but motilin does not affect gastrin release. Fatty acids are not thought to stimulate somatostatin release.

    TMP12 780

53. **C)** Hirschsprung disease results from the absence of parasympathetic ganglion cells in the myenteric and submucosal plexus of the rectum and/or colon. Congenital aganglionosis begins with the anus, which is always involved, and continues proximally for a variable distance. Both the myenteric (Auerbach) and submucosal (Meissner) plexus are absent, resulting in reduced bowel peristalsis and function. The precise mechanism underlying the development of Hirschsprung disease is unknown. It should be clear that an absence of lymphatic endothelial cells, capillary endothelial cells, or red blood cells would not affect colonic motility. Smooth muscle cells are present in Hirschsprung disease.

    TMP12 802

54. **A)** Mass movements force feces into the rectum. When the walls of the rectum are stretched by the feces, the defecation reflex is initiated and a bowel movement follows when this is convenient. Mass movements do not affect gastric motility. Haustrations are bulges in the large intestine caused by contraction of adjacent circular and longitudinal smooth muscle. It should be clear that mass movements in the colon do not affect esophageal contractions or pharyngeal peristalsis.

    TMP12 770–771

55. **A)** Celiac sprue is a chronic disease of the digestive tract that interferes with the absorption of nutrients from food. The mucosal lesions seen on upper GI biopsy are the result of an abnormal, genetically determined, cell-mediated immune response to gliadin, a constituent of the gluten found in wheat. A similar response occurs to comparable proteins found in rye and barley. Gluten is not found in oats, rice, and maize. When affected individuals ingest gluten, the mucosa of their small intestine is damaged by an immunologically mediated inflammatory response, resulting in malabsorption and maldigestion at the brush border. Digestion of fat is normal in celiac sprue because the pancreas which secretes lipase still functions normally. Because celiac sprue causes malabsorption it should be clear that the stool content of carbohydrates, fat, and nitrogen is increased.

    TMP12 801

56. E) ZES is typically caused by a gastrin-secreting tumor that is located in the pancreas, duodenal wall, or in lymph nodes. The most simple and reliable test for ZES is secretin injection. Secretin inhibits antral gastrin, but it simulates gastrin secretion in patients with ZES (gastrinoma). Two units of secretin per kilogram body weight are injected intravenously. Serum gastrin levels are measured at various times for 30 min after injection. An increase in serum gastrin of more than 200 ng/mL is diagnostic for ZES. The physiological mechanism of the secretin test remains unclear; however, it is the most important diagnostic test to exclude other conditions associated with increased acid secretion. CCK, GLIP, motilin, and pentagastrin have minimal effects on gastrin secretion and are not diagnostic for gastrinoma.

TMP12 758

57. A) Intrinsic factor is a glycoprotein secreted from parietal cells (i.e., acid secreting cells in the stomach) that is necessary for absorption of vitamin B12. The patient has a diminished capacity to secrete acid because of chronic gastritis. Because acid and intrinsic factor are both secreted by parietal cells, a diminished capacity to secrete acid is usually associated with diminished capacity to secrete intrinsic factor. Ptyalin, also known as salivary amylase, is an enzyme that begins carbohydrate digestion in the mouth. The secretion of ptyalin is not affected by gastritis. Rennin, known also as chymosin, is a proteolytic enzyme synthesized by chief cells in the stomach. Its role in digestion is to curdle or coagulate milk in the stomach, a process of considerable importance in very young animals. It should be clear that saliva secretion is not affected by gastritis. Trypsin is a proteolytic enzyme secreted by the pancreas.

TMP12 778

58. C) Gastrin, acetylcholine, and histamine can directly stimulate parietal cells to secrete acid. These three secretagogues also have a multiplicative effect on acid secretion such that inhibition of one secretagogue reduces the effectiveness of the remaining two secretagogues. Acetylcholine also has an indirect effect to increase acid secretion by stimulating gastrin secretion from G cells. Somatostatin inhibits acid secretion.

TMP12 758, 778, 780

59. D) Duodenal ulcer patients have about 2 billion parietal cells and can secrete about 40 mEq H^+ per hour. Normal individuals have about 50% of these values. Plasma gastrin levels are related inversely to acid secretory capacity because of a feedback mechanism whereby antral acidification inhibits gastrin release. Thus, plasma gastrin levels are reduced in duodenal ulcer patients. Maximal acid secretion and plasma gastrin levels are not diagnostic for duodenal ulcer disease because of significant overlap with the normal population among individuals in each group.

TMP12 800–801

60. E) A proton pump inhibitor such as omeprazole inhibits all acid secretion by directly inhibiting the H^+, K^+-ATPase (H^+ pump). The parietal cell has receptors for secretagogues such as gastrin, acetylcholine, and histamine. Therefore, antigastrin antibodies, atropine, and histamine H_2 blockers can reduce the secretion of acid, but none of these can totally eliminate acid secretion. Antacids neutralize gastric acid once it has entered the stomach, but they cannot inhibit acid secretion from parietal cells.

TMP12 779, 801

61. B) Secretin inhibits gastrin release from the antrum of the stomach, but it stimulates gastrin secretion from a gastrinoma. Thus, patients with a gastrinoma have increased serum gastrin levels within 30 min after secretin administration; whereas secretin decreases serum gastrin levels in normal subjects. Secretin injection is the most simple and reliable test for gastrinoma; however, the physiological mechanism of the secretin test is poorly understood. Secretin normally inhibits gastric acid secretion, but it could conceivably increase acid secretion in patients with gastrinoma because of the increase in gastrin secretion that occurs. Secretin can inhibit gastric emptying when pharmacological doses are given, but this is not diagnostic for gastrinoma. Secretin has a normal physiological effect to stimulate pancreatic $HCO3^-$ secretion, which is independent of gastrinoma.

TMP12 758, 801

62. D) The discovery of *H. pylori* and its association with peptic ulcer disease, adenocarcinoma, gastric lymphoma, and other diseases make it one of the most significant medical discoveries of this century. In the United States, about 26 million people will suffer from ulcer disease in their lifetime and up to 90% will likely be due to *H. pylori*. *H. pylori* is a gram-negative bacterium with high urease activity, an enzyme that catalyzes the formation of ammonia from urea. The ammonia (NH_3) is converted to ammonium (NH_4^+) in the acid environment of the stomach. The ammonium damages the gastric mucosal barrier because it damages epithelial cells. *H. pylori* also increases gastric acid secretion, possibly by increasing parietal cell mass. This combination of increased acid secretion along with damage to the gastric mucosal barrier promotes the development of gastric ulcer. Bile salts can damage the gastric mucosal barrier, but they do not have a clinically significant effect on acid secretion. Epidermal growth factor, gastrin, and mucous strengthen the gastric mucosal barrier.

TMP12 801

63. B) Antral peristalsis pushes chyme toward the pylorus and thus promotes gastric emptying. Other factors that promote gastric emptying include (a) decreased compliance of the stomach, (b) relaxation of the pylorus, and (c) an absence of segmentation contractions in the small bowel. Gastric emptying is thought to be slow in eating disorders such as anorexia nervosa, bulimia nervosa, and obesity. Scleroderma is a systemic disease that affects many organ systems. The symptoms result from progressive tissue fibrosis and occlusion of the microvasculature by excessive production and deposition of types I and III collagens. Deposition of fibrous tissues in the pylorus reduces gastric emptying. Gastroparesis (paralysis of the stomach) occurs in about 20% of type I diabetics. The high blood glucose is thought to damage the vagus nerve and thereby reduce gastric emptying.

TMP12 758, 768

64. **C)** Pancreatitis is inflammation of the pancreas. The pancreas secretes digestive enzymes into the small intestine that are essential in the digestion of fats, proteins, and carbohydrates. Reduced secretion of fluid into the pancreatic ducts in cystic fibrosis cause these digestive enzymes to accumulate in the ducts. The digestive enzymes then become activated in the pancreatic ducts (which typically would not occur) and can begin to "digest" the pancreas, leading to inflammation and a myriad of other problems (cysts and internal bleeding). Enterokinase is located at the brush border of intestinal enterocytes where it normally activates trypsin from its precursor, trypsinogen. Trypsin inhibitor is normally present in the pancreatic ducts where it prevents trypsin from being activated, and thus prevents autodigestion of the pancreas. When the ducts are blocked in cystic fibrosis, the available trypsin inhibitor is insufficient to prevent trypsin from being activated. Excessive secretion of CCK does not occur in cystic fibrosis. Gallstone obstruction can lead to pancreatitis (by autodigestion) when the obstruction prevents pancreatic juice from entering the intestine, but this is unrelated to cystic fibrosis.

TMP12 801

65. **C)** The cephalic phase of gastric secretion is mediated entirely by the vagus nerve: vagotomy abolishes the response. The vagus also mediates a significant portion of the gastric phase of gastric secretion. Vagal stimulation increases acid secretion by a direct action of parietal cells as well as by stimulating gastrin secretion. Vagal stimulation increases gastrin secretion by (a) directly stimulating G cells, which secrete gastrin, and (b) inhibiting somatostatin cells from secreting somatostatin, which would otherwise inhibit G cells from secreting gastrin. Gastrin releasing peptide (GRP) is the neurotransmitter released from interneurons that stimulate G cells to secrete gastrin.

TMP12 758, 779–780

66. **E)** Following a meal, the pH of the gastric contents increases because the food buffers the acid in the stomach. This increase in pH suppresses the release of somatostatin from delta cells in the stomach (hydrogen ions stimulate the release of somatostatin). Because somatostatin inhibits secretion of both gastrin and gastric acid, the fall in somatostatin levels leads to an increase in acid secretion. The increase in acid secretion causes the pH of the gastric contents to decrease. As the pH of the gastric contents decreases, the rate of acid secretion also decreases.

TMP12 777–778

67. **C)** About 20% of persons older than 65 years have gallstones (cholelithiasis) in the United States, and 1 million newly diagnosed cases of gallstones are reported each year. Gallstones are the most common cause of biliary obstruction. Regardless of the cause of gallstones, serum bilirubin values (especially direct or conjugated) are usually elevated. Indirect or unconjugated bilirubin values are usually normal or only slightly elevated. Only answer C shows a high level of direct bilirubin (conjugated bilirubin) compared to the level of indirect bilirubin (unconjugated bilirubin).

TMP12 786

Metabolism and Temperature Regulation

1. Fatty acid degradation in mitochondria produces which of the following two-carbon substances?

   A) Acetyl coenzyme A
   B) Carnitine
   C) Glycerol
   D) Glycerol 3-phosphate
   E) Oxaloacetic acid

2. The hypothalamic set-point temperature normally averages about 98.6°F. Which of the following factors can alter the set-point level for core temperature control?

	Skin temperature	Pyrogens	Antipyretics	Thyroxin
A)	No	Yes	Yes	No
B)	No	Yes	Yes	Yes
C)	Yes	Yes	Yes	Yes
D)	Yes	No	No	Yes
E)	Yes	Yes	Yes	No

3. A 54-year-old man consumes a meal containing a large amount of fat. At which of the locations in the following figure is bile salts most likely to be absorbed by an active transport process?

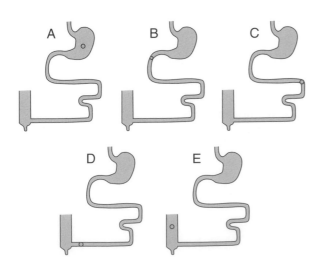

4. A 69-year-old woman has a 30-year history of alcoholism and liver disease. She visits her physician because of

swelling in the abdomen. An increase in which of the following is the most likely cause of the ascites?

   A) Hepatic artery pressure
   B) Hepatic vein pressure
   C) Hydrostatic pressure of peritoneal fluid
   D) Plasma albumin concentration
   E) Portal vein pressure

5. The first stage in using triglycerides for energy is hydrolysis of the triglycerides to which of the following substance(s)?

   A) Acetyl coenzyme A and glycerol
   B) Cholesterol and fatty acids
   C) Glycerol 3-phosphate and cholesterol
   D) Glycerol and fatty acids
   E) Phospholipids and glycerol

6. Most of the heat loss from an unclothed person at room temperature occurs by which of the following mechanisms?

   A) Conduction to air
   B) Conduction to objects
   C) Convection
   D) Evaporation
   E) Radiation

7. The increase in serum bilirubin levels in patients with alcoholic cirrhosis most often results from which of the following?

   A) Decreased excretion of bilirubin into bile
   B) Increased uptake of bilirubin by hepatocytes
   C) Enhanced conjugation of bilirubin
   D) Excessive hemolysis

8. A 65-year-old man has a 25-year history of alcoholism and liver disease. He visits his physician because of swelling in his legs. A decrease in which of the following is likely to contribute to the development of edema in his legs?

   A) Capillary hydrostatic pressure
   B) Femoral vein pressure
   C) Interstitial fluid hydrostatic pressure
   D) Liver lymph flow
   E) Plasma albumin concentration

9. A 45-year-old African-American man is admitted to the emergency department because of upper right quadrant pain. The man has a history of sickle-cell disease. Laboratory tests show that plasma bilirubin levels are three times greater compared to normal. Ultrasound studies confirm the presence of gallstones. Which of the following is the most likely composition of the gallstones in this patient?

A) Bile pigments
B) Calcium
C) Cholesterol
D) Fatty acids
E) Sugar

Questions 10 and 11
Refer to the following figure to answer questions 10 and 11.

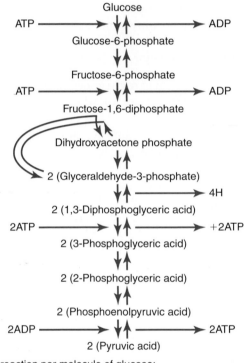

Glucose

ATP ⟶ ↓↑ ⟶ ADP

Glucose-6-phosphate

↓↑

Fructose-6-phosphate

ATP ⟶ ↓↑ ⟶ ADP

Fructose-1,6-diphosphate

↓↑

Dihydroxyacetone phosphate

↓↑

2 (Glyceraldehyde-3-phosphate)

↓↑ ⟶ 4H

2 (1,3-Diphosphoglyceric acid)

2ATP ⟶ ↓↑ ⟶ +2ATP

2 (3-Phosphoglyceric acid)

↓↑

2 (2-Phosphoglyceric acid)

↓↑

2 (Phosphoenolpyruvic acid)

2ADP ⟶ ↓↑ ⟶ 2ATP

2 (Pyruvic acid)

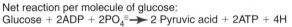

Net reaction per molecule of glucose:
Glucose + 2ADP + 2PO$_4^{\equiv}$ ⟶ 2 Pyruvic acid + 2ATP + 4H

10. Abundant amounts of adenosine triphosphate (ATP) in the cytoplasm of the cell inhibit which of the following steps in glycolysis?

A) Conversion of glucose to glucose-6-phosphate
B) Conversion of fructose-6-phosphate to fructose-1,6-diphosphate
C) Conversion of 1,3-diphosphoglyceric acid to 3-phosphoglyceric acid
D) Conversion of phosphoenolpyruvic acid to pyruvic acid

11. Abundant amounts of adenosine diphosphate (ADP) or adenosine monophosphate (AMP) stimulate which of the following steps in glycolysis?

A) Conversion of glucose to glucose-6-phosphate
B) Conversion of fructose-6-phosphate to fructose-1,6-diphosphate
C) Conversion of 1,3-diphosphoglyceric acid to 3-phosphoglyceric acid
D) Conversion of phosphoenolpyruvic acid to pyruvic acid

12. The transport of glucose through the membranes of most tissue cells occurs by which of the following processes?

A) Facilitated diffusion
B) Primary active transport
C) Secondary active co-transport
D) Secondary active countertransport
E) Simple diffusion

13. Which of the following mechanisms causes heat loss from a normal person when the environmental temperature is 106°F and the relative humidity is less than 10%?

A) Conduction
B) Convection
C) Evaporation
D) Radiation

14. About 75% of the blood flowing through the liver is from the portal vein, and the remainder is from the hepatic artery during resting conditions. Which of the following best describes the liver circulation in terms of resistance, pressure, and flow?

	Resistance	Pressure	Flow
A)	High	High	High
B)	High	Low	High
C)	Low	High	Low
D)	Low	Low	High
E)	Low	Low	Low

15. A scuba diver explores an underwater lava flow where the water temperature is 102°F. Which of the following profiles best describes the mechanisms of heat loss that are effective in this man?

	Evaporation	Radiation	Convection	Conduction
A)	No	No	No	Yes
B)	No	No	No	No
C)	Yes	Yes	No	Yes
D)	No	Yes	No	Yes
E)	Yes	Yes	Yes	Yes

16. A 57-year-old obese woman on hormone replacement therapy develops gallstones. Her gallstones are most likely composed of which of the following substances?

    A) Bile salts
    B) Bilirubin
    C) Calcium salts
    D) Cholesterol
    E) Free fatty acids

17. Deamination means removal of the amino groups from the amino acids. Which of the following substances is produced when deamination occurs by transamination?

    A) Acetyl coenzyme A
    B) Ammonia
    C) Citrulline
    D) Ornithine
    E) α-ketoglutaric acid

18. Most of the energy released from the glucose molecule occurs by which of the following processes?

    A) Citric acid cycle
    B) Glycogenesis
    C) Glycogenolysis
    D) Glycolysis
    E) Oxidative phosphorylation

19. A 30-year-old man runs on an inclined treadmill until near exhaustion for an experiment examining anaerobic exercise conditioning. All of the following statements concerning the conversion of pyruvic acid to lactic under anaerobic conditions are true EXCEPT one. Which one is this EXCEPTION?

    A) Conversion of pyruvic acid to lactic acid provides a sinkhole into which the end-products of glycolysis can disappear
    B) Pyruvic acid combines with NAD^+ to produce lactic acid and NADH
    C) The NAD^+ produced by the conversion of pyruvic acid to lactic acid can combine with two hydrogen atoms and allow glycolysis to continue
    D) Under the above conditions, the heart can use lactic acid as an energy source

20. A 45-year-old man is admitted to the emergency department after he was found lying in the street in an inebriated state. He is markedly pale with icteric conjunctivae and skin. His abdomen is distended, and there is shifting dullness, indicating ascites. The liver is enlarged about 5 centimeters below the right costal margin and tender. The spleen cannot be palpated. There is bilateral edema of his legs and feet. Which of the following values of direct and indirect bilirubin (in milligrams per deciliter) are most likely to be present in this man's plasma?

	Direct	Indirect
A)	1.1	1.2
B)	1.7	5.4
C)	2.4	2.5
D)	5.2	1.8
E)	5.8	7.2

Questions 21–23

Use the following figure to answer questions 21 to 23. The diagram shows the effects of changing the set-point of the hypothalamic temperature controller. The red line indicates the body temperature, and the blue line represents the hypothalamic set-point temperature.

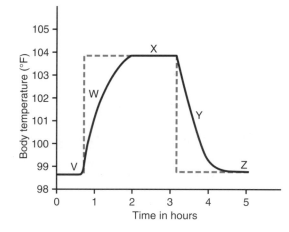

21. Which of the following sets of changes occurs at point W, compared with point V?

	Shivering	Sweating	Vasoconstriction	Vasodilation
A)	No	No	No	No
B)	No	Yes	No	Yes
C)	No	Yes	Yes	No
D)	Yes	No	No	Yes
E)	Yes	No	Yes	No
F)	Yes	Yes	Yes	Yes

22. Which of the following sets of changes occurs at point Y, compared with point V?

	Shivering	Sweating	Vasoconstriction	Vasodilation
A)	No	No	No	No
B)	No	Yes	No	Yes
C)	No	Yes	Yes	No
D)	Yes	No	No	Yes
E)	Yes	No	Yes	No
F)	Yes	Yes	Yes	Yes

23. Which of the following sets of changes occurs at point X, compared with point V?

	Shivering	Sweating	Vasoconstriction	Vasodilation
A)	No	No	No	No
B)	No	Yes	No	Yes
C)	No	Yes	Yes	No
D)	Yes	No	No	Yes
E)	Yes	No	Yes	No
F)	Yes	Yes	Yes	Yes

24. Which of the following is the most abundant source of high-energy phosphate bonds in the cells?

A) Adenosine triphosphate (ATP)
B) Phosphocreatine
C) Adenosine diphosphate (ADP)
D) Creatine
E) Creatinine

25. A 54-year-old man is admitted to the emergency department after being found lying in his yard near a running lawnmower on a hot summer day. His body temperature is 106°F, blood pressure is normal, and heart rate is 160 beats/min. Which of the following sets of changes is most likely to be present in this man?

	Sweating	Hyperventilation	Vasodilation of skin
A)	No	No	No
B)	No	Yes	Yes
C)	Yes	No	Yes
D)	Yes	Yes	No
E)	Yes	Yes	Yes

26. Which of the following accounts for the largest component of daily energy expenditure in a sedentary individual?

A) Basal metabolic rate
B) Maintaining body posture
C) Nonshivering thermogenesis
D) Thermic effect of food

27. Most of the energy for strenuous exercise that lasts for more than 5 to 10 seconds but less than 1 to 2 minutes comes from which of the following sources?

A) Adenosine triphosphate (ATP)
B) Anaerobic glycolysis
C) Oxidation of carbohydrates
D) Oxidation of lactic acid
E) Conversion of lactic acid into pyruvic acid

28. The ammonia released during deamination of amino acids is removed from the blood almost entirely by conversion into which of the following substances?

A) Ammonium
B) Carbon dioxide
C) Citrulline
D) Ornithine
E) Urea

29. Erythrocytes are constantly dying and being replaced. Heme from the hemoglobin is converted to which of the following substances before being eliminated from the body?

A) Bilirubin
B) Cholesterol
C) Cholic acid
D) Globin
E) Verdigarbin

30. Which of the following best describes the process by which glucose can be formed from amino acids?

A) Gluconeogenesis
B) Glycogenesis
C) Glycogenolysis
D) Glycolysis
E) Hydrolysis

31. A 32-year-old pregnant woman in the third trimester is admitted to the emergency department because of severe upper right quadrant pain following a meal of chicken fried steak. Her blood pressure is 130/84 mm Hg, heart rate is 105 beats/min, and respirations are 30/min. Body mass index before pregnancy was 45 kg/m². Physical examination shows abdominal guarding and diaphoresis. Serum bilirubin levels and white cell count are both normal. This patient is most likely suffering from which of the following conditions?

A) Cholelithiasis
B) Constipation
C) Hepatitis
D) Pancreatitis
E) Peritonitis

32. An experimental device containing hepatocytes is developed to provide effective support for patients with hepatic failure pending liver regeneration or liver transplantation. Hepatocyte viability is best documented by an increase in which of the following?

A) Lactate dehydrogenase (LDH) uptake
B) Ethanol output
C) Albumin output
D) Glucuronic acid uptake
E) Oxygen output
F) Carbon dioxide uptake

33. The metabolic rate of a person is normally expressed in terms of the rate of heat liberation that results from the chemical reactions of the body. Metabolic rate can be estimated with reasonable accuracy from the oxygen consumption of a person. Which of the following factors tends to increase or decrease the metabolic rate of a person?

	Growth hormone	Fever	Sleep	Malnutrition
A)	Decrease	Decrease	Decrease	Decrease
B)	Decrease	Increase	Decrease	Increase
C)	Increase	Increase	Increase	Increase
D)	Increase	Increase	Decrease	Increase
E)	Increase	Increase	Decrease	Decrease

34. Urinary nitrogen excretion measured in a patient is 16.0 g in 24 hr. What is the approximate amount of protein breakdown in this patient for 24 hr in grams?

    A) 16.0
    B) 17.6
    C) 100
    D) 110
    E) 120

35. A deficiency of which of the following proteins would be most likely to cause increased appetite?

    A) Melanin concentrating hormone
    B) NPY
    C) Ghrelin
    D) Orexin A
    E) Leptin
    F) Agouti-related peptide

36. In a person with type 1 diabetes who is not receiving insulin therapy and who has a fasting blood glucose of 400mg/100 mL, what would you expect the respiratory quotient (RQ) to be 2 hr after eating a light meal containing 60% carbohydrates, 20% protein, and 20% fat?

    A) 0.5
    B) 0.7
    C) 0.9
    D) 1.0
    E) 1.2

37. A gene mutation which reduces formation of which of the following proteins would be most likely to cause early onset, morbid obesity?

    A) NPY
    B) Ghrelin
    C) Melanin concentrating hormone
    D) Melanocortin 4 receptor
    E) Agouti-related peptide
    F) Orexin A

38. Deficiency of which of the following would cause "night blindness" in humans?

    A) Vitamin A
    B) Vitamin B_1
    C) Vitamin B_6
    D) Vitamin B_{12}
    E) Vitamin C
    F) Niacin

39. Which of the following changes would be expected to stimulate hunger in a person who has not eaten for 24 hours?

    A) increased neuropeptide Y in hypothalamus
    B) increased leptin secretion
    C) increased peptide YY secretion
    D) decreased ghrelin secretion
    E) activation of hypothalamic pro-opiomelanocortin (POMC) neurons
    F) increased cholescystokinin secretion

40. Deficiency of which of the following would cause *pellagra* in humans or *black tongue* in canines?

    A) Vitamin A
    B) Vitamin B_1
    C) Vitamin B_{12}
    D) Vitamin C
    E) Niacin

41. Deficiency of which of the following vitamins is the main cause of beriberi?

    A) Vitamin A
    B) Thiamine (vitamin B_1)
    C) Riboflavin (vitamin B_2)
    D) Vitamin B_{12}
    E) Pyridoxine (vitamin B_6)

1. **A)** Fatty acids are degraded in mitochondria by the progressive release of two-carbon segments in the form of acetyl coenzyme A. This is called the beta-oxidation process for degradation of fatty acids.

      TMP12 822

2. **E)** Pyrogens released from toxic bacteria or degenerating tissues of the body can increase the set-point temperature of the hypothalamic thermostat. Fever-reducing medications such as aspirin, ibuprofen, and Tylenol are called "antipyretics" (meaning "against fire"). These medications can reduce body temperature and alleviate fever. Thyroxin can increase metabolic rate and therefore increase the rate of heat production by the body, but thyroxin does not change the set-point temperature of the hypothalamic thermostat. A decrease in skin temperature causes the set-point temperature to increase, and the set-point temperature decreases when the skin is hot.

      TMP12 875–876

3. **D)** About 95% of bile salts is reabsorbed from the small intestine; about half of this occurs by diffusion through the mucosa in the early portions of the small intestine, and the remainder by an active transport process through the intestinal mucosa in the distal ileum. The bile salts then enter the portal blood and pass back to the liver. This recirculation of bile salts is called the enterohepatic circulation.

      TMP12 829

4. **E)** When liver parenchymal cells are destroyed, they are replaced with fibrous tissue that eventually contracts around the blood vessels, thereby greatly impeding the flow of portal blood through the liver. This increase in vascular resistance leads to an increase in portal vein pressure, which in turn raises the capillary pressure of the splanchnic organs, causing excess amounts of fluid transudate to enter the abdomen.

      TMP12 838

5. **D)** Triglycerides are hydrolyzed to glycerol and fatty acids which, in turn, are oxidized to provide energy. Almost all cells, with the exception of some brain tissue, can use fatty acids almost interchangeably with glucose for energy.

      TMP12 819–820

6. **E)** About 60% of the body heat is lost by radiation. Loss of heat by radiation means loss in the form of infrared heat waves, which is a type of electromagnetic wave. All objects radiate heat waves; thus, heat waves are radiated from the walls of rooms and other objects toward the body, and the body radiates heat waves to all surrounding objects. If the temperature of the body is greater than the temperature of surrounding objects, more heat radiates from the body than is radiated to the body.

      TMP12 868–869

7. **A)** Damage to hepatic cells in cirrhosis of the liver leads to the development of obstructive jaundice. The rate of bilirubin formation is normal, and free bilirubin enters the liver cells and becomes conjugated in the normal way. However, the conjugated bilirubin is then returned to the blood, probably by rupture of the congested bile cannaliculi and direct emptying of the bile into the lymph leaving the liver.

      TMP12 841–842

8. **E)** Essentially all the albumin in the plasma is formed in the liver. One of the complications of cirrhosis is the failure of liver parenchymal cells to produce adequate amounts of albumin, thus leading to decreased plasma colloid osmotic pressure and generalized edema. Under normal conditions, about 75% of the plasma colloid osmotic pressure can be attributed to albumin produced in the liver.

      TMP12 833–834

9. **A)** Hemolytic diseases, such as sickle-cell disease, result in the premature destruction of erythrocytes. Excessive amounts of hemoglobin released from the red blood cells lead to overproduction of bilirubin by phagocytes. This increase in bilirubin production can lead to the development of pigment stones in the gallbladder that are composed primarily of bilirubin.

      TMP12 840–842

10. **B)** Continual release of energy from glucose when energy is not needed by the cells would be an extremely wasteful process. Both ATP and adenosine diphosphate (ADP) control the rate of chemical reactions in the energy metabolism sequence. When ATP is abundant within the cell, it helps control energy metabolism by inhibiting the conversion of fructose-6-phosphate to fructose-1,6-diphosphate. It does so by inhibiting the enzyme phosphofructokinase.

      TMP12 815

11. **B)** Both ADP and AMP increase the activity of the enzyme phosphofructokinase and increase the conversion of fructose-6-phosphate to fructose-1,6-diphosphate.
    TMP12 812

12. **A)** The transport of glucose through the membranes of most cells is different from that which occurs through the gastrointestinal membrane or through the epithelium of the renal tubules. In both these latter cases, the glucose is transported by the mechanism of secondary active co-transport, in which active transport of sodium provides energy for absorbing glucose against a concentration difference. This sodium co-transport mechanism functions only in certain special epithelial cells that are specifically adapted for active absorption of glucose. At all other cell membranes, glucose is transported only from higher concentrations toward lower concentrations by facilitated diffusion made possible by the special binding properties of membrane glucose carrier protein.
    TMP12 810–811

13. **C)** Evaporation is the only mechanism of heat loss when the air temperature is greater than the body temperature. Each gram of water that evaporates from the surface of the body causes 0.58 kilocalorie of heat to be lost from the body. Even when a person is not sweating, water still evaporates insensibly from the skin and lungs at a rate of 450 to 600 mL/day, which amounts to about 12 to 16 kilocalories of heat loss per hour.
    TMP12 869

14. **D)** The liver has a high blood flow, low vascular resistance, and low blood pressure. During resting conditions, about 27% of the cardiac output flows through the liver, yet the pressure in the portal vein leading into the liver averages only 9 mm Hg. This high flow and low pressure indicate that the resistance to blood flow through the hepatic sinusoids is normally very low.
    TMP12 838

15. **B)** None of the mechanisms of heat loss are effective when a person is placed in water that has a temperature greater than body temperature. Instead, the body will continue to gain heat until the body temperature becomes equal to the water temperature.
    TMP12 868–869

16. **D)** Under abnormal conditions, the cholesterol present in bile may precipitate, resulting in the formation of cholesterol gallstones. These account for about 80% of all gallstones. Some of the risk factors for cholesterol gallstones include obesity, excess estrogen from pregnancy or hormone replacement, and gender. Women between 20 and 60 years of age are twice as likely to develop gallstones as are men.
    TMP12 No discussion

17. **B)** The degradation of amino acids occurs almost entirely in the liver, and it begins with deamination, which occurs mainly by the following transamination schema: The amino group from the amino acid is transferred to α-ketoglutaric acid, which then becomes glutamic acid. The glutamic acid then transfers the amino group to still other substances or releases it in the form of ammonia. In the process of losing the amino group, the glutamic acid once again becomes α-ketoglutaric acid, so that the cycle can repeat again and again.
    TMP12 834

18. **E)** About 90% of the total adenosine triphosphate (ATP) produced by glucose metabolism is formed during oxidation of the hydrogen atoms released during the early stages of glucose degradation. This process is called oxidative phosphorylation. Only two ATP molecules are formed by glycolysis, and another two are formed in the citric acid cycle. ATP is not formed by glycogenesis or glycogenolysis.
    TMP12 814

19. **B)** The two end-products of glycolysis—pyruvic acid and hydrogen atoms—combine with NAD^+ to form NADH and H^+. The buildup of either or both of these products would stop the glycolytic process and prevent the formation of ATP. Under anaerobic conditions, the majority of pyruvic acid is converted to lactic acid. Therefore, lactic acid represents a type of sinkhole into which the glycolytic end-products can disappear.
    TMP12 816

20. **D)** This man has cirrhosis of the liver. In this condition, the rate of bilirubin production is normal, and the free bilirubin still enters the liver cells and becomes conjugated in the usual way. The conjugated bilirubin (direct) is mostly returned to the blood, probably by rupture of congested bile cannaliculi, so that only small amounts enter the bile. The result is elevated levels of conjugated (direct) bilirubin in the plasma, with normal or near-normal levels of unconjugated (indirect) bilirubin.
    TMP12 840–841

21. **E)** When the hypothalamic set-point temperature is greater than the body temperature, the person feels cold, and exhibits responses that lead to an elevation of body temperature. These responses include shivering and vasoconstriction as well as piloerection and epinephrine secretion. Shivering increases heat production. The increase in epinephrine secretion causes an immediate increase in the rate of cellular metabolism, which is an effect called *chemical thermogenesis*. Vasoconstriction of the skin blood vessels decreases heat loss through the skin.
    TMP12 876

22. **B)** When the hypothalamic set-point temperature is lower than the body temperature, the person feels hot, and exhibits responses that cause body temperature to decrease. These responses include sweating and vasodilation. Sweating increases heat loss from the body by evaporation. Vasodilation of skin blood vessels facilitates heat loss from the body by increasing the skin blood flow.
    TMP12 876

23. **A)** When the hypothalamic set-point temperature is equal to the body temperature, the body exhibits neither heat loss nor heat conservation mechanisms, even when the body temperature is far above normal. Therefore, the person does not feel hot even when the body temperature is 104°F.
    TMP12 876

24. **B)** Phosphocreatine contains high-energy phosphate bonds and is three to eight times as abundant as ATP or ADP in a cell. Creatine does not contain high-energy phosphate bonds. Creatinine is a breakdown product of creatine phosphate in muscle.
    TMP12 860

25. **B)** This patient is suffering from heatstroke. Patients with heatstroke commonly exhibit tachypnea and hyperventilation caused by direct central nervous system stimulation, acidosis, or hypoxia. The blood vessels in the skin are vasodilated, and the skin is warm. Sweating ceases in patients with true heatstroke, most likely because the high temperature itself causes damage to the anterior hypothalamic-preoptic area. The nerve impulses from this area are transmitted in the autonomic pathways to the spinal cord and then through sympathetic outflow to the skin to cause sweating.
    TMP12 869, 876

26. **A)** Basal metabolic rate counts for about 50% to 70% of the daily energy expenditure in most sedentary individuals. Non-exercise activity, such as fidgeting or maintaining posture, accounts for approximately 7% of daily energy expenditure, and the thermic effect of food accounts for about 8%. Nonshivering thermogenesis can occur in response to cold stress, but the maximal response in adults is less than 15% of the total metabolic rate.
    TMP12 863

27. **B)** Most of the extra energy required for strenuous activity that lasts for more than 5 to 10 sec but less than 1 to 2 min is derived from anaerobic glycolysis. Release of energy by glycolysis occurs much more rapidly than oxidative release of energy, which is much too slow to supply the needs of the muscle in the first few minutes of exercise. ATP and phosphocreatine already present in the cells are rapidly depleted in less than 5 to 10 sec. After the muscle contraction is over, oxidative metabolism is used to reconvert much of the accumulated lactic acid into glucose; the remainder becomes pyruvic acid, which is degraded and oxidized in the citric acid cycle.
    TMP12 860–861

28. **E)** Two molecules of ammonia and one molecule of carbon dioxide combine to form one molecule of urea and one molecule of water. Essentially all urea formed in the human body is synthesized in the liver. In the absence of the liver or in serious liver disease, ammonia accumulates in the blood. The ammonia is toxic to the brain, often leading to a state called *hepatic coma*.
    TMP12 835

29. **A)** Hemoglobin is metabolized by tissue macrophages (also called the reticuloendothelial system). The hemoglobin is first split into globin and heme, and the heme ring is opened to produce free iron and a straight chain of four pyrrole nuclei, from which bilirubin will eventually be formed. The free bilirubin is taken up by hepatic cells, and most of it is conjugated with glucuronic acid; the conjugated bilirubin passes into the bile cannaliculi and then into the intestines.
    TMP12 840

30. **A)** When the body's stores of carbohydrates decrease below normal, moderate quantities of glucose can be formed from amino acids and the glycerol portion of fat. This process is called gluconeogenesis. Glycogenesis is the formation of glycogen. Glycogenolysis means the breakdown of the cell's stored glycogen to re-form glucose in the cells. Glycolysis means splitting of the glucose molecule to form two molecules of pyruvic acid. Hydrolysis is a process in which a molecule is split into two parts by the addition of a water molecule.
    TMP12 817

31. **A)** Cholelithiasis is the presence of gallstones (choleliths) in the gallbladder or bile ducts. This patient exhibits typical symptoms caused by gallstones.
    TMP12 No discussion

32. **C)** Hepatocytes produce essentially all the albumin normally present in blood. Viable hepatocytes use oxygen and produce carbon dioxide. Glucuronic acid produced by hepatocytes is used to conjugate bilirubin forming bilirubin glucuronide. Lactate dehydrogenase is an enzyme that converts pyruvic acid to lactic acid under anaerobic conditions.
    TMP12 833

33. **E)** Growth hormone can increase the metabolic rate 15% to 20% as a result of direct stimulation of cellular metabolism. Fever, regardless of its cause, increases the chemical reactions of the body by an average of about 120% for every 10°C rise in temperature. The metabolic rate decreases 10% to 15% below normal during sleep. Prolonged malnutrition can decrease the metabolic rate 20% to 30%, presumably due to the paucity of food substances in the cells.
    TMP12 863–864

34. **D)** The rate of protein metabolism can be estimated by measuring the nitrogen in the urine, then adding 10% (since about 90% of the nitrogen in proteins is excreted in the urine) and multiplying by 6.25 (100/16) since the average protein contains about 16% nitrogen.
    TMP12 845

35. **E)** Leptin is an anorexigenic hormone which powerfully reduces appetite. Therefore, deficiency of leptin causes voracious feeding. All of the other neurotransmitters and hormones stimulate feeding and deficiency would tend to reduce appetite.
    TMP12 846–849, Table 71-2

36. **B)** Type I diabetes is characterized by lack of insulin. In the absence of adequate insulin, little carbohydrate can be used by the body's cells and the respiratory quotient remains near that for fat metabolism (0.70).
    TMP12 845

37. **D)** Activation of the melanocortin 4 receptor suppresses food intake and deficiency of this receptor causes excessive feeding and early onset, morbid obesity. All of the other neurotransmitters and hormones listed in this question have the opposite effect and their deficiency would tend to reduce appetite.
    TMP12 846--847

38. **A)** One of the basic functions of Vitamin A is in the formation of retinal pigments and therefore the prevention of night blindness.
    TMP12 853

39. **A)** Neuropeptide Y is an orexigenic neurotransmitter that stimulates feeding and is increased during food deprivation. Leptin, peptide YY, cholecystokinin, and activation of POMC neurons are all reduced by fasting. Ghrelin is increased, not decreased, by fasting.
    TMP12 846–849, Table 71-2

40. **F)** Niacin, also called nicotinic acid, functions as a coenzyme and combines with hydrogen atoms as they remove food substrates by various types of dehydrogenases. When a deficiency of niacin exists, the normal rate of dehydrogenation is reduced, and oxidation and delivery of energy from foodstuffs cannot occur at a normal rate. This causes dermatitis, inflammation of the mucous membranes, and psychic disturbances, as well as other disorders of the clinical entity called pellagra in humans and black tongue in canines.
    TMP12 853–854

41. **B)** Thiamine is needed for the final metabolism of carbohydrates and amino acids. Decreased utilization of these nutrients secondary to thiamine deficiency is responsible for many of the characteristics of beriberi, including peripheral vasodilation and edema, lesions of the central and peripheral nervous system, and gastrointestinal tract disturbances.
    TMP12 875, 876

Endocrinology and Reproduction

1. Seven days after ovulation, pituitary secretion of luteinizing hormone (LH) decreases rapidly. What is the cause of this decrease in secretion?

   A) The anterior pituitary gland becomes unresponsive to the stimulatory effect of gonadotropin-releasing hormone (GnRH)

   B) Estrogen from the developing follicles exerts a feedback inhibition on the hypothalamus

   C) The rise in body temperature inhibits hypothalamic release of GnRH

   D) Secretion of estrogen and progesterone by the corpus luteum suppresses hypothalamic secretion of GnRH and pituitary secretion of LH

   E) None of the above

2. Which of the following is inconsistent with the diagnosis of Graves' disease?

   A) Increased heart rate

   B) Exophthalmos

   C) Increased plasma levels of triiodothyronine (T_3)

   D) Increased plasma levels of thyroxine (T_4)

   E) Increased plasma levels of thyroid-stimulating hormone

3. Which of the following statements about antidiuretic hormone is true?

   A) It is synthesized in the posterior pituitary gland

   B) It increases salt and water reabsorption in the collecting tubules and ducts

   C) It stimulates thirst

   D) It has opposite effects on urine and plasma osmolality

4. After menopause, hormone replacement therapy with estrogen-like compounds is effective in preventing the progression of osteoporosis. What is the mechanism of their protective effect?

   A) They stimulate the activity of osteoblasts

   B) They increase absorption of calcium from the gastrointestinal tract

   C) They stimulate calcium reabsorption by the renal tubules

   D) They stimulate parathyroid hormone secretion by the parathyroid gland

5. Within minutes following a normal delivery, flow through the foramen ovale decreases dramatically. What is the cause of this change?

   A) Increased formation of prostaglandin E_2 in the endocardium

   B) Increased rate of flow through the pulmonary artery

   C) Increased left atrial pressure

   D) Increased right atrial pressure

   E) Increased P_{O_2}

Questions 6–8

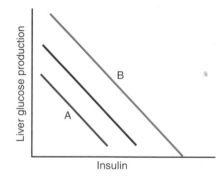

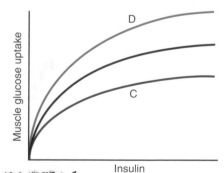

The red lines in the figure above illustrate the normal relationships between plasma insulin concentration and glucose production by the liver and between plasma insulin concentration and glucose uptake in muscle.

6. In the figure, which lines most likely illustrate these relationships in a patient with type 2 diabetes?

    A) A and C
    B) A and D
    C) B and C
    D) B and D

7. In the figure, which lines most likely illustrate these relationships in a patient with acromegaly?

    A) A and C
    B) A and D
    C) B and C
    D) B and D

8. In the figure, line D most likely illustrates the influence of which of the following?

    A) Exercise
    B) Obesity
    C) Growth hormone
    D) Cortisol
    E) Glucagon

9. One treatment for erectile dysfunction requires the injection of a substance into the corpora cavernosa of the penis. The injection of which of the following causes an erection?

    A) Norepinephrine
    B) A substance that inhibits formation of nitric oxide
    C) Thromboxane A_2, which is a vasoconstrictor prostaglandin
    D) Angiotensin II
    E) None of the above

10. A baby is born with a penis, a scrotum with no testes, no vagina, and XX chromosomes. This condition is referred to as hermaphroditism. Which of the following could cause this abnormality?

    A) Abnormally high levels of human chorionic gonadotropin production by the trophoblast cells
    B) The presence of a testosterone-secreting tumor in the mother's right adrenal gland
    C) Abnormally high levels of luteinizing hormone in the maternal blood
    D) Abnormally low levels of testosterone in the maternal blood
    E) Abnormally low rates of estrogen production by the placenta

11. A young woman is given daily injections of a substance beginning on the 16th day of her normal menstrual cycle and continuing for 3 weeks. As long as the injections continue, she does not menstruate. The injected substance could be which of the following?

    A) Testosterone
    B) FSH
    C) An inhibitor of progesterone's actions
    D) A prostaglandin E_2 inhibitor
    E) HCG

12. Which of the following could inhibit the initiation of labor?

    A) Administration of an antagonist of the actions of progesterone
    B) Administration of luteinizing hormone
    C) Administration of an antagonist of prostaglandin E_2 effects
    D) Mechanically dilating and stimulating the cervix
    E) Administration of oxytocin

13. Exposure to UV light directly facilitates which of the following?

    A) Conversion of cholesterol to 25-hydroxycholicalciferol
    B) Conversion of 25-hydroxycholicalciferol to 1,25-dihydroxycholicalciferol
    C) Transport of calcium into the extracellular fluid
    D) Formation of calcium binding protein
    E) Storage of vitamin D_3 in the liver

14. After birth, the pressure in the pulmonary artery decreases greatly. What is the cause of this?

    A) Systemic arterial pressure increases
    B) Ductus arteriosus closes
    C) Left ventricular pressure increases
    D) Pulmonary vascular resistance decreases

15. If a radioimmunoassay is properly conducted and the amount of radioactive hormone bound to antibody is low, this would indicate which of the following?

    A) Plasma levels of endogenous hormone are high
    B) Plasma levels of endogenous hormone are low
    C) More antibody is needed
    D) Less radioactive hormone is needed

16. Spermatogenesis is regulated by a negative feedback control system in which follicle-stimulating hormone (FSH) stimulates the steps in sperm cell formation. What is the negative feedback signal associated with sperm cell production that inhibits pituitary formation of FSH?

    A) Testosterone
    B) Inhibin
    C) Estrogen
    D) Luteinizing hormone

17. During the 12-hr period preceding ovulation, which of the following is true?

    A) The plasma concentration of estrogen is rising
    B) A surge of luteinizing hormone is secreted from the pituitary
    C) The surge occurs immediately after the formation of the corpus luteum
    D) The surge is followed immediately by a fall in the plasma concentration of progesterone
    E) The number of developing follicles is increasing

18. When do progesterone levels rise to their highest point during the female hormonal cycle?

    A) Between ovulation and the beginning of menstruation
    B) Immediately before ovulation
    C) When the blood concentration of luteinizing hormone is at its highest point
    D) When 12 primary follicles are developing to the antral stage

19. Some cells secrete chemicals into the extracellular fluid that act on cells in the same tissue. Which of the following refers to this type of regulation?

    A) Neural
    B) Endocrine
    C) Neuroendocrine
    D) Paracrine
    E) Autocrine

20. Which of the following pairs is an example of the type of regulation referred to in question 19?

    A) Somatostatin—growth hormone secretion
    B) Somatostatin—insulin secretion
    C) Dopamine—prolactin secretion
    D) Norepinephrine—corticotropin-releasing hormone secretion
    E) Corticotropin-releasing hormone—adrenocorticotropic hormone secretion

21. Estrogen is required for normal reproductive function in the male. Where is the principal site of estrogen synthesis in the male?

    A) Leydig cells
    B) Osteoblasts
    C) Liver cells
    D) Prostate cells

22. A professional athlete in her mid-20s has not had a menstrual cycle for 5 years, although a bone density scan revealed normal skeletal mineralization. Which of the following facts elicited during the taking of her medical history may explain these observations?

    A) She consumes a high-carbohydrate diet
    B) Her grandmother suffered a hip fracture at age 79
    C) Her blood pressure is greater than normal
    D) Her plasma estrogen concentration is very low
    E) She has been taking anabolic steroid supplements for 5 years

23. In the circulatory system of a fetus, which of the following is greater before birth than after birth?

    A) Arterial P_{O_2}
    B) Right atrial pressure
    C) Aortic pressure
    D) Left ventricular pressure

Questions 24–26

Match each of the patients described in questions 24 to 26 with the correct set of plasma values listed in the table below. Normal values are as follows: plasma aldosterone concentration, 10 ng/dL; plasma cortisol concentration, 10 mg/dL; plasma potassium concentration, 4.5 mEq/L.

	Aldosterone concentration	Cortisol concentration	Potassium concentration
A)	10.0	2.0	4.5
B)	2.0	2.0	6.0
C)	40.0	30.0	2.0
D)	40.0	10.0	4.5
E)	40.0	10.0	2.0

24. A patient with Addison's disease

25. A patient with Conn's syndrome

26. A patient on a low-sodium diet

27. In the following figure, which lines most likely reflect the responses in a patient with nephrogenic diabetes insipidus?

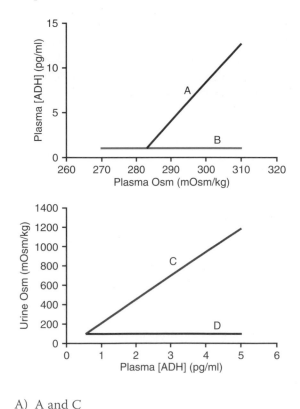

A) A and C
B) A and D
C) B and C
D) B and D

28. Which of the following is greater after birth than before birth?

    A) Flow through the foramen ovale
    B) Pressure in the right atrium
    C) Flow through the ductus arteriosus
    D) Aortic pressure

29. Parathyroid hormone directly

    A) controls the rate of 25-hydroxycholicalciferol formation
    B) controls the rate of calcium transport in the mucosa of the small intestine
    C) controls the rate of formation of calcium binding protein
    D) controls the rate of formation of 1, 25-dihydroxy-cholicalciferol
    E) stimulates renal tubular phosphate reabsorption

30. Which of the following is most likely to produce the greatest increase in insulin secretion?

    A) Amino acids
    B) Amino acids and glucose
    C) Amino acids and somatostatin
    D) Glucose and somatostatin

31. In order for male differentiation to occur during embryonic development, testosterone must be secreted from the testes. What stimulates the secretion of testosterone during embryonic development?

    A) Luteinizing hormone from the maternal pituitary gland
    B) Human chorionic gonadotropin
    C) Inhibin from the corpus luteum
    D) Gonadotropin-releasing hormone from the embryo's hypothalamus

32. A patient has an elevated plasma thyroxine (T_4) concentration, a low plasma thyroid-stimulating hormone (TSH) concentration, and a thyroid gland that is smaller than normal. Which of the following is the most likely explanation for these findings?

    A) Patient has a lesion in the anterior pituitary that prevents TSH secretion
    B) Patient is taking propylthiouracil
    C) Patient is taking thyroid extract
    D) Patient is consuming large amounts of iodine
    E) Patient has Graves disease

33. Extracellular ionic calcium activity will be decreased within 1 min by which of the following?

    A) Increase in extracellular phosphate ion activity
    B) Increase in extracellular pH
    C) Decrease in extracellular P_{CO_2}
    D) All of the above
    E) None of the above

34. As menstruation ends estrogen levels in the blood rise rapidly. What is the source of the estrogen?

    A) Corpus luteum
    B) Developing follicles
    C) Endometrium
    D) Stromal cells of the ovaries
    E) Anterior pituitary gland

35. Which of the following anterior pituitary hormones plays a major role in the regulation of a nonendocrine target gland?

    A) Adrenocorticotropic hormone
    B) Thyroid-stimulating hormone
    C) Prolactin
    D) Follicle-stimulating hormone
    E) Luteinizing hormone

36. An experiment is conducted in which antidiuretic hormone (ADH) is administered at hour 3 to four subjects (A to D). In the following figure, which lines most likely reflect the response to ADH administration in a normal patient and in a patient with central diabetes insipidus?

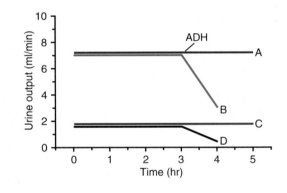

	Normal	Central diabetes insipidus
A)	B	A
B)	B	D
C)	D	A
D)	D	B

37. A female athlete who took testosterone-like steroids for several months stopped having normal menstrual cycles. What is the best explanation for this observation?

    A) Testosterone stimulates inhibin production from the corpus luteum
    B) Testosterone binds to receptors in the endometrium, resulting in the endometrium's failure to develop during the normal cycle
    C) Testosterone binds to receptors in the anterior pituitary that stimulate the secretion of follicle-stimulating hormone (FSH) and luteinizing hormone (LH)
    D) Testosterone inhibits the hypothalamic secretion of gonadotropin-releasing hormone and the pituitary secretion of LH and FSH

38. Which of the following would be expected in a patient with a genetic deficiency in 11β-hydroxysteroid dehydrogenase type 2?

    A) Increased mineralocorticoid activity
    B) Increased glucocorticoid activity
    C) Hyperkalemia
    D) Decreased blood pressure
    E) Hypoglycemia

39. Which of the following decreases the resistance in the arteries leading to the sinuses of the penis?

    A) Stimulation of the sympathetic nerves innervating the arteries
    B) Nitric oxide
    C) Inhibition of activity of the parasympathetic nerves leading to the arteries
    D) All of the above

40. A patient has a goiter associated with high plasma levels of both thyrotropin-releasing hormone (TRH) and thyroid-stimulating hormone (TSH). Her heart rate is elevated. This patient most likely has which of the following?

    A) Endemic goiter
    B) Hypothalamic tumor secreting large amounts of TRH
    C) Pituitary tumor secreting large amounts of TSH
    D) Graves' disease

41. A 40-year-old woman comes to the emergency room with a fracture in the neck of the femur. Radiographs reveal generalized demineralization of the bone in the area. Her plasma calcium ion concentration is significantly greater than normal: 12.2 mg/dL. Which of the following conditions is consistent with this presentation?

    A) Osteoporosis
    B) Rickets
    C) Hyperparathyroidism
    D) Renal failure

42. A man eats a low carbohydrate meal rich in proteins containing the amino acids that stimulate insulin secretion. Which of the following responses accounts for the absence of hypoglycemia?

    A) Suppression of growth hormone
    B) Suppression of somatomedin C secretion
    C) Stimulation of cortisol secretion
    D) Stimulation of glucagon secretion
    E) Stimulation of epinephrine secretion

43. A 46-year-old man has "puffy" skin and is lethargic. His plasma thyroid-stimulating hormone concentration is low and increases markedly when he is given thyrotropin-releasing hormone. Which of the following is the most likely diagnosis?

    A) Hyperthyroidism due to a thyroid tumor
    B) Hyperthyroidism due to an abnormality in the hypothalamus
    C) Hypothyroidism due to an abnormality in the thyroid
    D) Hypothyroidism due to an abnormality in the hypothalamus
    E) Hypothyroidism due to an abnormality in the pituitary

44. Which of the following hormones is both synthesized and stored in the pituitary gland?

    A) Growth hormone (GH)
    B) GH releasing hormone (GHRH)
    C) ADH
    D) Somatostatin
    E) Somatomedin

45. A man is taking a number of medications, one of which appears to be interfering with the emission phase of the sexual act. Which of the following medications could cause this problem?

    A) A medication that prolongs the duration of action of nitric oxide
    B) A medication that blocks the smooth muscle receptors for nitric oxide
    C) A medication that increases the release of nitric oxide
    D) A testosterone-like androgen compound
    E) An inhibitor of beta-adrenergic nervous system receptors

46. In controlling aldosterone secretion, angiotensin II acts on which of the following structures?

    A) Zona glomerulosa
    B) Zona fasciculata
    C) Zona reticularis
    D) Adrenal medulla

47. Giving prostaglandin E_2 (PGE_2) to a pregnant woman may result in an abortion. What is the best explanation for this finding?

    A) PGE_2 strongly stimulates uterine contraction
    B) PGE_2 causes constriction of the arteries leading to the placenta
    C) PGE_2 stimulates the release of oxytocin from the posterior pituitary
    D) PGE_2 increases the secretion of progesterone from the corpus luteum

48. During the first few years after menopause, follicle-stimulating hormone (FSH) levels are normally extremely high. A 56-year-old woman completed menopause 3 years ago. However, she is found to have low levels of FSH in her blood. Which of the following is the best explanation for this finding?

    A) She has been receiving hormone replacement therapy with estrogen and progesterone since she completed menopause
    B) Her adrenal glands continue to produce estrogen
    C) Her ovaries continue to secrete estrogen
    D) She took birth control pills for 20 years before menopause

49. Which of the following pairs of hormones and the corresponding action is incorrect?

    A) Glucagon—increased glycogenolysis in liver
    B) Glucagon—increased glycogenolysis in skeletal muscle
    C) Glucagon—increased gluconeogenesis
    D) Cortisol—increased gluconeogenesis
    E) Cortisol—decreased glucose uptake in muscle

50. A large dose of insulin is administered intravenously to a patient. Which of the following sets of hormonal changes is most likely to occur in the plasma in response to the insulin injection?

	Growth hormone	Glucagon	Epinephrine
A)	↑	↓	↔
B)	↔	↑	↑
C)	↑	↑	↑
D)	↓	↑	↑
E)	↓	↓	↔

51. Delayed breathing at birth is a common danger faced by newborn infants. What is a frequent cause of delayed breathing?

    A) Fetal hypoxia during the birth process
    B) Maternal hypoxia during the birth process
    C) Fetal hypercapnia
    D) Maternal hypercapnia

52. Which of the following hormones is largely unbound to plasma proteins?

    A) Cortisol
    B) Thyroxine (T_4)
    C) Antidiuretic hormone
    D) Estradiol
    E) Progesterone

53. A 3-week-old infant is brought to the emergency room in a comatose condition. The history reveals that her parents have been feeding her concentrated, undiluted formula for 5 days. (Infant formula preparations are often sold in concentrated forms that must be properly diluted with water before feeding.) The infant's plasma osmolality is 352 mOsm/L (normal is 280 to 300 mOsm/L), and the osmolality of the urine is 497 mOsm/L. What is the explanation for the hyperosmotic condition of the plasma?

    A) The infant has inappropriate antidiuretic hormone regulation
    B) The infant has excessive secretion of aldosterone
    C) The infant is unable to form urine sufficiently concentrated to excrete the solute load from the formula without losing more water than required to maintain normal plasma osmolality
    D) The infant has a renal collecting duct abnormality that prevents it from forming concentrated urine

54. Why is milk produced only after delivery, not before?

    A) Levels of luteinizing hormone and follicle-stimulating hormone are too low during pregnancy to support milk production
    B) High levels of progesterone and estrogen during pregnancy suppress milk production
    C) The alveolar cells of the breast do not reach maturity until after delivery
    D) High levels of oxytocin are required for milk production to begin, and oxytocin is not secreted until the baby stimulates the nipple

55. In an experiment, patients in group 1 are given compound X, and patients in group 2 are given compound Y. After 1 week, group 1 patients have a lower metabolic rate and a larger thyroid gland than group 2 patients do. Identify compounds X and Y. (T_4, thyroxine; TRH, thyrotropin-releasing hormone; TSH, thyroid-stimulating hormone)

	Compound X	Compound Y
A)	TSH	Placebo
B)	T_4	Placebo
C)	Placebo	TSH
D)	Placebo	T_4
E)	Placebo	TRH

56. Which of the following increases the rate of excretion of calcium ions by the kidney?

    A) Decrease in calcitonin concentration in the plasma
    B) Increase in phosphate ion concentration in the plasma
    C) Decrease in the plasma level of parathyroid hormone
    D) Metabolic alkalosis

57. A patient has hyperthyroidism due to a pituitary tumor. Which of the following sets of physiological changes would be expected?

	Thyroglobulin synthesis	Heart rate	Exopthalomos
A)	↑	↑	+
B)	↑	↑	−
C)	↑	↓	+
D)	↓	↓	+
E)	↓	↓	−
F)	↓	↑	−

58. A 25-year-old man is severely injured when hit by a speeding vehicle and loses 20% of his blood volume. Which of the following sets of physiological changes would be expected to occur in response to the hemorrhage? (ADH, antidiuretic hormone)

	Atrial stretch receptor activity	Arterial baroreceptor activity	ADH secretion
A)	↓	↓	↑
B)	↓	↓	↓
C)	↔	↑	↑
D)	↑	↑	↑
E)	↑	↑	↓

59. A patient with normal thyroid function has been given the wrong medication. Which of the following sets of changes would most likely be reported if this patient took propylthiouracil for several weeks? (T_4, thyroxine; TSH, thyroid-stimulating hormone)

	Thyroid size	Plasma T_4 concentration	Plasma TSH concentration
A)	↓	↓	↓
B)	↓	↓	↑
C)	↑	↓	↓
D)	↑	↓	↑
E)	↑	↑	↑

60. If a woman has a tumor secreting large amounts of estrogen from the adrenal gland, which of the following will occur?

A) Progesterone levels in the blood will be very low
B) Her luteinizing hormone secretion rate will be totally suppressed
C) She will not have normal menstrual cycles
D) Her bones will be normally calcified
E) All of the above

61. In a normal young man, what is the maximum pressure that can be achieved within the corpora cavernosa during a sexual experience?

A) 20 to 40 mm Hg
B) 60 to 80 mm Hg
C) 150 to 250 mm Hg
D) 400 to 600 mm Hg

Questions 62 and 63

	Hepatic glucose uptake	Muscle glucose uptake	Hormone-sensitive lipase activity
A)	↑	↑	↑
B)	↑	↓	↑
C)	↓	↑	↓
D)	↑	↑	↓
E)	↓	↑	↑

62. When compared with the postabsorptive state, which of the previous sets of metabolic changes would most likely occur during the postprandial state?

63. When compared with resting conditions, which of the previous sets of metabolic changes would most likely occur during exercise?

64. Very early in embryonic development, testosterone is formed within the male embryo. What is the function of this hormone at this stage of development?

A) Stimulation of bone growth
B) Stimulation of development of male sex organs
C) Stimulation of development of skeletal muscle
D) Inhibition of luteinizing hormone secretion

65. Which of the following changes would be expected to occur with increased binding of a hormone to plasma proteins?

A) Increase in plasma clearance of the hormone
B) Decrease in half-life of the hormone
C) Increase in hormone activity
D) Increase in degree of negative feedback exerted by the hormone
E) Increase in plasma reservoir for rapid replenishment of free hormone

66. A patient arrives in the emergency room apparently in cardiogenic shock due to a massive heart attack. His initial arterial blood sample reveals the following concentrations of ions:

Sodium	137 mmol/L
Bicarbonate	14 mmol/L
Free calcium	2.8 mmol/L
Potassium	4.8 mmol/L
pH	7.16

To correct the acidosis, the attending physician begins an infusion of sodium bicarbonate and after 1 hr takes another blood sample, which reveals the following values:

Sodium	138 mmol/L
Bicarbonate	22 mmol/L
Free calcium	2.3 mmol/L
Potassium	4.5 mmol/L
pH	7.34

What is the cause of the decrease in calcium ion concentration?

A) The increase in arterial pH resulting from the sodium bicarbonate infusion inhibited parathyroid hormone secretion

B) The increase in pH resulted in the stimulation of osteoblasts, which removed calcium from the circulation

C) The increase in pH resulted in an elevation in the concentration of HPO_4^-, which shifted the equilibrium between HPO_4^- and Ca^{++} toward $CaHPO_4$

D) The increase in arterial pH stimulated the formation of 1,25-dihydroxycholecalciferol, which resulted in an increased rate of absorption of calcium from the gastrointestinal tract

67. A 30-year-old woman is breast-feeding her infant. During suckling, which of the following hormonal responses is expected?

A) Increased secretion of antidiuretic hormone (ADH) from the supraoptic nuclei

B) Increased secretion of ADH from the paraventricular nuclei

C) Increased secretion of oxytocin from the paraventricular nuclei

D) Decreased secretion of neurophysin

E) Increased plasma levels of both oxytocin and ADH

68. A 30-year-old man has Conn's syndrome. Which of the following sets of physiological changes is most likely to occur in this patient compared with a healthy person?

	Arterial pressure	Extracellular fluid volume	Sodium excretion
A)	↔	↔	↔
B)	↑	↔	↔
C)	↑	↑	↔
D)	↔	↑	↓
E)	↑	↑	↓

69. Why is it important to feed newborn infants every few hours?

A) The hepatic capacity to store and synthesize glycogen and glucose is not adequate to maintain the plasma glucose concentration in a normal range for more than a few hours after feeding

B) If adequate fluid is not ingested frequently, the plasma protein concentration will rise to greater than normal levels within a few hours

C) The function of the gastrointestinal system is poorly developed and can be improved by keeping food in the stomach at all times

D) The hepatic capacity to form plasma proteins is minimal and requires the constant availability of amino acids from food to avoid hypoproteinemic edema

70. Which of the following would be associated with parallel changes in aldosterone and cortisol secretion?

A) Addison's disease

B) Cushing's disease

C) Cushing's syndrome (adrenal tumor)

D) A low sodium diet

E) Administration of a converting enzyme inhibitor

71. RU486 causes abortion if it is administered before or soon after implantation. What is the specific effect of RU486?

A) It binds to luteinizing hormone receptors, stimulating the secretion of progesterone from the corpus luteum

B) It blocks progesterone receptors so that progesterone has no effect within the body

C) It blocks the secretion of follicle-stimulating hormone by the pituitary

D) It blocks the effects of oxytocin receptors in the uterine muscle

72. Following ejaculation, arterial blood flow into the corpora cavernosa decreases back to the normal resting level resulting in the flaccid state. What is the best explanation for this decrease in blood flow?

A) Systemic arterial pressure decreases due to absence of sexual stimulation

B) The level of sympathetic stimulation to the arterioles supplying the corpora cavernosa decreases

C) Resistance of the arterioles supplying the corpora cavernosa increases

D) Formation of nitric oxide in the endothelial cells of the arterioles supplying the corpora cavernosa is stimulated by the increase in parasympathetic nervous system activity

E) Resistance of the venules draining the sinuses of the corpora cavernosa increases

73. Which of the following decreases the rate of urinary excretion of calcium ions by the kidney?

A) Increase in calcitonin concentration in the plasma

B) Decrease in phosphate ion concentration in the plasma

C) Increase in the plasma level of parathyroid hormone

D) Metabolic acidosis

E) Increase in calcium ion activity in the plasma

74. A 55-year-old man has developed the syndrome of inappropriate antidiuretic hormone secretion due to carcinoma of the lung. Which of the following physiological responses would be expected?

A) Increased plasma osmolality

B) Inappropriately low urine osmolality (relative to plasma osmolality)

C) Increased thirst

D) Decreased secretion of antidiuretic hormone from the pituitary gland

75. During pregnancy, the uterine smooth muscle is quiescent. During the 9th month of gestation the uterine muscle becomes progressively more excitable. What factors contribute to the increase in excitability?

   A) Placental estrogen synthesis rises to high rates
   B) Progesterone synthesis by the placenta decreases
   C) Uterine blood flow reaches its highest rate
   D) Prostaglandin E_2 synthesis by the placenta decreases
   E) Activity of the fetus falls to low levels

76. A 40-year-old man who is sodium-depleted is administered an angiotensin-converting enzyme (ACE) inhibitor for 2 weeks. Which of the following sets of physiological changes would most likely occur in this patient after taking the ACE inhibitor for 2 weeks?

	Plasma aldosterone concentration	Plasma cortisol concentration	Sodium excretion
A)	↔	↔	↔
B)	↔	↓	↔
C)	↓	↔	↑
D)	↓	↓	↑
E)	↓	↔	↔

77. A 20-year-old woman is not having menstrual cycles. Her plasma progesterone concentration is found to be minimal. What is the explanation for the low level of progesterone?

   A) LH secretion rate is elevated
   B) LH secretion rate is suppressed
   C) FSH secretion rate is suppressed
   D) No corpus luteum is present
   E) High inhibin concentration in the plasma has suppressed progesterone synthesis

78. Before the preovulatory surge in luteinizing hormone, granulosa cells of the follicle secrete which of the following?

   A) Testosterone
   B) Progesterone
   C) Estrogen
   D) Inhibin

Questions 79 and 80

79. Based on the following figure, which set of curves most likely reflects the responses in a healthy individual and in patients with type 1 and type 2 diabetes mellitus (DM)?

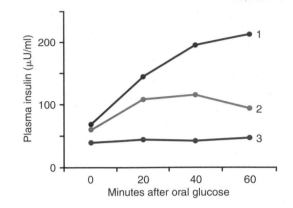

	Healthy	Type 1 DM	Type 2 DM
A)	3	2	1
B)	1	2	3
C)	1	3	2
D)	2	1	3
E)	2	3	1

80. Based on the figure above, which set of curves most likely reflects the responses in a healthy individual and in a patient in the early stages of Cushing's syndrome?

	Healthy	Cushing's syndrome
A)	3	2
B)	1	2
C)	1	3
D)	2	1
E)	2	3

81. Neonates that are kept in 100% oxygen incubators for several days become blind when they are removed from the incubator, a condition referred to as retrolental fibroplasia. What is the explanation for the loss of sight?

   A) The high concentration of oxygen stimulates the growth of fibrous tissue into the retina
   B) The high concentration of oxygen causes rupture of blood vessels in the retina, resulting in fibrous infiltration of the vitreous humor
   C) The high concentration of oxygen retards the growth of blood vessels in the retina, but when the oxygen therapy is stopped, the fall in oxygen concentration stimulates an overgrowth of blood vessels in the retina and vitreous humor, which later become densely fibrous and block the light from the pupil
   D) The high concentration of oxygen destroys the retinal neurons

82. Which of the following hormones activate enzyme-linked receptors?

    A) ADH
    B) Insulin
    C) ACTH
    D) PTH
    E) Aldosterone

83. Which of the following is produced by the trophoblast cells during the first 3 weeks of pregnancy?

    A) Estrogen
    B) Luteinizing hormone
    C) Oxytocin
    D) Human chorionic gonadotropin
    E) None of the above

84. Which of the following findings is most likely in a patient who has myxedema?

    A) Somnolence
    B) Palpitations
    C) Increased respiratory rate
    D) Increased cardiac output
    E) Weight loss

85. At birth, a large, well-nourished baby is found to have a plasma glucose concentration of 17 mg/dL (normal is 80 to 100 mg/dL) and a plasma insulin concentration twice the normal value. What is the explanation for these findings?

    A) Neonate suffered from in utero malnutrition
    B) Mother was malnourished during pregnancy
    C) Mother is diabetic, with poorly controlled hyperglycemia
    D) Mother is obese

86. Which of the following stimulates the secretion of parathyroid hormone (PTH)?

    A) Increase in extracellular calcium ion activity above the normal value
    B) Increase in calcitonin concentration
    C) Respiratory acidosis
    D) Increased secretion of PTH-releasing hormone from the hypothalamus
    E) None of the above

87. A 40-year-old woman is placed on a high-potassium diet for several weeks. Which of the following hormonal changes is most likely to occur?

    A) Increased secretion of dehydroepiandrosterone
    B) Increased secretion of cortisol
    C) Increased secretion of aldosterone
    D) Increased secretion of adrenocorticotropic hormone
    E) Decreased secretion of corticotropin-releasing hormone

88. Which of the following sets of physiological changes is most likely to occur in a patient in the early stages of acromegaly?

	Somatomedin C production	Somatostatin secretion	Insulin secretion
A)	↑	↓	↔
B)	↑	↑	↓
C)	↑	↑	↑
D)	↓	↓	↔
E)	↓	↑	↑

89. If a woman hears her baby cry, she may experience milk ejection from the nipples even before the baby is placed to the breast. What is the explanation for this?

    A) The sound of the hungry baby's cry elicits secretion of oxytocin from the posterior pituitary, which reaches the breast and causes contraction of the myoepithelial cells
    B) The sound of the hungry baby's cry causes a reflex relaxation of the myoepithelial cells, allowing the milk to flow
    C) The sound of the hungry baby's cry elicits a surge of prolactin from the anterior pituitary, which promptly stimulates milk production from the breast
    D) The sound of the hungry baby's cry elicits sympathetic nervous system discharge that causes contraction of the myoepithelial cells

90. Which of the following hormones is not stored in its endocrine-producing gland?

    A) T_4
    B) PTH
    C) Aldosterone
    D) ACTH
    E) Insulin

91. A young woman comes to the emergency room with a vertebral compression fracture. Radiographs of the spine indicate generalized demineralization. She is vegetarian, does not smoke or drink alcohol, has normal plasma potassium concentration of 5.4 mEq/L, sodium concentration of 136 mEq/L, plasma calcium concentration is 7.0 mg/dL. Her vitamin D3 value is several times greater than normal, although her 1,25-dihydroxycholecalciferol concentration is at the lower limit of detectability. She has been in renal failure for the last 5 years and undergoes hemodialysis three times each week. What is the cause of her low 1,25-dihydroxycholecalciferol level?

    A) Metabolic acidosis
    B) Metabolic alkalosis
    C) She is unable to form 1,25-dihydroxycholecalciferol because of her extensive kidney disease
    D) She is being dialyzed with a dialysis fluid without calcium
    E) She is not receiving calcium supplements

92. A neonate develops a jaundice condition with a bilirubin concentration of 10 mg/dL on day 2 (normal is 3 mg/dL at 2 days old). The neonatologist can be confident that the condition is not erythroblastosis fetalis if which of the following is true?

    A) Bilirubin concentration rises no further
    B) Hematocrit falls only slightly
    C) Mother, father, and neonate are all Rh-negative
    D) Mother has no history of hepatic dysfunction

93. Which of the following findings would likely be reported in a patient with a deficiency in iodine intake?

    A) Weight loss
    B) Nervousness
    C) Increased sweating
    D) Increased synthesis of thyroglobulin
    E) Tachycardia

94. Before intercourse, a woman irrigates her vagina with a solution that lowers the pH of the vaginal fluid to 4.5. What will be the effect on sperm cells in the vagina?

    A) Metabolic rate will increase
    B) Rate of movement will decrease
    C) Formation of prostaglandin E_2 will increase
    D) Rate of oxygen consumption will increase

95. Which of the following hormonal responses would be expected after a meal high in protein?

	Insulin	Glucagon	Growth hormone
A)	↑	↑	↓
B)	↑	↑	↑
C)	↑	↓	↓
D)	↓	↓	↑
E)	↓	↑	↑

96. Men who take large doses of testosterone-like androgenic steroids for long periods are sterile in the reproductive sense of the word. What is the explanation for this finding?

    A) High levels of androgens bind to testosterone receptors in the Sertoli cells, resulting in overstimulation of inhibin formation
    B) Overstimulation of sperm cell production results in the formation of defective sperm cells
    C) High levels of androgen compounds inhibit the secretion of gonadotropin-releasing hormone by the hypothalamus, resulting in the inhibition of luteinizing hormone and follicle-stimulating hormone release by the anterior pituitary
    D) High levels of androgen compounds produce hypertrophic dysfunction of the prostate gland

97. A 30-year-old woman is administered cortisone for the treatment of an autoimmune disease. Which of the following is most likely to occur?

    A) Increased adrenocorticotropic hormone secretion
    B) Increased cortisol secretion
    C) Increased insulin secretion
    D) Increased muscle mass
    E) Hypoglycemia between meals

98. The function of which of the following is increased by an elevated parathyroid hormone concentration?

    A) Osteoclasts
    B) Hepatic formation of 25-hydroxycholecalciferol
    C) Phosphate reabsorptive pathways in the renal tubules
    D) All of the above

99. Which of the following statements about peptide or protein hormones is usually true?

    A) They have longer half-lives than steroid hormones
    B) They have receptors on the cell membrane
    C) They have a slower onset of action than both steroid and thyroid hormones
    D) They are not stored in endocrine-producing glands

100. Which of the following sets of physiological changes would be most likely to occur in a patient with acromegaly?

	Pituitary mass	Kidney mass	Femur length
A)	↓	↓	↑
B)	↓	↑	↑
C)	↑	↔	↔
D)	↑	↑	↔
E)	↑	↑	↑

101. Cortisol and growth hormone are most dissimilar in their metabolic effects on which of the following?

    A) Protein synthesis in muscle
    B) Glucose uptake in peripheral tissues
    C) Plasma glucose concentration
    D) Mobilization of triglycerides

102. Infants of mothers who had adequate nutrition during pregnancy do not require iron supplements or a diet rich in iron until about 3 months of age. Why is this?

    A) Growth of the infant does not require iron until after the 3rd month
    B) The fetal liver stores enough iron to meet the infant's needs until the third month
    C) Synthesis of new red blood cells begins after 3 months
    D) Muscle cells that develop before the 3rd month do not contain myoglobin

103. Which of the following would least likely be associated with thyrotoxicosis?

    A) Tachycardia
    B) Increased appetite
    C) Somnolence
    D) Increased sweating
    E) Muscle tremor

104. Where does fertilization normally take place?

    A) Uterus
    B) Cervix
    C) Ovary
    D) Ampulla of the fallopian tubes

105. A patient comes to the emergency room and is found to have a slightly below-normal concentration of calcium in the blood (calcium ion activity = 0.9 mmol/L), a phosphate concentration approximately 50% below normal (HPO_4^- = 0.5 mmol/L), and undetectable amounts of calcium ion in the urine. Which of the following would one expect to find in this patient?

    A) Above normal calcitonin concentration in the blood
    B) Greater than normal parathyroid hormone concentration in the blood
    C) Suppressed osteoclastic activity in the bone
    D) Below normal blood pH

106. Which of the following findings is most likely to occur in a patient who has uncontrolled type 1 diabetes mellitus?

    A) Decreased plasma osmolality
    B) Increased plasma volume
    C) Increased plasma pH
    D) Increased release of glucose from the liver
    E) Decreased rate of lipolysis

107. Growth hormone secretion would most likely be suppressed under which of the following conditions?

    A) Acromegaly
    B) Gigantism
    C) Deep Sleep
    D) Exercise
    E) Acute hyperglycemia

108. Two days before the onset of menstruation, secretions of follicle-stimulating hormone (FSH) and luteinizing hormone (LH) reach their lowest levels. What is the cause of this low level of secretion?

    A) The anterior pituitary gland becomes unresponsive to the stimulatory effect of gonadotropin-releasing hormone (GnRH)
    B) Estrogen from the developing follicles exerts a feedback inhibition on the hypothalamus
    C) The rise in body temperature inhibits hypothalamic release of GnRH
    D) Secretion of estrogen, progesterone, and inhibin by the corpus luteum suppresses hypothalamic secretion of GnRH and pituitary secretion of FSH

109. Which of the following would most likely occur in the earliest stages of type II diabetes?

    A) Increased insulin sensitivity
    B) High circulating levels of C-peptide
    C) Decreased hepatic glucose output
    D) Metabolic acidosis
    E) Hypovolemia

110. A baby is born with a penis, a scrotum with no testes, no vagina, and XX chromosomes. This condition is referred to as hermaphroditism. Which of the following could cause this abnormality?

    A) Abnormally high levels of human chorionic gonadotropin production by the trophoblast cells
    B) Abnormally low rates of estrogen production by the placenta
    C) Abnormally high levels of luteinizing hormone in the maternal blood
    D) Abnormally high levels of testosterone in the maternal blood

111. Which of the following contributes to "sodium escape" in Conn's syndrome?

    A) Decreased plasma levels of atrial natriuretic peptide
    B) Increased plasma levels of angiotensin II
    C) Decreased sodium reabsorption in the collecting tubules
    D) Increased arterial pressure

112. A scientist studying developmental physiology performs an experiment in which a substance is given to pregnant rats that give birth to pups that have XY chromosomes but female genital organs. What was the substance given to the rats?

    A) An antibody that blocked the effect of human chorionic gonadotropin in the embryo and fetus
    B) A large quantity of estrogen-like compounds
    C) Follicle-stimulating hormone
    D) Testosterone

113. An experiment is conducted in which patients in group 1 are given compound X, and patients in group 2 are given compound Y. After 3 weeks, studies show that patients in group 1 have a higher rate of adrenocorticotropic hormone (ACTH) secretion and a lower blood glucose concentration than those in group 2. Identify compounds X and Y.

	Compound X	Compound Y
A)	Cortisone	Placebo
B)	Cortisol	Placebo
C)	Placebo	Cortisol
D)	ACTH	Placebo
E)	Placebo	ACTH

114. A 30-year-old woman reports to the clinic for a routine physical examination. The examination reveals that she is pregnant. Plasma levels of TSH are high but total T_4 concentration (protein bound and free) is normal. Which of the following best reflects this patient's clinical state?

    A) Graves' disease
    B) Hashimoto's disease
    C) Pituitary tumor secreting TSH
    D) Hypothalamic tumor secreting TRH
    E) Patient is taking thyroid extract

115. Which of the following metabolic substrates is preferentially metabolized by growth hormone?

    A) Fats
    B) Proteins
    C) Glycogen
    D) Glucose

116. A man suffers from a disease that destroyed only the motor neurons of the spinal cord below the thoracic region. Which aspect of sexual function would not be possible?

    A) Arousal
    B) Erection
    C) Lubrication
    D) Ejaculation

117. A sustained program of lifting heavy weights will increase bone mass. What is the mechanism of this effect of weightlifting?

    A) Elevated metabolic activity stimulates parathyroid hormone secretion
    B) Mechanical stress on the bones increases the activity of osteoblasts
    C) Elevated metabolic activity results in an increase in dietary calcium intake
    D) Elevated metabolic activity results in stimulation of calcitonin secretion

118. Levels of transcortin are elevated in a pregnant woman. Which of the following laboratory findings would be expected in this patient?

    A) Increased total (protein-bound plus free) plasma cortisol concentration
    B) Increased free (non–protein-bound) plasma cortisol concentration
    C) Decreased total plasma cortisol concentration
    D) Decreased free plasma cortisol concentration
    E) Little or no change in total plasma cortisol concentration

119. Birth control pills containing combinations of synthetic estrogen and progesterone compounds given for the first 21 days of the menstrual cycle are effective in preventing pregnancy. What is the explanation for their efficacy?

    A) Prevention of the preovulatory surge of luteinizing hormone secretion from the pituitary gland
    B) Prevention of development of the ovarian follicles
    C) Suppressing function of the corpus luteum soon after it forms
    D) Prevention of normal development of the endometrium

120. Which of the following physiological responses is greater for triiodothyronine (T_3) than for thyroxine (T_4)?

    A) Secretion rate from the thyroid
    B) Plasma concentration
    C) Plasma half-life
    D) Affinity for nuclear receptors in target tissues
    E) Latent period for onset of action in target tissues

121. A "birth control" compound for men has been sought for several decades. Which of the following would provide effective sterility?

    A) Substance that mimics the actions of luteinizing hormone
    B) Substance that blocks the actions of inhibin
    C) Substance that blocks the actions of follicle-stimulating hormone
    D) Substance that mimics the actions of gonadotropin-releasing hormone

122. In order for milk to flow from the nipple of the mother into the mouth of the nursing infant, which of the following must occur?

    A) Myoepithelial cells must relax
    B) Prolactin levels must fall
    C) Oxytocin secretion from the posterior pituitary must take place
    D) The baby's mouth must develop a strong negative pressure over the nipple
    E) All of the above

123. Failure of the ductus arteriosus to close is a common developmental defect. Which of the following would likely be present in a 12-month-old infant with patent ductus arteriosus?

    A) Below-normal arterial P_{O_2}
    B) Below-normal arterial P_{CO_2}
    C) Greater than normal arterial blood pressure
    D) Lower than normal pulmonary arterial pressure

124. Which of the following sets of physiological changes would be expected in a non-diabetic patient with Cushing's disease?

	Plasma aldosterone	Plasma cortisol	Plasma insulin
A)	↑	↑	↑
B)	↑	↑	↔
C)	↑	↔	↔
D)	↔	↔	↑
E)	↔	↑	↔
F)	↔	↑	↑

125. The placenta does which of the following?

    A) Develops from the granulosa cells
    B) Secretes luteinizing hormone
    C) Secretes estrogen
    D) Allows direct mixing of maternal and fetal blood
    E) None of the above

126. Why is osteoporosis much more common in elderly women than in elderly men?

    A) Men continue to produce testosterone throughout their lifetime, whereas women cease estrogen production after menopause
    B) Women consume less dietary calcium than men
    C) Gastrointestinal absorption of calcium is more effective in men than in women
    D) The bones of women contain less calcium than those of men even before menopause

127. When compared with the late-evening values typically observed in normal subjects, plasma levels of both adrenocorticotropic hormone and cortisol would be expected to be higher in which of the following individuals?

    A) Normal subjects after waking in the morning
    B) Normal subjects administered dexamethasone
    C) Patients with Cushing's syndrome (adrenal adenoma)
    D) Patients with Addison's disease
    E) Patients with Conn's syndrome

128. Which of the following conditions or hormones would most likely increase growth hormone secretion?

    A) Hyperglycemia
    B) Exercise
    C) Somatomedin
    D) Somatostatin
    E) Aging

129. Which blood vessel in the fetus has the highest P_{O_2}?

    A) Ductus arteriosus
    B) Ductus venosus
    C) Ascending aorta
    D) Left atrium

130. A 59-year-old woman has osteoporosis, hypertension, hirsutism, and hyperpigmentation. Magnetic resonance imaging indicates that the pituitary gland is not enlarged. Which of the following conditions is most consistent with these findings?

    A) Pituitary adrenocorticotropic hormone (ACTH)–secreting tumor
    B) Ectopic ACTH-secreting tumor
    C) Inappropriately high secretion rate of corticotropin-releasing hormone
    D) Adrenal adenoma
    E) Addison's disease

131. Which of the following is an inappropriate hypophysial hormone response to the hypothalamic hormone listed? (ACTH, adrenocorticotropic hormone; CRH, corticotropin-releasing hormone; GH, growth hormone; GnRH, gonadotropin-releasing hormone; LH, luteinizing hormone; TRH, thyrotropin-releasing hormone; TSH, thyroid-stimulating hormone)

	Hypothalamic hormone secretion	Hypophysial hormone
A)	Somatostatin	↓ GH
B)	Dopamine	↑ Prolactin
C)	GnRH	↑ LH
D)	TRH	↑ TSH
E)	CRH	↑ ACTH

132. Extracellular calcium concentration remains only slightly below normal for many months even when dietary calcium intake is minimal. What accounts for this ability to maintain calcium concentration in the extracellular fluid?

A) Only a slight reduction in plasma calcium concentration stimulates large, sustained increases in parathyroid hormone secretion
B) Osteoclasts stimulated by high levels of parathyroid hormone remove calcium from the large quantity stored in the bone, thereby maintaining the near-normal extracellular calcium level
C) Renal excretion of calcium is greatly reduced under the influence of high concentrations of parathyroid hormone
D) All of the above

133. A patient is administered sufficient thyroxine (T_4) to increase plasma levels of the hormone several-fold. Which of the following sets of changes is most likely in this patient after several weeks of T_4 administration?

	Respiratory rate	Heart rate	Plasma cholesterol concentration
A)	↑	↑	↑
B)	↑	↑	↓
C)	↑	↓	↑
D)	↓	↓	↑
E)	↓	↑	↓

134. During the latter stages of pregnancy, many women experience an increase in body hair growth in a masculine pattern. What is the explanation for this?

A) The ovaries secrete some testosterone along with the large amounts of estrogen produced late in pregnancy
B) The fetal ovaries and testes secrete androgenic steroids
C) The maternal and fetal adrenal glands secrete large amounts of androgenic steroids that are used by the placenta to form estrogen
D) The placenta secretes large amounts of estrogen, some of which is metabolized to testosterone

135. What is the cause of menopause?

A) Reduced levels of gonadotropic hormones secreted from the anterior pituitary gland
B) Reduced responsiveness of the follicles to the stimulatory effects of gonadotropic hormones
C) Reduced rate of secretion of progesterone from the corpus luteum
D) Reduced numbers of follicles available in the ovary for stimulation by gonadotropic hormones

136. Release of which of the following hormones is an example of neuroendocrine secretion?

A) Growth hormone
B) Cortisol
C) Oxytocin
D) Prolactin
E) Adrenocorticotropic hormone

137. During the week following ovulation, the endometrium increases in thickness to 5 to 6 millimeters. What stimulates this increase in thickness?

A) Luteinizing hormone
B) Estrogen from the corpus luteum
C) Progesterone from the corpus luteum
D) Follicle-stimulating hormone

138. Which of the following metabolic responses would be expected during the postabsorptive period, compared to the postprandial state?

	Glucagon secretion	Hormone-sensitive lipase	Adipocyte α-glycerol phosphate
A)	↑	↑	↓
B)	↑	↑	↑
C)	↑	↓	↓
D)	↓	↓	↑
E)	↓	↑	↑
F)	↓	↓	↓

139. Inhibition of the iodide pump would be expected to cause which of the following changes?

A) Increased synthesis of thyroxine (T_4)
B) Increased synthesis of thyroglobulin
C) Increased metabolic rate
D) Decreased thyroid-stimulating hormone secretion
E) Extreme nervousness

140. Before implantation, the blastocyst obtains its nutrition from the uterine endometrial secretions. How does the blastocyst obtain nutrition during the first week after implantation?

A) It continues to derive nutrition from endometrial secretions
B) The cells of the blastocyst contain stored nutrients that are metabolized for nutritional support
C) The placenta provides nutrition derived from maternal blood
D) The trophoblast cells digest the nutrient-rich endometrial cells and then absorb their contents for use by the blastocyst

141. Which of the following increases the rate of deposition and decreases the rate of absorption of bone?

A) Elevation of parathyroid hormone concentration
B) Elevation of estrogen concentration
C) Elevation of extracellular hydrogen ion concentration
D) Reduction in mechanical stress on the bone

142. Which of the following pituitary hormones has a chemical structure most similar to that of antidiuretic hormone?

A) Oxytocin
B) Adrenocorticotropic hormone
C) Thyroid-stimulating hormone
D) Follicle-stimulating hormone
E) Prolactin

143. What is the most common cause of respiratory distress syndrome in neonates born at 7 months gestation?

A) Pulmonary edema due to pulmonary arterial hypertension
B) Formation of a hyaline membrane over the alveolar surface
C) Failure of the alveolar lining to form adequate amounts of surfactant
D) Excessive permeability of the alveolar membrane to water

144. Which of the following steroid hormones is not synthesized to any appreciable degree in the zona fasciculata?

A) Aldosterone
B) Cortisol
C) Corticosterone
D) Dehydroepiandrosterone
E) Deoxycorticosterone

145. A 45-year-old woman has a mass in the sella turcica that compresses the portal vessels, disrupting pituitary access to hypothalamic secretions. The secretion rate of which of the following hormones would most likely increase in this patient?

A) Adrenocorticotropic hormone
B) Growth hormone
C) Prolactin
D) Luteinizing hormone
E) Thyroid-stimulating hormone

146. A man who has been exposed to high levels of gamma radiation is sterile due to destruction of the germinal epithelium of the seminiferous tubules, although he has normal levels of testosterone. Which of the following would be found in this patient?

A) Normal secretory pattern of gonadotropin-releasing hormone
B) Normal levels of inhibin
C) Suppressed levels of follicle-stimulating hormone
D) Absence of Leydig cells

147. A patient has hypothyroidism due to a primary abnormality in the thyroid gland. Increased plasma levels of which of the following would most likely be reported?

A) Cholesterol
B) Thyroxine-binding globulin
C) Reverse triiodothyronine (RT_3)
D) Diiodotyrosine
E) Iodide

Questions 148 and 149
An experiment was conducted in which rats were injected with one of two hormones or saline (control) for 2 weeks. Autopsies were then performed, and organ weights were measured (in milligrams)

	Control	Hormone 1	Hormone 2
Pituitary	12.9	8.0	14.5
Thyroid	250	500	245
Adrenal glands	40	37	85
Body weight	300	152	175

148. Hormone 1 is which of the following?

A) Thyroid-releasing hormone
B) Thyroid-stimulating hormone (TSH)
C) Thyroxine (T_4)
D) Adrenocorticotropic hormone (ACTH)
E) Cortisol

149. Hormone 2 is which of the following?

A) TSH
B) T_4
C) Corticotropin-releasing hormone
D) ACTH
E) Cortisol

1. **D)** Estrogen and progesterone are formed in large amounts by the mature corpus luteum that has formed by 7 days following ovulation, causing negative feedback inhibition of LH secretion from the anterior pituitary.

2. **E)** In Graves' disease, thyroid-stimulating immunoglobulins bind to cell membrane receptors, causing the thyroid to produce excessive amounts of thyroid hormones (T_3 and T_4). As a result of negative feedback, increased plasma levels of T_3 and T_4 suppress the secretion of thyroid-stimulating hormone. In addition, increased plasma levels of immunoglobulins often cause exophthalmos, and an increased heart rate is a common response to high circulating levels of thyroid hormones.
   TMP12 916

3. **D)** Antidiuretic hormone (ADH) increases the permeability of the collecting tubules and ducts to water, but not to sodium, which in turn increases water reabsorption and decreases water excretion. As a result, urine concentration increases, and the retained water dilutes the plasma. ADH is synthesized in the supraoptic and paraventricular nuclei of the hypothalamus and has no direct effect on the thirst center.
   TMP12 348–350, 358, 904–905

4. **A)** Estrogen compounds are believed to have an osteoblast-stimulating effect. When the amount of estrogen in the blood falls to very low levels after menopause, the balance between the bone-building activity of the osteoblasts and the bone-degrading activity of the osteoclasts is tipped toward bone degradation. When estrogen compounds are added as part of hormone replacement therapy, the bone-building activity of the osteoblasts is increased to balance the osteoclastic activity.
   TMP12 904, 994

5. **C)** Following birth, systemic arterial resistance increases dramatically due to loss of the placental vasculature. Consequently, arterial pressure, left ventricular pressure, and left atrial pressure all increase. At the same time pulmonary vascular resistance decreases due to expansion of the lungs, pulmonary artery pressure, right ventricular pressure and right atrial pressure all fall. Blood flow through the foramen is a function of the pressure gradient, which after birth favors flow from the left to the right atrium, but most of the flow is blocked by the septal flap on the septal wall of the left atrium.

6. **C)** Type 2 diabetes mellitus is characterized by diminished sensitivity of target tissues to the metabolic effects of insulin; that is, there is insulin resistance. As a result, hepatic uptake of glucose is impaired, and glucose release is enhanced. In muscle, the uptake of glucose is impaired.
   TMP12 941–942, 951

7. **C)** In acromegaly, high plasma levels of growth hormone cause insulin resistance. Consequently, there is increased glucose production by the liver and impaired glucose uptake by peripheral tissues.
   TMP12 951

8. **A)** During exercise, glucose utilization by muscle is increased, which is largely independent of insulin.
   TMP12 941

9. **E)** Erection requires dilation of the vascular smooth muscle of the resistance vessels leading to the corpora cavernosa. All of the substance listed are vasoconstrictors and would prevent erection.

10. **B)** Very high concentration of testosterone in a female embryo will induce formation of male genitalia. An adrenal tumor in the mother synthesizing testosterone at a high, uncontrolled rate could produce the masculinizing effect.

11. **E)** HCG has the same stimulatory effect as LH on the corpus luteum. Administration of HCG would cause the corpus luteum to continue to secrete estrogen and progesterone, preventing degradation of the endometrium and onset of menstruation.

12. **C)** Antagonism of progesterone's effects, dilation of the cervix, and oxytocin all increase uterine smooth muscle excitability and will facilitate contractions and onset of labor. LH would have no effect. PGE_2 strongly stimulates uterine smooth muscle contraction and is formed in increasing rate by the placenta late in gestation.

13. **A)** Ultraviolet light absorbed by the skin directly facilitates conversion of cholesterol to 25-hydroxycholesterol.

14. **D)** The pulmonary vascular resistance greatly decreases as a result of expansion of the lungs. In the unexpanded fetal lungs, the blood vessels are compressed because of the small volume of the lungs. Immediately on expansion, these vessels are no longer

compressed, and the resistance to blood flow decreases several-fold.
TMP12 1023

15. **A)** In a radioimmunoassay, there is too little antibody to bind completely the radioactively tagged hormone and the hormone in the fluid (plasma) to be assayed. Thus, there is completion between the labeled and endogenous hormone for binding sites on the antibody. Consequently, if the amount of radioactive hormone bound to antibody is low, this would indicate that plasma levels of endogenous hormone are high.
TMP12 891–892

16. **B)** The Sertoli cells of the seminiferous tubules secrete inhibin at a rate proportional to the rate of production of sperm cells. Inhibin has a direct inhibitory effect on anterior pituitary secretion of FSH. FSH binds to specific receptors on the Sertoli cells, causing the cells to grow and secrete substances that stimulate sperm cell production. The secretion of inhibin thereby provides the negative feedback control signal from the seminiferous tubules to the pituitary gland.
TMP12 984

17. **B)** Ovulation will not take place unless a surge of LH precedes it. Immediately prior to ovulation the number of follicles is decreasing due to normal attrition of all but one follicle, and consequently estrogen synthesis by the ovary is decreasing. Progesterone synthesis is stimulated by the LH surge.

18. **A)** The corpus luteum is the only source of progesterone production, except for minute quantities secreted from the follicle before ovulation. The corpus luteum is functional between ovulation and the beginning of menstruation, during which time the concentration of luteinizing hormone (LH) is suppressed below the level achieved during the preovulatory LH surge.
TMP12 995

19. **D)** Paracrine communication refers to cell secretions that diffuse into the extracellular fluid to affect neighboring cells.
TMP12 881

20. **B)** The delta cells of the pancreas secrete somatostatin, which inhibits the secretion of insulin and glucagon from the pancreatic beta and alpha cells, respectively. Choice D is an example of neural communication, and the remaining choices are examples of neuroendocrine communication.
TMP12 881, 949

21. **C)** Large amounts of estrogen are formed from testosterone and androstanediol in the liver, accounting for as much as 80% of the total male estrogen production.
TMP12 980

22. **E)** Anabolic steroids bind to testosterone receptors in the hypothalamus, providing feedback inhibition of normal ovarian cycling and preventing menstrual cycling, as well as stimulation of osteoblastic activity in the bones.

23. **B)** Right atrial pressure falls dramatically after the onset of breathing due to a reduction in pulmonary vascular resistance, pulmonary arterial pressure, and right ventricular pressure.
TMP12 1023

24. **B)** Secretion of adrenal cortical hormones is deficient in patients with Addison's disease. Consequently, low plasma levels of both aldosterone and cortisol would be reported. As a result of the low plasma levels of aldosterone, plasma potassium concentration would be increased.
TMP 934

25. **E)** Patients with Conn's syndrome have tumors of the zona glomerulosa that secrete large amounts of aldosterone. Consequently, plasma levels of aldosterone are elevated, causing hypokalemia. The secretion of cortisol from the zona fasciculata is normal.
TMP 936

26. **D)** Aldosterone secretion is elevated when dietary sodium intake is low, but cortisol secretion is normal. Although aldosterone increases the rate of potassium secretion by the principal cells of the collecting tubules, this effect is offset by a low distal tubular flow rate. Consequently, there is little change in either potassium excretion or plasma potassium concentration.
TMP 364–366, 927

27. **B)** In patients with nephrogenic diabetes insipidus, the kidneys do not respond appropriately to antidiuretic hormone (ADH), and the ability to form concentrated urine is impaired. In contrast, there is a normal ADH secretory response to changes in plasma osmolality.
TMP 354–355, 904–905

28. **D)** Owing to the loss of blood flow through the placenta, systemic vascular resistance doubles at birth. This increases the aortic pressure as well as the pressure in the left ventricle and left atrium.
TMP12 1023

29. **D)** Parathyroid hormone acts in the renal cortex to stimulate the reaction forming 1, 25-dihydroxycholicalciferol from 25-hydroxycholicalciferol. It has no effects on the other reactions.

30. **B)** Both amino acids and glucose stimulate insulin secretion. Further, amino acids strongly potentiate the glucose stimulus for insulin secretion. Somatostatin inhibits insulin secretion.
TMP12 946–947, 949

31. **B)** Human chorionic gonadotropin also binds to luteinizing hormone receptors on the interstitial cells of the testes of the male fetus, resulting in the production of testosterone in male fetuses up to the time of birth. This small secretion of testosterone is what causes the fetus to develop male sex organs instead of female sex organs.

    TMP12 1008

32. **C)** If a subject were taking sufficient amounts of exogenous thyroid extract to increase plasma levels of T_4 above normal, feedback would cause TSH secretion to decrease. Low plasma levels of TSH would result in atrophy of the thyroid gland. In Graves' disease, the same changes in plasma levels of T_4 and TSH would be present, but the thyroid gland would not be atrophied. In fact, goiter is often present in patients with Graves' disease. A lesion in the anterior pituitary that prevents TSH secretion or the taking of propylthiouracil or large amounts of iodine would be associated with low plasma levels of T_4.

    TMP12 915–916

33. **D)** Choices A to C all will shift the mass action balance toward the side favoring association of ionic calcium with phosphate compounds or other anionic compounds, resulting in reduced levels of free ionic calcium.

34. **B)** In the non-pregnant female, the only significant source of estrogen is ovarian follicles or corpus luteae. Menstruation begins when the corpus luteum degenerates. Menstruation ends when developing follicles secrete estrogen sufficiently to raise circulating concentration to a level that stimulates regrowth of the endometrium.

35. **C)** The major target tissue for prolactin is the breast, where it stimulates the secretion of milk. The other anterior pituitary hormones (adrenocorticotropic hormone, thyroid-stimulating hormone, follicle-stimulating hormone, and luteinizing hormone) stimulate hormones from endocrine glands.

    TMP 883

36. **D)** In patients with central diabetes insipidus, there is an inappropriately low secretion rate of ADH in response to changes in plasma osmolality, but there is no impairment in the renal response to ADH. Because plasma levels of ADH are depressed, there is an impaired ability to concentrate urine, and a large volume of dilute urine is excreted. Loss of water tends to increase plasma osmolality, which stimulates the thirst center. This leads to a very high rate of water turnover.

    TMP12 354, 358, 904–905

37. **D)** The cells of the anterior pituitary that secrete LH and FSH, and the cells of the hypothalamus that secrete gonadotropin-releasing hormone, are inhibited by both estrogen and testosterone. The steroids taken by the woman caused sufficient inhibition to result in cessation of the monthly menstrual cycle.

    TMP12 984, 996–997

38. **A)** The enzyme 11β-hydroxysteroid dehydrogenase type 2 is present in renal tubular cells and converts cortisol to cortisone, which does not readily bind to mineralocorticoid receptors. When this enzyme is deficient, cortisol, which is present in the plasma in considerably higher concentrations than aldosterone, binds the mineralocorticoids receptor and exerts mineralocorticoid effects. Hyperkalemia and decreased blood pressure reflect mineralocorticoid deficiency.

    TMP12 926

39. **B)** Nitric oxide is the vasodilator that is normally released, causing vasodilatation in these arteries.

    TMP12 979

40. **B)** A hypothalamic tumor secreting large amounts of TRH would stimulate the pituitary gland to secrete increased amounts of TSH. As a result, the secretion of thyroid hormones would increase, and this would result in an elevated heart rate. In comparison, a patient with either a pituitary tumor secreting large amounts of TSH or Graves' disease would have low plasma levels of TRH because of feedback. Both TRH and TSH levels would be elevated in endemic goiter, but the heart rate would be depressed because of the low rate of T_4 secretion.

    TMP12 913–918

41. **C)** Demineralization of the bone could be caused by any of the choices, but only an elevated parathyroid hormone concentration would result in both demineralization and elevated plasma calcium concentration. The elevated parathyroid hormone concentration results in overstimulation of the osteoclasts, loss of calcium from bone, stimulation of calcium absorption from the renal tubular fluid and inhibition of calcium excretion, and stimulation of the formation of 1,25-dihydroxycholecalciferol, which increases the rate of calcium absorption from the gastrointestinal tract.

42. **D)** Consumption of amino acids stimulates both growth hormone and glucagon secretion. Increased glucagon secretion tends to increase blood glucose concentration and thus opposes the effects of insulin to cause hypoglycemia.

    TMP12 947–948

43. **D)** Lethargy and myxedema are signs of hypothyroidism. Low plasma levels of thyroid-stimulating hormone indicate that the abnormality is in either the hypothalamus or the pituitary gland. Because the pituitary was responsive to the administration of

thyrotropin-releasing hormone (TRH), this suggests that pituitary function is normal and that the hypothalamus is producing insufficient amounts of TRH.
TMP12 914–917

44. **A)** GH and ADH are stored in the anterior and posterior lobes of the pituitary gland, respectively. However, although GH is also synthesized in the (anterior) pituitary gland, this is not the case for ADH. ADH and the hypothalamic releasing (GHRH) and hypothalamic inhibitory hormones (somatostatin) are synthesized in the hypothalamus. Somatomedins are growth factors (small proteins) that stimulate growth in bone and peripheral tissues. One of the most important somatomedins is somatomedin C, which is produced by the liver in response to GH. Somatomedin C stimulates all aspects of bone growth.
TMP12 895–898, 900–901

45. **E)** Emission is elicited by reflexes mediated by the beta-adrenergic nervous system. Beta adrenergic antagonists interfere with the reflex. None of the other choices is involved.

46. **A)** The cells of the zona glomerulosa secrete most of the aldosterone. These cells have receptors for angiotensin II, which is a major controller of aldosterone secretion.
TMP12 927

47. **A)** The fetal portion of the placenta releases prostaglandins in high concentrations at the time of labor. This release is associated with deterioration of the placenta. Prostaglandins, especially PGE_2, strongly stimulate uterine smooth muscle.
TMP12 1012

48. **A)** After menopause, the absence of feedback inhibition by estrogen and progesterone results in extremely high rates of FSH secretion. Women taking estrogen as part of hormone replacement therapy for symptoms associated with postmenopausal conditions have suppressed levels of FSH owing to the inhibitory effect of estrogen.
TMP12 999

49. **B)** Glucagon stimulates glycogenolysis in the liver, but it has no physiological effects in muscle. Both glucagon and cortisol increase gluconeogenesis, and cortisol impairs glucose uptake by muscle.
TMP12 928–929, 948

50. **C)** Injection of insulin leads to a decrease in blood glucose concentration. Hypoglycemia stimulates the secretion of growth hormone, glucagon, and epinephrine, all of which have counter regulatory effects to increase glucose levels in the blood.
TMP12 901, 948–949

51. **A)** Prolonged fetal hypoxia during delivery can cause serious depression of the respiratory center. Hypoxia may occur during delivery because of compression of the umbilical cord, premature separation of the placenta, excessive contraction of the uterus, or excessive anesthesia of the mother.
TMP12 1021

52. **C)** In general, peptide hormones are water soluble and are not highly bound by plasma proteins. Antidiuretic hormone, a neurohypophysial peptide hormone, is virtually unbound by plasma proteins. In contrast, steroid and thyroid hormones are highly bound to plasma proteins.
TMP12 885–886

53. **C)** Functional development of the kidneys is not complete until about the end of the 1st month of life. The kidneys of a neonate can concentrate urine to only about 1.5 times the osmolality of plasma (in contrast to three to four times plasma osmolality in an adult). If the undiluted formula had a very high osmotic concentration, the neonate would be unable to excrete the solute in sufficiently concentrated urine to prevent the development of hyperosmolality of the plasma.
TMP12 1024

54. **B)** Although estrogen and progesterone are essential for the physical development of the breast during pregnancy, a specific effect of both these hormones is to inhibit the actual secretion of milk. Even though prolactin levels are increased 10- to 20-fold at the end of pregnancy, the suppressive effects of estrogen and progesterone prevent milk production until after the baby is born. Immediately after birth, the sudden loss of both estrogen and progesterone secretion from the placenta allows the lactogenic effect of prolactin to promote milk production.
TMP12 1014

55. **D)** Administration of T_4 in amounts that increase plasma levels of the hormone above normal would be expected to increase the metabolic rate and decrease TSH secretion. Decreased plasma levels of TSH lead to atrophy of the thyroid gland. Thus, patients in group 1 would have a lower metabolic rate and a larger thyroid than patients in group 2, who were administered T_4.
TMP12 911, 915–916

56. **C)** The concentration of parathyroid hormone strongly regulates the absorption of calcium ion from the renal tubular fluid. A reduction in hormone concentration reduces calcium reabsorption and increases the rate of calcium excretion in the urine. The other choices have little effect on or decrease calcium excretion.
TMP12 964

57. **B)** A pituitary tumor secreting increased amounts of TSH would be expected to stimulate the thyroid gland to secrete increased amounts of thyroid hormones. TSH stimulates several steps in the synthesis of thyroid hormones, including the synthesis of thyroglobulin. Increased heart rate is among the many physiological responses to high plasma levels of thyroid hormones. However, high plasma levels of thyroid hormones do not cause exophthalmos. Immunoglobulins cause exophthalmos in Graves' disease, the most common form of hyperthyroidism.

   TMP12 908, 913, 916

58. **A)** Hemorrhage decreases the activation of stretch receptors in the atria and arterial baroreceptors. Decreased activation of these receptors increases ADH secretion.

   TMP12 357, 905

59. **D)** Propylthiouracil blocks several of the early steps in the synthesis of thyroid hormones but does not prevent the formation of thyroglobulin in follicular cells. Therefore, if propylthiouracil were administered to a normal patient, plasma levels of T_4 would fall, and decreased feedback inhibition would lead to an increase in TSH secretion. High plasma levels of TSH would cause hypertrophy of the thyroid gland, even though the production of thyroid hormones is depressed.

   TMP12 915

60. **E)** Choices A to D are true: LH secretion will be suppressed (B) by the negative feedback effect of the estrogen from the tumor; consequently, she will not have menstrual cycles (C); since she will not have normal cycles, no corpus luteae will develop so no progesterone will be formed (A). The high levels of estrogen produced by the tumor will provide stimulation of osteoblastic activity to maintain normal bone activity (D).

61. **C)** Arterial resistance leading into the corpora cavernosa is greatly reduced during erection, while venous resistance leading from the sinuses is extremely high due to compression of the veins against the fibrous tissue surrounding the sinuses. Therefore, pressure in the sinuses during erection is at least equal to systolic arterial pressure. However, contraction of the skeletal muscles in the floor of the perineum that overlies portions of the corpora cavernosa can compress the sinuses, increasing the pressure to levels that are substantially higher than systolic pressure.

   TMP12 979

62. **D)** After eating a meal, insulin secretion is increased. As a result, there is an increased rate of glucose uptake by both the liver and muscle. Insulin also inhibits hormone-sensitive lipase, which decreases hydrolysis of triglycerides in fat cells.

   TMP12 941–943, 947

63. **E)** During exercise, glucose uptake by muscle is enhanced, which tends to decrease the blood glucose concentration. Insulin secretion is depressed during exercise, whereas the secretion of glucagon and epinephrine is elevated. Therefore, hepatic glucose uptake is impaired, and the activity of hormone-sensitive lipase is increased.

   TMP12 941–943, 947

64. **B)** The primary function of testosterone in the embryonic development of males is to stimulate formation of the male sex organs.

   TMP12 981

65. **E)** Protein-bound hormones are biologically inactive and cannot be metabolized. Thus, an increase in protein binding would tend to decrease hormone activity and plasma clearance and increase the half-life of the hormone. Free hormone is also responsible for negative feedback inhibition of hormone secretion. Therefore, a sudden increase in hormone binding to plasma proteins would decrease negative feedback. Protein binding of hormones does, however, provide a reservoir for the rapid replacement of free hormone.

   TMP12 885–886

66. **C)** The reduction in hydrogen ion indicated by the elevation in pH increases the concentration of negatively charged phosphate ion species available for ionic combination with calcium ions. Consequently, free calcium ion concentration is reduced.

   TMP12 966–967

67. **C)** During suckling, stimulation of receptors on the nipples increases neural input to both the supraoptic and paraventricular nuclei. Activation of these nuclei leads to the release of oxytocin and neurophysin from secretion granules in the posterior pituitary gland. Suckling does not stimulate the secretion of appreciable amounts of ADH.

   TMP12 904–905

68. **C)** In Conn's syndrome, large amounts of aldosterone are secreted. Because aldosterone causes sodium retention, hypertension is a common finding in patients with this condition. However, the degree of sodium retention is modest, as is the resultant increase in extracellular fluid volume. This occurs because the rise in arterial pressure offsets the sodium-retaining effects of aldosterone, limiting sodium retention and permitting daily sodium balance to be achieved.

   TMP12 925, 936

69. **A)** Because the liver functions imperfectly during the first weeks of life, the glucose concentration in the blood is unstable and falls to very low levels within a few hours after feeding.

   TMP12 1023

70. **A)** In Addison's disease, there is diminished secretion of both glucocorticoids (cortisol) and mineralocorticoids (aldosterone). In Cushing's disease and Cushing's syndrome, cortisol secretion is elevated but aldosterone secretion is normal. A low sodium diet is associated with a high rate of aldosterone secretion but a secretion rate of cortisol that is normal. By inhibiting the generation of ANG II and thus the stimulatory effects of ANG II on the zona glomerulosa, administration of a converting enzyme inhibitor would decrease aldosterone secretion without altering the rate of cortisol secretion.
     TMP12 927, 934–935

71. **B)** Progesterone is required to maintain the decidual cells of the endometrium. If progesterone levels fall, as they do during the last days of a nonpregnant menstrual cycle, menstruation will follow within a few days, with loss of pregnancy. Administration of a compound that blocks the progesterone receptor during the first few days after conception will terminate the pregnancy.
     TMP12 1008

72. **C)** The only true choice is the increase in arteriolar resistance in the vasculature supplying the corpora (C). The others will tend to maintain erection (B, D, E). (A), reduction in arterial pressure, will have a negligible effect.

73. **C)** Parathyroid hormone strongly stimulates calcium ion absorption from the tubular fluid, decreasing calcium excretion. The other choices have either no effect or tend to increase calcium excretion.

74. **D)** An inappropriately high rate of antidiuretic hormone (ADH) secretion from the lung promotes excess water reabsorption, which tends to produce concentrated urine and a decrease in plasma osmolality. Low plasma osmolality suppresses both thirst and ADH secretion from the pituitary gland.
     TMP12 375–376, 905

75. **B)** Very high plasma concentration of progesterone maintains the uterine muscle in a quiescent state during pregnancy. In the final month of gestation the concentration of progesterone begins to decline, increasing the excitability of the muscle.

76. **E)** During sodium depletion, the renin-angiotensin system is activated, and the high levels of circulating angiotensin II stimulate the adrenal glands to secrete increased amounts of aldosterone. In contrast, angiotensin II has no effect on cortisol secretion, and sodium depletion is associated with normal plasma levels of cortisol. Consequently, reducing plasma levels of angiotensin II by administering an ACE inhibitor would decrease plasma aldosterone to normal levels but would have no effect on plasma cortisol concentration. Because high plasma levels of aldosterone promote sodium retention, reducing aldosterone levels by administering an ACE inhibitor would tend to produce a natriuresis and a decrease in arterial pressure. In time, the opposing effects of reduced arterial pressure and aldosterone secretion on sodium excretion would offset each other, and sodium balance would eventually be achieved at a lower arterial pressure.
     TMP12 925, 927–928

77. **D)** The corpus luteum is the only source of progesterone, and if she is not having menstrual cycles no corpus luteum is present.

78. **C)** Follicle-stimulating hormone stimulates the granulosa cells of the follicle to secrete estrogen.
     TMP12 989

79. **E)** In response to increased blood levels of glucose, plasma insulin concentration normally increases during the 60-minute period following oral intake of glucose. In type 1 diabetes mellitus, insulin secretion is depressed. In contrast, in type 2 diabetes mellitus, insulin resistance is a common finding and, at least in the early stages of the disease, there is an abnormally high rate of insulin secretion.
     TMP12 952–953

80. **D)** In Cushing's syndrome, high plasma levels of cortisol impair glucose uptake in peripheral tissues, which tends to increase plasma levels of glucose. As a result, the insulin response to oral intake of glucose is enhanced.
     TMP 952–953

81. **C)** Too much oxygen in the incubator stops the growth of new blood vessels in the retina. Then when oxygen therapy is stopped, an overgrowth of blood vessels occurs, with a great mass of vessels growing all through the vitreous humor. Later the vessels are replaced by a mass of fibrous tissue, causing permanent blindness.
     TMP12 1027

82. **B)** In general, protein hormones cause physiological effects by binding to receptors on the cell membrane. However, of the four protein hormones indicated, only insulin activates an enzyme-linked receptor. Aldosterone is a steroid hormone and enters the cytoplasm of the cell before binding to its receptor.
     TMP12 888

83. **D)** Human chorionic gonadotropin is secreted from the trophoblast cells beginning shortly after the blastocyst implants in the endometrium.
     TMP12 1007–1008

84. **A)** Somnolence is a common feature of hypothyroidism. Palpitations, increased respiratory rate, increased cardiac output, and weight loss are all associated with hyperthyroidism.
    TMP12 913, 917–918

85. **C)** An infant born of an untreated diabetic mother will have considerable hypertrophy and hyperfunction of the islets of Langerhans in the pancreas. As a consequence, the infant's blood glucose concentration may fall to lower than 20 mg/dL shortly after birth.
    TMP12 1026

86. **E)** A to D would not stimulate PTH secretion: (A) (increase in Ca concentration) suppresses PTH secretion; (B) (calcitonin) has little to no effect on PTH secretion; (C) (acidosis) would increase free Ca in the extracellular fluid, thereby inhibiting PTH secretion; and there is no such thing as (D) (PTH-releasing hormone).

87. **C)** Potassium is a potent stimulus for aldosterone secretion, as is angiotensin II. Therefore, a patient consuming a high-potassium diet would exhibit high circulating levels of aldosterone.
    TMP12 927

88. **C)** The adult form of excess growth hormone secretion is called acromegaly and is usually associated with a pituitary tumor. Increased plasma levels of growth hormone stimulate the liver and other tissues to produce somatomedin C. As a result of feedback, increased plasma levels of somatomedin C cause the hypothalamus to increase the secretion of growth hormone–inhibiting hormone, somatostatin. Elevated plasma levels of growth hormone also tend to increase plasma glucose concentration, which favors an increase in insulin secretion.
    TMP12 899–902

89. **A)** Neural projections from higher centers of the brain to the hypothalamus can elicit the secretion of oxytocin into the blood from the posterior pituitary gland. Upon reaching the breast, oxytocin stimulates contraction of the myoepithelial cells, forcing milk from the alveoli and ducts to the nipple.
    TMP12 1015–1016

90. **C)** Steroid hormones are not stored to any appreciable extent in their endocrine producing glands. This is true for aldosterone, which is produced in the adrenal cortex. In contrast, there are appreciable stores of thyroid hormones and peptide hormones in their endocrine-producing glands.
    TMP12 882

91. **C)** 1,25-dihydroxycholecalciferol is formed only in the renal cortex. Extensive renal disease reduces the amount of cortical tissue, eliminating the source of the active calcium regulating hormone, 1,25-dihydroxycholecalciferol.

92. **C)** In order for erythroblastosis fetalis to occur, the baby must inherit Rh-positive red blood cells from the father. If the mother is Rh-negative, she then becomes immunized against the Rh-positive antigen in the red blood cells of the fetus, and her antibodies destroy fetal red blood cells, releasing large quantities of bilirubin into the fetus's plasma.
    TMP12 1024

93. **D)** Because iodine is needed to synthesize thyroid hormones, the production of thyroid hormones is impaired if iodine is deficient. As a result of feedback, plasma levels of thyroid-stimulating hormone increase and stimulate the follicular cells to increase the synthesis of thyroglobulin. This results in a goiter. Increased metabolic rate, sweating, nervousness, and tachycardia are all common features of hyperthyroidism, not hypothyroidism due to iodine deficiency.
    TMP12 917–918, 932–933

94. **B)** Sperm cell motility decreases as pH is reduced below 6.8. At a pH of 4.5, sperm cell motility is significantly reduced. However, the buffering effect of sodium bicarbonate in the prostatic fluid raises the pH somewhat, allowing the sperm cells to regain some mobility.
    TMP12 976

95. **B)** A protein meal stimulates all three of the hormones indicated.
    TMP12 901, 913, 946, 948

96. **C)** Testosterone secreted by the testes in response to luteinizing hormone (LH) inhibits hypothalamic secretion of gonadotropin-releasing hormone (GnRH), thereby inhibiting anterior pituitary secretion of LH and follicle-stimulating hormone. Taking large doses of testosterone-like steroids also suppresses the secretion of GnRH and the pituitary gonadotropic hormones, resulting in sterility.
    TMP12 984

97. **C)** Steroids with potent glucocorticoid activity tend to increase plasma glucose concentration. As a result, insulin secretion is stimulated. Increased glucocorticoid activity also diminishes muscle protein. Because of feedback, cortisone administration leads to a decrease in adrenocorticotropic hormone secretion and, therefore, a decrease in plasma cortisol concentration.
    TMP12 928–929

98. A) An increase in the concentration of parathyroid hormone results in the stimulation of existing osteoclasts and, over longer periods, increases the number of osteoclasts present in the bone.
TMP12 964

99. B) In general, peptide hormones produce biological effects by binding to receptors on the cell membrane. Peptide hormones are stored in secretion granules in their endocrine-producing cells and have relatively short half-lives because they are not highly bound to plasma proteins. Protein hormones often have a rapid onset of action because, unlike steroid and thyroid hormones, protein synthesis is usually not a prerequisite to produce biological effects.
TMP12 882, 885–888

100. D) A pituitary tumor secreting growth hormone is likely to present as an increase in pituitary gland size. The anabolic effects of excess growth hormone secretion lead to enlargement of the internal organs, including the kidneys. Because acromegaly is the state of excess growth hormone secretion after epiphyseal closure, increased femur length does not occur.
TMP12 903

101. A) Growth hormone and cortisol have opposite effects on protein synthesis in muscle. Growth hormone is anabolic and promotes protein synthesis in most cells of the body, whereas cortisol decreases protein synthesis in extrahepatic cells, including muscle. Both hormones impair glucose uptake in peripheral tissues and, therefore, tend to increase plasma glucose concentration. Both hormones also mobilize triglycerides from fat stores.
TMP12 899–900, 928–929

102. B) If the mother has had adequate amounts of iron in her diet, the infant's liver usually has enough stored iron to form blood cells for 4 to 6 months after birth. However, if the mother has had insufficient iron, the infant may develop severe anemia after about 3 months of life.
TMP12 1020, 1025

103. C) Thyrotoxicosis indicates the effects of thyroid hormone excess. Thyroid hormone excites synapses. In contrast, somnolence is characteristic of hypothyroidism. Tachycardia, increased appetite, increased sweating, and muscle tremor are all signs of hyperthyroidism.
TMP12 913, 916

104. D) Fertilization of the ovum normally takes place in the ampulla of one of the fallopian tubes.
TMP12 1003

105. B) The below-normal plasma calcium concentration in this patient would be expected to strongly stimulate the secretion of parathyroid hormone, which in turn would be expected to increase the rate of excretion of phosphate ions by the kidney and reduce the rate of calcium ion excretion into the urine. Therefore, all the findings can be attributed to a greater than normal parathyroid hormone concentration.
TMP12 966

106. D) Because insulin secretion is deficient in type 1 diabetes mellitus, there is increased (not decreased) release of glucose from the liver. Low plasma levels of insulin also lead to a high rate of lipolysis; increased plasma osmolality, hypovolemia, and acidosis are all symptoms of uncontrolled type 1 diabetes mellitus.
TMP12 950–951

107. E) Under acute conditions, an increase in blood glucose concentration will decrease growth hormone secretion. Growth hormone secretion is characteristically elevated in the chronic pathophysiological states of Acromegaly and Gigantism. Deep sleep and exercise are stimuli that increase growth hormone secretion.
TMP12 901–902

108. D) Estrogen and, to a lesser extent, progesterone secreted by the corpus luteum during the luteal phase have strong feedback effects on the anterior pituitary gland to maintain low secretory rates of both FSH and LH. In addition, the corpus luteum secretes inhibin, which inhibits the secretion of FSH.
TMP12 991

109. B) The early stages of type II are associated with diminished sensitivity of target tissues to the metabolic effects of insulin, a condition referred to as insulin resistance. Decreased insulin sensitivity tends to increase plasma glucose concentration, in part by promoting hepatic release of glucose. Increased plasma glucose concentration leads to a compensatory increase in the secretion of insulin and C-peptide, which is a cleavage product of proinsulin. Metabolic acidosis and hypovolemia occur in type I diabetes but are not present in the early stages of type II diabetes.
TMP12 940, 951, 952

110. D) If a pregnant woman bearing a female child has high blood levels of androgenic hormones early in pregnancy, the child will be born with male genitalia, resulting in a type of hermaphroditism.
TMP12 1026

111. **D)** Under chronic conditions, the effects of high plasma levels of aldosterone to promote sodium reabsorption in the collecting tubules are sustained. However, persistent sodium retention does not occur, because of concomitant changes that promote sodium excretion. These include increased arterial pressure and increased plasma levels of atrial natriuretic peptide and decreased plasma angiotensin II concentration.
TMP12 925, 936

112. **A)** In order for a male embryo to develop male genitalia, testosterone must be present in the embryo. Normally, human chorionic gonadotropin (HCG) secreted by the trophoblast cells stimulates testosterone secretion from the testes. Giving an antibody that blocks HCG would prevent testosterone secretion, resulting in the development of female genitalia in a male fetus.
TMP12 980

113. **C)** Increased plasma levels of cortisol tend to increase plasma glucose concentration and inhibit adrenocorticotropic hormone (ACTH) secretion. Therefore, if cortisol were administered to patients in group 2, the patients in group 1 would have lower plasma glucose concentrations and higher plasma levels of ACTH.
TMP12 928, 932–933

114. **B)** Circulating levels of free T_4 exert biological effects and are regulated by feedback inhibition of TSH secretion from the anterior pituitary gland. Protein bound T_4 is biologically inactive. Circulating T_4 is highly bound to plasma proteins, especially to thyroid-binding globulin (TBG), which increases during pregnancy. An increase in TBG tends to decrease free T_4, which then leads to an increase in TSH secretion, causing the thyroid to increase thyroid hormone secretion. Increased secretion of thyroid hormones persists until free T_4 returns to normal levels, at which time there is no longer a stimulus for increased TSH secretion. Therefore, in a chronic steady-state condition associated with elevated TBG, high plasma total T_4 (bound and free) and normal plasma TSH levels would be expected. In this pregnant patient, the normal levels of total T_4 along with high plasma levels of TSH would indicate an inappropriately low plasma level of free T_4. Deficient thyroid hormone secretion in this patient would be consistent with Hashimoto's disease, the most common form of hypothyroidism.
TMP12 910, 914–917

115. **A)** Fats are readily oxidized by growth hormone. In contrast, growth hormone decreases carbohydrate utilization and promotes the incorporation of amino acids into proteins.
TMP12 899–900

116. **D)** The motor neurons of the spinal cord of the thoracic and lumbar regions are the sources of innervation for the skeletal muscles of the perineum involved in ejaculation.
TMP12 978

117. **B)** Bone is deposited in proportion to the compressional load that the bone must carry. Continual mechanical stress stimulates osteoblastic deposition and calcification of bone.
TMP12 958

118. **A)** Cortisol is highly bound to plasma proteins, particularly transcortin. Increased plasma levels of transcortin, such as occur during pregnancy, tend to decrease free cortisol concentration, but feedback results in increased adrenocorticotropic hormone secretion, which stimulates cortisol secretion until free plasma levels of the steroid return to normal levels. Thus, in a steady state, total plasma cortisol concentration (bound plus free) is elevated, but free cortisol concentration is normal.
TMP12 923, 931–932

119. **A)** Administration of either estrogen or progesterone in appropriate quantities during the first half of the menstrual cycle can inhibit ovulation by preventing the preovulatory surge of luteinizing hormone secretion by the anterior pituitary gland, which is essential for ovulation.
TMP12 998, 1001

120. **D)** In target tissues, nuclear receptors for thyroid hormones have a greater affinity for T_3 than for T_4. The secretion rate, plasma concentration, half-life, and onset of action are all greater for T_4 than for T_3.
TMP12 909–910

121. **C)** Blocking the action of follicle-stimulating hormone on the Sertoli cells of the seminiferous tubules interrupts the production of sperm. Choice C is the only option that is certain to provide sterility.
TMP12 984

122. **C)** Oxytocin is secreted from the posterior pituitary gland and carried in the blood to the breast, where it causes the cells that surround the outer walls of the alveoli and ductile system to contract. Contraction of these cells raises the hydrostatic pressure of the milk in the ducts to 10 to 20 mm Hg. Consequently, milk flows from the nipple into the baby's mouth.
TMP12 1015–1016

123. **A)** If the ductus arteriosus remains patent, poorly oxygenated blood from the pulmonary artery flows into the aorta, giving the arterial blood an oxygen level that is below normal.
TMP12 1023

124. **F)** In Cushing's disease, there is a high rate of corti-sol secretion, but aldosterone secretion is normal. High plasma levels of cortisol tend to increase plasma glucose concentration by impairing glucose uptake in peripheral tissues and by promoting gluconeogene-sis. However, at least in the early stages of Cushing's disease, the tendency for glucose concentration to increase appreciably is counteracted by increased insulin secretion.
     TMP12 927, 935–936

125. **C)** The placenta secretes both estrogen and proges-terone from the trophoblast cells.
     TMP12 1005

126. **A)** Testosterone stimulates the cellular functions of bone that lead to bone formation. Testosterone se-cretion from the interstitial cells declines with age, but it continues at sufficient levels to stimulate bone formation throughout a man's lifetime. Conversely, estrogen production in women falls to zero after menopause, leaving the bones without the stimula-tory effect of estrogen. As a result, osteoporosis is common in women after menopause.
     TMP12 969

127. **A)** In healthy patients, the secretory rates of adreno-corticotropic hormone (ACTH) and cortisol are low in the late evening but high in the early morning. In patients with Cushing's syndrome (adrenal adenoma) or in patients administered dexamethasone, plasma levels of ACTH are very low and are certainly not higher than normal early-morning values. In patients with Addison's disease, plasma levels of ACTH are elevated as a result of deficient adrenal secretion of cortisol. The secretion of ACTH and cortisol would be expected to be normal in Conn's syndrome.
     TMP12 933–936

128. **B)** Exercise stimulates GH secretion. Hyperglyce-mia, somatomedin, and the hypothalamic inhibitory hormone somatostatin all inhibit GH secretion. GH secretion also decreases in aging.
     TMP12 901

129. **B)** Blood returning from the placenta through the umbilical vein passes through the ductus venosus. The blood coming from the placenta has the highest concentration of oxygen found in the fetus.
     TMP12 1022

130. **B)** Osteoporosis, hypertension, hirsutism, and hy-perpigmentation are all symptoms of Cushing's syn-drome associated with high plasma levels of ACTH. If the high plasma ACTH levels were the result of either a pituitary adenoma or an abnormally high rate of corticotropin-releasing hormone secretion from the hypothalamus, the patient would likely have an enlarged pituitary gland. In contrast, the pituitary gland would not be enlarged if an ectopic tumor were secreting high levels of ACTH.
     TMP12 934–935

131. **B)** Prolactin secretion is inhibited, not stimulated, by the hypothalamic release of dopamine into the median eminence. Growth hormone is inhibited by the hypothalamic inhibiting hormone somatostatin. The secretion of luteinizing hormone, thyroid-stimu-lating hormone, and adrenocorticotropic hormone are all under the control of the releasing hormones indicated.
     TMP12 898

132. **D)** During prolonged calcium deficiency, the plasma calcium concentration begins to fall. However, as it falls, parathyroid hormone secretion increases sharply, thereby stimulating osteoclastic degradation of bone and liberating calcium to the extracellular fluid. At the same time, the elevated parathyroid hor-mone concentration strongly stimulates calcium re-absorption from the tubular fluid of the kidneys and reduces calcium excretion to very low levels.
     TMP12 967

133. **B)** Increased heart rate, increased respiratory rate, and decreased cholesterol concentration are all re-sponses to excess thyroid hormone.
     TMP12 912–913

134. **C)** Estrogen secreted by the placenta is not synthe-sized from basic substrates in the placenta. Instead, it is formed almost entirely from androgenic steroid compounds that are formed in both the mother's and the fetus's adrenal glands. These androgenic com-pounds are transported by the blood to the placenta and converted by the trophoblast cells to estrogen compounds. Their concentration in the maternal blood may also stimulate hair growth on the body.
     TMP12 1008

135. **D)** By age 45 years, only a few primordial follicles remain in the ovaries to be stimulated by gonado-tropic hormones, and the production of estrogen decreases as the number of follicles approaches zero. When estrogen production falls below a critical value, it can no longer inhibit the production of go-nadotropic hormones from the anterior pituitary. Follicle-stimulating hormone and luteinizing hor-mone are produced in large quantities, but as the remaining follicles become atretic, production by the ovaries falls to zero.
     TMP12 999

136. **C)** The secretion of chemical messengers (neuro-hormones) from neurons into the blood is referred to as neuroendocrine secretion. Thus, in contrast to the local actions of neurotransmitters at nerve endings,

neurohormones circulate in the blood before producing biological effects at target tissues. Oxytocin is synthesized from magnocellular neurons whose cell bodies are located in the paraventricular and supraoptic nuclei and whose nerve terminals terminate in the posterior pituitary gland. Target tissues for circulating oxytocin are the breast and uterus, where the hormone plays a role in lactation and parturition, respectively.
TMP12 904–906

137. **C)** Progesterone secreted in large quantities from the corpus luteum causes marked swelling and secretory development of the endometrium.
TMP12 995

138. **A)** Several hours after eating a meal (the postabsorptive period), plasma glucose concentration tends to fall. As a result, insulin secretion decreases. Because insulin inhibits hormone sensitive lipase in adipocytes, the activity of this enzyme increases in response to the declining plasma levels of insulin. This leads to increased hydrolysis of triglycerides. A fall in insulin concentration also diminishes glucose uptake in adipocytes, leading to decreased generation of α-glycerol phosphate, which is necessary to form triglycerides from fatty acids. Both of these insulin-induced responses in adipocytes promote release of fatty acids into the circulation. As the postprandial period persists, reductions in plasma glucose concentration stimulate glucagon secretion, which tends to preserve glucose concentration by stimulating glycogenolysis and gluconeogenesis.
TMP12 943, 947

139. **B)** Inhibition of the iodide pump decreases the synthesis of thyroid hormones but does not impair the production of thyroglobulin by follicular cells. Decreased plasma levels of thyroid hormones result in a low metabolic rate and lead to an increase in thyroid-stimulating hormone (TSH) secretion. Increased plasma levels of TSH stimulate the follicular cells to synthesize more thyroglobulin. Nervousness is a symptom of hyperthyroidism and is not caused by thyroid hormone deficiency.
TMP12 908, 911–912, 915

140. **D)** As the blastocyst implants, the trophoblast cells invade the decidua, digesting and imbibing it. The stored nutrients in the decidual cells are used by the embryo for growth and development. During the 1st week after implantation, this is the only means by which the embryo can obtain nutrients. The embryo continues to obtain at least some of its nutrition in this way for up to 8 weeks, although the placenta begins to provide nutrition after about the 16th day beyond fertilization (a little more than 1 week after implantation).
TMP12 1004

141. **B)** Elevation of estrogen concentration stimulates osteoblastic activity and reduces the rate of degradation of bone by osteoclasts.
TMP12 959, 994

142. **A)** Both antidiuretic hormone and oxytocin are peptides containing nine amino acids. Their chemical structures differ in only two amino acids.
TMP12 904

143. **C)** One of the most characteristic findings in respiratory distress syndrome is failure of the respiratory epithelium to secrete adequate quantities of surfactant into the alveoli. Surfactant decreases the surface tension of the alveolar fluid, allowing the alveoli to open easily during inspiration. Without sufficient surfactant, the alveoli tend to collapse, and there is a tendency to develop pulmonary edema.
TMP12 1022

144. **A)** The enzyme aldosterone synthase is not present in the zona fasciculata. Consequently, aldosterone is not synthesized in these cells of the adrenal cortex.
TMP12 921–922

145. **C)** The primary controllers of adrenocorticotropic hormone (ACTH), growth hormone, luteinizing hormone (LH), and thyroid-stimulating hormone (TSH) secretion from the pituitary gland are hypothalamic releasing hormones. They are secreted into the median eminence and subsequently flow into the hypothalamic-hypophysial portal vessels before bathing the cells of the anterior pituitary gland. Conversely, prolactin secretion from the pituitary gland is influenced primarily by the hypothalamic inhibiting hormone dopamine. Consequently, obstruction of blood flow through the portal vessels would lead to reduced secretion of ACTH, growth hormone, LH, and TSH, but increased secretion of prolactin.
TMP12 898

146. **A)** Gamma radiation destroys the cells undergoing the most rapid rates of mitosis and meiosis, the germinal epithelium of the testes. The man described is said to have normal testosterone levels, suggesting that the secretory patterns of gonadotropin-releasing hormone and luteinizing hormone are normal and that his interstitial cells are functional. Because he is not producing sperm, the levels of inhibin secreted by the Sertoli cells would be maximally suppressed, and his levels of follicle-stimulating hormone would be strongly elevated.
TMP11 984

147. **A)** Increased plasma cholesterol concentration is commonly observed in hypothyroidism.
TMP12 912

148. B) In this experiment, the size of the thyroid gland increased because thyroid-stimulating hormone (TSH) causes hypertrophy and hyperplasia of its target gland and increased secretion of thyroid hormones. Increased plasma levels of thyroid hormones inhibit the secretion of thyrotropin-releasing hormone, which decreases stimulation of the pituitary thyrotropes, resulting in a decrease in the size of the pituitary gland. Higher plasma levels of thyroid hormones also increase metabolic rate and decrease body weight.

TMP12 912, 914–915

149. C) In this experiment, the size of the pituitary and adrenal glands increased because corticotropin-releasing hormone stimulates the pituitary corticotropes to secrete adrenocorticotropic hormone, which in turn stimulates the adrenals to secrete corticosterone and cortisol. Higher plasma levels of cortisol increase protein degradation and lipolysis and, therefore, decrease body weight.

TMP12 928–929, 931–932

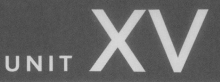

Sports Physiology

1. Which of the following sources can produce the greatest amount of ATP per minute over a short period of time?

   A) Aerobic system
   B) Phosphagen system
   C) Glycogen-lactic acid system
   D) Phosphocreatine system
   E) Stored ATP

2. What causes the excess muscle mass in the average male compared to a female?

   A) Increased testosterone secreted in the male
   B) Increased estrogen secreted by the female
   C) Higher exercise levels in the male
   D) Greater glycogen deposition by males

3. What is the definition of the strength of a muscle?

   A) Maximum weight it can lift
   B) Force required to stretch it after it has contracted
   C) Work that the muscle can perform per unit of time
   D) How long a muscle can lift a given amount of weight

4. Which of the following statements comparing slow-twitch and fast-twitch muscle fibers is most accurate?

   A) Fast-twitch fibers are less dependent on the phosphagen and glycogen-lactic acid systems
   B) Slow-twitch fibers have more mitochondria surrounding them
   C) Slow-twitch fibers have less myoglobin
   D) Number of capillaries surrounding slow-twitch fibers is less
   E) Fast-twitch fibers are smaller in diameter

5. Olympic athletes who run marathons or perform cross-country skiing have much higher maximum cardiac outputs than non-athletes. Which of the following statements about the hearts of these athletes compared to non-athletes is most accurate?

   A) Stroke volume in the Olympic athletes is about 5% greater at rest
   B) Percentage increase in heart rate during maximal exercise is much greater in the Olympic athletes
   C) Maximum cardiac output is only 3% to 4% greater in the Olympic athletes
   D) Resting heart rate in the Olympic athletes is significantly higher

6. Which of the following statements about respiration in exercise is most accurate?

   A) Maximum oxygen consumption of a male marathon runner is less than that of an untrained average male
   B) Maximum oxygen consumption can be increased about 100% by training
   C) Maximum oxygen diffusing capacity of a male marathon runner is much greater than that of an untrained average male
   D) Blood levels of oxygen and carbon dioxide are abnormal during exercise

7. Which of the following athletes is able to exercise the longest before exhaustion occurs?

   A) One on a high-fat diet
   B) One on a high-carbohydrate diet
   C) One on a mixed carbohydrate–fat diet
   D) One on a high-protein diet
   E) One on a mixed protein–fat diet

8. If muscle strength is increased with resistive training, which of the following conditions will most likely occur?

   A) Decrease in the number of myofibrils
   B) Increase in mitochondrial enzymes
   C) Decrease in the components of the phosphagen energy system
   D) Decrease in stored triglycerides

9. Tobacco smoking causes which of the following effects on the pulmonary system?

   A) Dilation of terminal bronchioles
   B) Decreased airflow resistance
   C) Decreased fluid secretion in the bronchial tree
   D) Paralyzed cilia on the respiratory epithelial cells

10. In athletes who use androgens to increase performance experience, which of the following would most likely occur?

    A) Decreased high-density blood lipoproteins
    B) Decreased low-density blood lipoproteins
    C) Increased testicular function
    D) Decreased incidence of hypertension

249

1. B) Over a short period of time the phosphagen system can produce 4 moles of ATP/min. The phosphagen system comprises the ATP and phosphocreatine system combined. However, when a person runs a long distance race, such as a 10-km race, the phosphagen system can supply energy for 8 to 10 sec only. The glycogen-lactic acid system supplies energy can produce 2.5 moles of ATP per minute. Therefore, the aerobic system, which consists of metabolism of glucose, fats, and amino acids, can produce 1 mole of ATP/min.

TMP12 1033

2. A) The increased muscle mass in a male is caused by testosterone, which is secreted by the male testes. This causes a powerful anabolic effect causing greatly increased deposition of protein everywhere in the body, but especially in the muscles. Estrogen in the female causes a greater deposition of fat but not protein.

TMP12 1031

3. A) The strength is determined by the maximum amount of weight that can be lifted. Muscle power is the work the muscle can perform in a unit of time. This is determined not only by the strength of the muscle contraction but also by the distance of contraction and the number of times it contracts each minute. The power is generally measured in kilogram-meters per minute. This is equivalent to a muscle lifting 1 kg to a height of 1 m in 1 min.

TMP12 1032

4. B) The basic differences between the fast-twitch and slow-twitch in the fibers are the following: Fast-twitch fibers are more dependent on anaerobic metabolism and slow-twitch fibers are more dependent on aerobic metabolism. In fast-twitch fibers, the dependence on phosphagen and glycogen-lactic acid systems is much greater than in the fast-twitch fibers. The slow-twitch fibers are organized for endurance and are dependent upon aerobic metabolism; therefore, they have many more mitochondria and myoglobin, which combines with oxygen in the muscle fiber. The number of capillaries that supply the oxygen is much greater in the vicinity of slow-twitch fibers than in the vicinity of fast-twitch fibers.

TMP12 1036

5. B) When comparing Olympic athletes and non-athletes, we find that there are several differences in the responses of the heart. Stroke volume is much higher at rest in the Olympic athlete and heart rate is much lower. The heart rate can increase approximately 270% in the Olympic athlete during maximal exercise, which is a much greater percentage than occurs in a non-athlete. In addition, the maximal increase in cardiac output is approximately 30% greater in the Olympic athlete.

TMP12 1039

6. C) During exercise the maximum oxygen consumption of a male marathon runner is much greater than that of an untrained average male. However, athletic training increases the maximum oxygen consumption by only about 10%. Therefore, the maximum oxygen consumption in marathon runners is probably partly genetically determined. These runners also have a large increase in maximum oxygen diffusing capacity, and their blood levels of oxygen and carbon dioxide remain relatively normal during exercise.

TMP12 1036–1037

7. B) An athlete on a high-carbohydrate diet will store nearly twice as much glycogen in the muscles compared to an athlete on a mixed carbohydrate–fat diet. This glycogen is converted to lactic acid and supplies four ATP molecules for each molecule of glucose. It also forms ATP 2.5 times as fast as oxidative metabolism in the mitochondria. This extra energy from glycogen significantly increases the time an athlete can exercise.

TMP12 1035

8. B) During resistive training the muscles that are contracted with at least a 50% maximal force for at least three times a week experience an optimal increase in muscle strength. This causes muscle hypertrophy and several changes occur. There will be an increase in the number of myofibrils and up to a 120% increase in mitochondrial enzymes. As much as a 60% to 80% increase in the components of the phosphagen energy system can occur, and up to a 50% increase in stored glycogen can occur. Also, as much as a 75% to 100% increase in stored triglycerides can occur.

TMP12 1035–1036

9. D) Tobacco smoking decreases an athlete's pulmonary ventilatory ability. This is true for several reasons. First, nicotine constricts the terminal bronchioles of the lungs, which increases the resistance to air flow in and out of the lungs. Second, the smoke has an irritating effect in the bronchiolar trees which increases fluid secretion. Third, nicotine paralyzes the cilia on the surfaces of the respiratory epithelial cells that normally beat continually to remove excess fluid and foreign particles.

TMP12 1037–1038

10. A) Use of male sex hormones (androgens) or other anabolic steroids to increase muscle strength increases athletic performances under some conditions but can have adverse effects on the body. Anabolic steroids increase the risk of cardiovascular damage, because they increase the instance of hypertension, decrease high-density blood lipoproteins, and increase low-density blood lipoproteins. These factors all promote heart attacks and strokes. These androgenic substances also decrease testicular function which decreases the formation of sperm and the body's own production of natural testosterone.

TMP12 1040